SPIN DOCTORS

SPIN DOCTORS
The Chiropractic Industry Under Examination

Paul Benedetti & Wayne MacPhail

THE DUNDURN GROUP
TORONTO · OXFORD

Copy-Editor: Andrea Pruss
Design: Scott Reid
Printer: Transcontinental

National Library of Canada Cataloguing in Publication Data

Benedetti, Paul
Spin doctors : the chiropractic industry under examination/Paul Benedetti, Wayne MacPhail.

Includes bibliographical references.
ISBN 1-55002-406-X

1. Chiropractic–Evaluation. 2. Chiropractic–Complications. I. MacPhail, Wayne, 1955- II. Title.

RZ242.B45 2002   615.5'34   C2002-904310-7

1   2   3   4   5   06   05   04   03   02

We acknowledge the support of the **Canada Council for the Arts** and the **Ontario Arts Council** for our publishing program. We also acknowledge the financial support of the **Government of Canada** through the **Book Publishing Industry Development Program** and **The Association for the Export of Canadian Books**, and the **Government of Ontario** through the **Ontario Book Publishers Tax Credit** program.

Care has been taken to trace the ownership of copyright material used in this book. The author and the publisher welcome any information enabling them to rectify any references or credit in subsequent editions.

J. Kirk Howard, President

Printed and bound in Canada.
Printed on recycled paper.
www.dundurn.com

Dundurn Press	Dundurn Press	Dundurn Press
8 Market Street	73 Lime Walk	2250 Military Road
Suite 200	Headington, Oxford,	Tonawanda NY
Toronto, Ontario, Canada	England	U.S.A. 14150
M5E 1M6	OX3 7AD	

CONTENTS

Dedication..6
Acknowledgements...7
Foreword..11
Introduction..15

1   A House Divided...25
2   The P.T. Barnum of Chiropractic...........................43
3   Subluxation: The Phantom Menace........................59
4   The Not-So-Well-Adjusted Child.............................81
5   Neck Manipulation and Stroke..............................117
6   The Forgotten Death of Lana Dale Lewis............153
7   Courting York — The Unsuitable Suitor.............171
8   Are Chiropractors Back Doctors?..........................185
9   So, How Did They Become Doctors Anyway?.....203
10   Gizmos, Parlour Tricks, and Nonsense.................209
11   A Profession Out of Control..................................229

Conclusion..267
Afterword..273
Notes..277

For my loving, and loved, wife, Barbara Ledger
Wayne MacPhail

For Mom and Dad, for everything
Paul Benedetti

ACKNOWLEDGEMENTS

This book couldn't have happened without remarkable contributions from dozens of our friends, colleagues, interview subjects, and others, who gave freely of their time, documents, expertise, and support.

This project began as a series of online features on canoe.ca. Those articles would never have seen the light of the screen without the commitment and encouragement of Hugh Stuart at @home Canada and Mike Simpson at canoe.ca. They both embraced the idea of online investigative journalism in a corporate climate that was anything but receptive to the idea. Mike Simpson, former executive producer at Canoe, is a strong proponent of solid journalism, and he just loves a good story. His support, both in terms of resources and leadership, was extremely valuable.

We were greatly assisted by excellent spadework and diligence by Anjali Kapoor at @Home Canada. At Canoe, reporter Tim Kran did valuable investigative fieldwork, as did Natasha Marko. Sharon Lem did excellent research on university affiliations. Online editor and reporter Diana Luciani was extremely helpful in putting the whole series online. Executive Producer of News Art Chamberlin used his substantial experience and editing skills to get our copy into shape.

An online series has to look as good as it reads, and Art Director Dan Clark made sure of that with his creative and highly functional interface. Thanks go as well to graphic artist Ayako Shimizu, who created the striking logos and banner for both online series.

Finally, Alan Shanoff put our series through a stringent legal filter, providing excellent advice, wise guidance, and a great deal of support both before and after the stories appeared. He is a fine lawyer and a solid journalist in his own right. We would also like to thank media lawyer Brian Rogers for his careful reading of the book and his sage advice, both legal and journalistic.

Thanks must go as well to Florence Sicoli, who cast an experienced editor's eye on a feature story Wayne wrote for the *Hamilton Spectator* that sprang out of our research into neck manipulation.

Our admiration and thanks go, of course, to the Lewis family, especially Mike and Judy Ford, who have shared their struggle with us while year after year carrying the crushing burden of Lana Dale's death and the questions surrounding it. The family's lawyer, Amani Oakley, despite the weight of her inquest responsibilities, was extremely helpful, responding to our frequent requests for information and documents quickly and with good humour.

We've both been impressed by the courage and generosity of the victims of neck manipulations: Kim Barton and Diane Rodrigue have both risen above misadventures that would have left lesser women defeated and silent. Similarly, Nilla Corvaro generously shared her story with us. We are also enormously indebted to Sharon Mathiason, who has suffered more loss than any human being deserves and still found time to answer our endless questions and reply to our frequent requests for documents and information. Her ongoing battle for truth and safety in health care is a tribute to her daughter, Laurie.

Through the years we've been chipping away at this story, Dr. Murray Katz has been a tireless aid. We can't thank him enough for the hours he's spent walking us through the medical jargon and sharing his documents selflessly with us. Though he has an active family and a busy practice, he has worked endless hours helping victims and families through terrible times. The chiropractic community sees Murray as the Great Satan, but we have found him to be a loyal, honest, and good-hearted *mensch*. Likewise, Dr. Stephen Barrett has been a great help over the years, as has his remarkable Web site, quackwatch.com. Dr. Barrett even took the time to cast an expert eye on some early drafts of chapters and made invaluable comments. Chiropractor Samuel Homola provided knowledgeable commentary on the profession, both in interviews and in his fine book. Third-generation chiropractor Charles DuVall Jr. kindly gave of his time and expertise to share his special insight into the profession. Dr. Marvin Levant responded to many requests for information and helped us understand the issues around chiropractic and x-ray. Thanks too to Dr. Terry Polevoy, a pediatrician with his finger on the pulse of chiropractic quackery in Canada. Terry tipped us off to some great stories. Dr. Tony Hammer, who showed stamina dealing with the College of Chiropractors of Ontario, also generously shared his travails with us. Physiotherapist Jeff Garrett deserves our thanks for his courage and his insights into manual therapy. Neurologist Dr. John Norris has also been very kind in sharing his stroke expertise with two simple-minded laymen. Of course, we're grateful to Dr. Brad Stewart, who wrote the powerful preface to this book and who has ably championed the cause of those harmed by chiropractors in Canada. Thanks must go as well to the men and women on Dr. Barrett's health fraud list, many of whom responded to our queries providing references and guidance.

Writing a book like this is a painstaking task that can smother you in data and detail. We were greatly assisted by our friend and researcher Deborah Jessop, who, armed with her information science skills, hunted down documents with tenacity and never failed to deliver gems every time we met.

We would be remiss not to thank our good friend and mentor Wilson Southam for his sage counsel, unwavering support, and occasional chauffeur service.

Wayne's wife, Barbara Ledger, spent several long days carefully reading and correcting our sorry drafts. She also had to put up with being in a confined space with both of us for hours and hours during the last, harried days of this book's creation. Thanks Barb, you did a remarkable job.

Paul's wife Marni and his three children, James, Matthew, and Ella, were unfailingly supportive, enthusiastic, and understanding about their father's long hours at the computer. They offered daily encouragement and the occasional cold drink.

Thanks too to the many friends who offered moral support and assistance as we pushed to the finish line. They include: Brent Wood and Brenda Flaherty, who lent us their home and air conditioning; Kevin von Appen, our dear friend, who mocked and cajoled us along; our good friend Wade Hemsworth, who offered advice and wisdom gained from writing his own books; Warren Barton, friend and mentor, who offered unstinting enthusiasm and support; Dave Estok, who gave his friendship and solid journalism advice; Brian Mather and Ruth Barker, who lent us encouragement and stroke data; Steven Toth and Sandra Makino and Lightning for the laser printer offer, fine dinners, and humour; Madelyn Herschorn and Gail Alexander at Centennial College for support, interest, and a life-saving library search; Anne Mullens for her advice on book writing; and Stephanie Ledger and Ron Van Logchem for their hospitality and encouragement. We would also like to thank our family and friends for their encouragement and support.

The making of a book is a team effort, and we would like to thank all the folks at Dundurn Press for having faith in us and for bringing the book to life.

We would like especially to show our appreciation of our agent, Kathryn Mulders, who believed in us and this book from day one, and who has had to put up with our unusual e-mails.

FOREWORD

I distinctly recall returning to Saskatoon in 1998 to the news that a young woman had suffered a stroke in a chiropractor's office and was in the intensive care unit, not expected to live. I spoke with the neurology resident who had recognized the stroke and had organized a desperate attempt to open up the blocked arteries in her brain. He told me that when the initial dose of the "clot buster" drug was given by the radiologist, the comatose patient had started to awaken and had to be paralyzed to allow the procedure to continue. Unfortunately, one of the arteries in her neck was so badly torn that it began to leak blood into her neck, bringing to a halt the efforts to save her life. Laurie Jean Mathiason died a few days later. She was, according to the chiropractic community, the first patient in Canada to die after suffering a stroke from a neck manipulation. This, of course, was pure fantasy.

The rhetoric that the chiropractic community espoused over the next while was disgusting at best and a series of well-constructed lies at worst. Representatives of the Canadian Chiropractic Association and the Canadian Memorial Chiropractic College went on national media stating that this was the first reported death in Canada, even though they were present at a meeting in 1996 where they were told that a forty-five-year-old woman had suffered a similar fate at the hands of a chiropractor. This was conveniently ignored, and the warning regarding the risk of stroke following neck manipulation that the chiropractic community was to distribute to potential chiropractic patients across Canada never materialized. One has to wonder if Laurie Jean Mathiason might be alive today had the chiropractors kept their word.

Since starting my training in neurology in 1993, I have seen virtually all the complications of chiropractic care that one can imagine. These include compressed spinal cords, crushed nerves in the neck and back, torn arteries and muscles in the neck, broken necks, a wide variety of strokes, and at least two deaths. I have also seen patients with huge tumours compressing their spinal cords, which their chiropractors were treating with a lengthy series of manipulations, needlessly delaying the urgent medical treatment that these patients required. My experience, unfortunately, is hardly unique. The vast majority of practicing clinical neurologists have similar stories to tell. The practice of chiropractic provides a steady stream of injured patients for an already grossly overworked medical community.

Much like the tobacco industry in the 1960s, the chiropractic community appears to feel that if they continue to deny virtually all complications arising from their treatment, the public will not listen to the warnings of medical doctors. Chiropractors state that they have an enviable record in treating patients when compared to mainstream medicine. As the vast majority of chiropractic complications occur in perfectly healthy people, comparing medical complications with chiropractic complications is a true "apples and oranges" scenario. Recent studies done by chiropractors and medical doctors alike (published in mainstream medical journals) have indicated that, at best, chiropractic has no effect upon patients, and, at worst, it increases the likelihood of them becoming chronically disabled. Mainstream chiropractic dismisses these studies as having been poorly designed, despite their involvement in the initial development.

For a number of reasons, Canadians are turning to alternative health care providers. They appear to believe that most alternative therapies are essentially risk-free and "natural." Chiropractors work very hard to nurture this benign image through endless television and newspaper ads. The notion that violent twisting of the neck is in any way natural or risk-free is simply not true. And any questions raised by medical doctors are dismissed by many patients and chiropractors alike. It mystifies me, however, why the public and the chiropractors dismiss our concerns. There is no reward, either financial or professional, for alerting people about the risks of non-scientific-based practice. There are, however, very real risks, as any doctor who stands up to the mythology of chiropractic will agree. Personal and legal threats are commonplace, though fortunately they have yet to lead anywhere.

As we move further into the twenty-first century, and the groups competing for health care dollars expand, it is essential that treatments provided are backed by scientific evidence. To continue to fund chiropractic therapy still desperately searching for validation after a hundred years is insulting to the public, the patients who attend chiropractors, and the medical doctors who are expected to clean up the wholly unjustifiable mistakes of the chiropractic community.

The work of Benedetti and MacPhail is an attempt to shine a bright light on areas that chiropractors have long hidden: their lack of scientific basis, their adherence to ridiculously antiquated notions, and their complete failure to accept the dangerous nature of the work they do. There is a straw that breaks the camel's back — perhaps this book will be it.

Dr. Brad Stewart, neurologist
Assistant Professor of Neurology, University of Alberta
Edmonton, Alberta
July 12, 2002

Introduction

WHY WE WROTE THIS BOOK

In a working class section of Toronto's Danforth Avenue, a small chiropractic office has wedged itself between a variety store and a take-out chicken restaurant. In its window, a large poster shows a side view of the human spine. The poster reads:

SUBLUXATIONS
are often present in
PAIN • SICKNESS • DISEASE

The picture of the spine shows just what a "subluxation" is. The middle vertebra in the poster looks a bit cockeyed, and the spinal nerve emerging from it is much thinner than the robust nerves above and below. The tilted vertebra is pinching the nerve, the poster explains, and that leads to the pain, sickness, and disease in the poster's heading. The sign in the window is a reproduction of a chiropractic ad from the 1920s. This explanation of how health and sickness are connected to the spine dates from the same era. But this is a typical chiropractic office at the beginning of the twenty-first century in Canada's largest city.

Inside, the walls of the chiropractor's office are decorated with inspirational slogans: "Expect a miracle today"; "Chiropractic first. Drugs second. Surgery Last." A bulky x-ray machine and a plastic model of the spine inhabit the narrow office's corners, and a black examining table takes centre stage.

Wayne, one of this book's authors, arrives complaining of allergies, but no back pain or spinal problems.

"Allergies and chiropractic, we go hand in hand," the gregarious, middle-aged chiropractor explains. How? Pinched nerves, he says. If nerves in the upper back are squeezed by a misaligned vertebra, it can decrease "nerve flow" and reduce the effectiveness of the immune system. The chiropractor, who wears a white lab coat and introduces himself as a doctor, explains that vertebrae can go out of alignment because of normal activity, stress, or chemicals in the environment. Subluxations can even be caused by the birth process, he explains.

Wayne asks the chiropractor for more details.

"It's very, very basic and simple," he says. "What chiropractors do, we mainly specialize in the spine. If anything is out of alignment, it can pinch the nerve and cause you to have symptoms. It could come in the form of allergies, it could come in the form of discomfort, it could come in the form of restricted movements or it could come in the form of you having no symptoms whatsoever. But it's in there, there are hidden dangers that haven't fully surfaced. So, I'm able to detect those kind of things."

What he's looking for are subluxations. He takes a brief history and checks Wayne's posture and leg lengths. Then, using his hands, he checks the position of each vertebra from the neck to the sacrum. "Yeah, just as I suspected," he says when his hands reach mid-back. He tells Wayne that his ninth thoracic vertebra is out of alignment and then, referring to the spine chart, explains how that could lead to allergies. He says an x-ray could confirm his diagnosis but proceeds to adjust Wayne's back. As he prepares to do the adjustment, he explains that treating allergies is something any chiropractor can do. "Every chiropractor has the same philosophy. I'm no different from any chiropractor, we're all the same."

He has Wayne lie back on the examining table, places one of his hands under Wayne's spine, and positions his legs in the air. "Okay, I'm going to give you an adjustment. You may hear a click, but it will feel comfortable. It will straighten out your spine and relieve the nerve irritation, and the healing's going to start. Your body's going to heal itself. Okay? Let's do it." The chiropractor performs a quick thrust, pressing Wayne's legs forward and driving his back against the chiropractor's hand. There's a popping sound.

"Great! Great! There. You can get up now, I'm finished. I'll give you some exercises along the way to improve your posture because you're slumping like this and you'll get the dowager's hump in the back also. I can prevent that from happening. I'm a specialist in posture."

Wayne asks if the bone isn't pinching the nerve anymore.

"That's right," the chiropractor says. "It's not pinching the nerve anymore. But the thing about it, Wayne, is, you're going to go to bed, you're going to get up, you're going to fight through traffic, you're going to bend down. It can occur again. It doesn't mean because I gave you just one treatment you're cured, you're finished. It's a series of treatments that you need. That took a long, long time to develop and it's going to take time to go away, just like your teeth when they're not straight. The dentist can't straighten out the teeth in one or two visits. It takes two or three years. I'm not saying you're going to take that long to correct, but it's like your teeth."

The chiropractor suggests that Wayne come for three treatments a week for three weeks and then two treatments a week for one week to see if the adjustments are effective. The session costs Wayne seventy-five dollars. And the chiropractor explains he'll also bill provincial government health insurance an additional eleven dollars for the visit.

The chiropractor was pleasant and the treatment was brief and painless. The problem? Everything the chiropractor told Wayne is wrong.

- Nerves cannot be pinched by misaligned vertebrae.
- Vertebrae don't go out of alignment during the activities of daily living.
- There is no evidence that subluxations exist.
- Even if they did exist, there is absolutely no scientific evidence that such a problem could result in the disease of any internal organ or cause allergies.
- The birth process does not create subluxations in newborns, and there is no evidence that chiropractic adjustment of children's spines is beneficial for anything.
- There is no evidence that chiropractors can detect subluxations or that they can correct them.
- There is no evidence that preventative or maintenance adjustments by chiropractors affect health in any way.
- Chiropractors are not licensed in any province in Canada to deal with allergies or any other non-musculoskeletal conditions.
- Chiropractors cannot bill provincial health plans for the treatment of non-musculoskeletal conditions. In billing the Ontario Health Insurance Plan (OHIP) for the treatment of allergies, the chiropractor committed fraud.

But is the Danforth chiropractor operating on the fringes of his profession? No, Wayne's visit is consistent with what a patient could expect walking into almost any chiropractic office in any city or town from Newfoundland to British Columbia. The equipment might be a little more up-to-date, the brochures glossier, the patter more polished and scientific-sounding, but the message would be the same: by adjusting the vertebrae of the human spine, chiropractors can affect general health by restoring, enhancing, and maintaining the body's natural ability to heal.

The truth is, they can't.

Every day, chiropractors are taking money from patients and health insurance plans to treat something — the subluxation — that doesn't exist. There is no evidence to support the way the majority of chiropractors in Canada practice. The profession is rooted in pseudo-science, and much of it is actively antiscientific. And the leading chiropractic organizations in Canada and the United States lie to the public and governments about the health benefits and scientific basis of chiropractic. Chiropractic in Canada is a "regulated health care profession" (it can govern itself and discipline its own members). But in practice, the profession is impossible to regulate and out of control. In dealing with the public and the media, chiropractic officials spin a story about the profession that bears little resemblance to reality.

It's taken us three years of research to uncover these facts. We began this journey in the fall of 1999, when we researched a feature about alternative medicine's quest for academic acceptance in Canada. We were both working in new media journalism and had planned to examine several proposed mergers and affiliations between Canadian universities and holistic health care training institutions. But when we looked into the claims made by the Canadian Memorial Chiropractic College (CMCC), Canada's only English school for chiropractors, we found more than enough material for a lengthy investigative report on chiropractic alone, which was first published on the Web site canoe.ca. Our investigation of that planned affiliation revealed that the CMCC had badly misled York University about the state of chiropractic in Canada. In turn, York had done a dreadful investigation, barely escaping what would have been a disastrous marriage.

The online series generated hundreds of letters to the editor, thousands of postings to Canoe's message boards, and more than a little consternation in the chiropractic profession worldwide. The letters and notes from the chiropractors criticizing the series revealed that we had barely scratched the surface of what was a seriously divided, dogmatic, and defensive profession. Throughout the next year, we spent another several months investigating the treatment of babies and children by chiropractors across Canada. We published a sequel to the first report in March 2001, again on canoe.ca. The series on pediatric chiropractic revealed a profession that produced and protected practitioners who set aside science and common sense to treat newborns and young children for a variety of disorders they had no business handling. In many cases, they even billed parents for spinal adjustments to babies and children with no symptoms, assuring the parents that chiropractic preventative treatment would keep their children healthy and disease-free.

These were not fringe practitioners. We discovered that the majority of Canadian chiropractors treat children. We found that many in the profession, including the leadership, promoted the notion that chiropractic adjustments could treat colic, bed-wetting, asthma, ear infections, respiratory problems, learning disabilities, scoliosis, attention deficit disorder, and much more. Furthermore, the profession actively promoted these treatments in their literature, Web sites, and marketing materials. As well, recruiting children is one of the focal points of practice building seminars attended by Canadian chiropractors. In the meantime, we found that governments — the bodies controlling both licensing and compensation — had no real idea what chiropractors were adjusting children for, but nevertheless paid out millions of dollars in public money for the treatments.

While we were developing these stories, we were also carefully watching and reporting on another controversy within chiropractic — the connection between stroke and chiropractic neck manipulation. We were the first to publish the story of a forty-six-year-old Toronto woman named Lana Dale Lewis, who died after having her neck adjusted by a chiropractor. Her family's multi-million dollar lawsuit and a coroner's inquest called in 2000 put the case and the issue of neck manipulation in the public eye. National media, including the *Globe and Mail,* CBC television and radio, and CTV's *Fifth Estate,* did feature reports on the controversial treatment.

Throughout the unfolding of these events, what we found most fascinating was the behaviour of chiropractors and their governing organizations. The face that they presented to the public and the media was a stark contrast to the reality we knew lay just beneath the surface. Chiropractors claimed that their profession was uniformly science-based, that their techniques were proven safe and effective, and that they embraced the scientific method and were striving to work hand in hand with the medical profession, which was growing more open to chiropractic every day.

We checked each of these claims and found each to be untrue.

Chiropractic is not based in science. Its philosophy has much more in common with magical and religious thinking than modern medicine. Chiropractic is a fractured, fragile profession, deeply divided along sectarian lines; some of the profession is openly hostile to science, and most of it is at least suspicious. In fact, when talking amongst themselves, some chiropractors claim their profession is beyond or above science. But despite the public rhetoric, chiropractic theory is utterly unproven after more than one hundred years. Parts of it, like some chiropractors' belief in "Innate Intelligence" in the body, are inherently untestable and unprovable. Though spinal manipulative therapy (SMT) may be modestly effective in the treatment of uncomplicated, acute low-back pain, chiropractic is not SMT. And though the profession has piggybacked on the evidence supporting SMT for some musculoskeletal problems, no manipulative technique exclusive to chiropractic has been shown to be effective for anything. On the contrary, one technique chiropractors commonly employ — high-neck manipulation — is increasingly shown to be far more dangerous than chiropractors will admit. As for the notion that chiropractors have been accepted by the medical community in universities and teaching hospitals across Canada, a close examination of those claims revealed the ties were far weaker and more informal than the public was led to believe.

Even more disturbing was our discovery that, despite the false face they present to the public and the media, chiropractic officials are fully aware that their fragile profession is in crisis. The schisms that cut to the core of chiropractic are now threatening to crack it apart. There's a well-known saying within the profession: "For every chiropractor there is an equal and opposite chiropractor." The witticism is frighteningly close to the truth. In the broadest sense, the major fissure is between a tiny minority of chiropractors, who are calling for a reformation to science-based practice, and the rest of the profession, which is hopelessly mired in its pseudo-scientific past. Within that larger group, it was surprising to us to discover the dizzying array of techniques — many of them mutually exclusive — practiced by chiropractors. Add to that a grab-bag of non-chiropractic alternative therapies such as applied kinesiology, cranial sacral therapy, homeopathy, herbalism, acupuncture, vitamin and supplement therapy, and much more. All of this turns chiropractic into the health care equivalent of Bits'n'Bites — you never know what you're going to get when you reach into the bag. In every Canadian province, the Yukon, and all American states, chiropractic is a regulated health care profession. In Canada, they can use the title "doctor," see patients without a referral, and discipline their own members. But, unlike any other regulated health care profession, chiropractors are incapable of unanimously defining what it is that they do. This is not a trivial, academic debate. In the real world, Canadians who walk into a chiropractor's office have no way of knowing what kind of chiropractic care they're going to get. Some chiropractors treat subluxations, some don't. Some use a variety of electronic gadgets, some don't. Most treat children, some don't. Many believe in maintenance adjustments for people with no symptoms, some don't. Will the real chiropractic please stand up?

Amongst themselves, chiropractors lament that the public is confused by them. In fact, they are confused by themselves. Their lack of consistency and cohesion makes it impossible to regulate the profession. And it is impossible for the profession as a whole to deliver responsible care to the public. These problems are rampant in Canada.

Simple searches on the Internet, random visits to chiropractic clinics, and a casual browse through brochures — even those produced by the leading chiropractic organizations in North America — reveal numerous unproven claims. We discovered flagrant violations of formal policies governing chiropractic's advertising, marketing, and scope of practice. It appears that these policies are toothless, and that chiropractic officials have spent more time convincing the public, governments, and the media that there are no problems than they have dealing with the horrendous incongruities and abuses right under the nose of anyone who cares to spend a little time investigating.

Until recently, chiropractic has been fairly effective at masking the realities of the profession. But, faced with tighter health care budgets, heightened scrutiny by the medical profession and the media, and an increased demand for accountability, chiropractic is losing ground. One strategy chiropractors have employed is to reposition themselves as leaders in the holistic and "wellness" health field. Unfortunately for chiropractic, there's no evidence that chiropractic adjustments promote overall wellness in any way. And the other things that some chiropractors offer — counselling on nutrition, exercise, and involving patients in their own wellness plans — are already being done by physicians, physiotherapists, dietitians, personal trainers, and others, who provide these services unencumbered by one hundred years of pseudo-scientific nonsense. While chiropractors remain isolated and mired in their own infighting, other health care practitioners are using the best evidence science can deliver to educate and treat their patients. On the other hand, chiropractic has only one treatment — the adjustment — for all problems and has been incapable of moving beyond it. One can legitimately ask, What's so holistic about a health care system based on a single therapy for everything?

Chiropractic's response to criticism of its anachronistic beliefs and its "one-trick" treatment method is to deny, lie, mislead, and attack. Legitimate questions by medical doctors about chiropractic are deflected by chiropractic officials as self-serving protectionism. Media exposés are denounced as hatchet jobs against chiropractic, and their findings are ignored or sometimes characterized as the product of some grand medical/pharmaceutical conspiracy. In general, chiropractors respond to such media attention with defensiveness and denials. Reports on chiropractic by *The Wall Street Journal, Consumer Reports* magazine, CBS's 20/20, CTV's *Fifth Estate*, and, most recently, the *Scientific American Frontiers* episode "A Different Way of Healing?" and our features on canoe.ca have all met with similar responses. In the case of Scientific American, chiropractic officials attempted to block the re-broadcast of the show on affiliate stations across the United States.

All critics of chiropractic — even those in their own ranks — are eventually described as "enemies of chiropractic" or "chiro bashers." Because of the stories we've written in the past, we've already had a deluge of criticism from chiropractors and their supporters, including hate mail, and we have no doubt this book will receive similar treatment.

But our hope with this book is to take readers on the same journey of discovery we've been on over the past three years. In that time, we've spent months reading chiropractic books and journals, days at the CMCC library, and hours and hours interviewing and visiting chiropractors, doctors, physiotherapists, lawyers, academics, and patients. We are not revealing anything that any well-read chiropractor doesn't (or shouldn't) already know, but we are doing the one thing they won't do — discussing it openly. Almost all the criticism that you will find in this book is not coming from doctors or scientists but from chiropractors themselves. A handful of courageous members of the chiropractic community, such as Joseph Keating Jr., Lon Morgan, and Joseph Donahue, have repeatedly pointed out that the emperor has few, if any, clothes. These writers show that there is no credible evidence for much of what chiropractors believe and practice. And they have warned the profession that its longstanding reliance on patient success stories and unprovable chiropractic philosophy to back up their claims of efficacy is no longer acceptable. For the most part, their warnings have been ignored or denounced as propaganda designed to make chiropractic more like mainstream medicine.

We found that most chiropractors have little time or patience for academics or science. In fact, chiropractic in general deals with scientific studies in a decidedly unscientific way. First, when they do their own research, they often focus on how subluxations might function, rather than whether they actually exist. For many chiropractors, the existence of subluxations is "received wisdom" and therefore above testing. Second, they treat all studies of chiropractic as potential marketing tools. Positive outcomes are trumpeted, negative outcomes are ignored or attacked, and some studies that have negative outcomes are misrepresented to the public and to governments as being supportive of chiropractic.

For example, during the recent Commission on the Future of Health Care in Canada, headed by former Saskatchewan premier Roy Romanov, the Canadian Chiropractic Association and the CMCC painted a rosy and inaccurate picture of the chiropractic profession in Canada. They grossly misled the commission about the evidence for the efficacy of chiropractic care for back pain, neck pain, and headache. In a report to the commission they wrote:

Evidence-based research supports the effectiveness of chiropractic in the treatment of low back pain, neck pain, and headaches. The results of more than 85 studies on manual therapy demonstrate efficacy and cost effectiveness with an admirable safety record for the treatment of neuromusculoskeletal pain syndromes.[1]

First, the authors of the report blur, within that one paragraph, the relationship between chiropractic care and manual therapy. They are not the same thing, a fact that has been repeatedly pointed out to chiropractic officials by the authors of some of the studies. While some studies have shown limited benefits from spinal manipulative therapy for some patients, there is no compelling evidence that chiropractic adjustments benefit patients with low-back pain. The evidence that mobilization or manipulation can treat headaches or neck pain is weak or non-existent. Second, the authors misrepresent, to their benefit, the conclusions of the studies they quote. Third, they pick and choose the studies they decide to present to the commission. This is not the way true scientists deal with evidence. Science is not a smorgasbord. You can't graze the studies, pile your plate with the ones you like, and ignore the rest. That's what marketers do with science.

A reasonable person reading the submission to the Commission might assume that chiropractic is a homogeneous, rational health care profession, not unlike dentistry, and that chiropractic practices and therapies are effective, economical, and fully backed by scientific research. This book will demonstrate that nothing could be further from the truth. Chiropractic is a chimera, and many of its claims are unsubstantiated quackery. A considerable element of its membership is anti-scientific, and the profession as a whole is mired in pseudo-science. Despite their claims that the profession is becoming more scientific and evidence-based, recent studies of CMCC students' attitudes and the marketing materials put out by chiropractic's major associations illustrate the opposite. In many ways, the profession has not moved significantly beyond the antiquated nineteenth-century concepts of chiropractic's founder, D.D. Palmer, and the excessive and unsubstantiated marketing claims and methods of his son, B.J. Palmer.

All of that is hard to believe, given that chiropractors are licensed health care professionals with the right to call themselves doctors. We recognize that. But as we take you on the journey that we've been on as we researched this book, we believe you'll draw the same disturbing conclusion: chiropractic is a fragile house of cards, built on an unsteady, irrational foundation that can no longer support it. While individual chiropractors may be well-meaning caregivers convinced that their therapies are helping their patients, chiropractic officials, who doubtless have read the same chiropractic reports, studies, and commentaries that we have, continue to mislead people about what chiro-practic really is and what little and limited proven benefit it provides.

What does all this mean to Canadians? Simply put, while chiropractors across Canada discreetly dicker and debate about what they do and about whether any of it does any good, individuals, governments, and private insurance companies pay them millions of dollars a year in good faith. Canadians have a right to expect that their governments are making sure that the health care they pay for and depend on is as safe, effective, and rational as it can be. It's reasonable for people to expect that health care professionals granted the right to call themselves doctors actually know what they're doing and that what they're doing makes sense. In the case of chiropractic, neither is true.

Paul Benedetti and Wayne MacPhail
Hamilton, 2002

1   Canadian Chiropractic Association & CMCC, "Sustaining and Improving Our Health Care: A Call for Action Submission to the Commission on the Future of Health Care in Canada," (January 2001), p. 7.

1

A HOUSE DIVIDED
How Canadian D.D. Palmer Built the Faulty Foundation of Modern Chiropractic

Old Dad Chiro

Chiropractors will proudly tell you that their form of "drugless health care" has been around for more than a century. They're much more secretive about how little it has changed in all those years. Chiropractic was born in the nine-teenth-century American midwest amidst a dust squall of religious revivalism, quackery, spiritualism, and anti-medical sentiment. It was invented by a deeply religious "magnetic healer," Daniel David Palmer, who mixed his religion with samplings of the folk medicine theories he experienced around him in Davenport, Ohio, on the banks of the Mississippi River. After dabbling in spiritualism, mesmerism, and even phrenology, he came to see the spine as a lightning rod for God's healing power. D.D. Palmer, as he is most commonly known, has become a cult hero of chiropractic. He's called "Old Dad Chiro"[1] even today. His writings are taken by many chiropractors as gospel truth. That's so much the case that it's really impossible to understand modern chiropractic without exploring the story of how Palmer came up with the "big idea" of chiropractic all those years ago. That story begins in Canada, near Port Perry, Ontario.

D.D. Palmer was born on March 7, 1845, in Brown's Corners, Ontario.[2] That tiny (now vanished) hamlet was a few kilometres from present-day Port Perry, just east of Toronto. Palmer's grandparents, Stephen and Abigail, had settled in the Toronto area decades earlier at a time when, as Palmer writes in

The Chiropractic Adjuster, "there was but one log house, the beginning of that great city. That region was known as 'away out west.'" Palmer's father, Thomas, was an Adventist, one of only about forty-two apocalyptic evangelicals in the area at that time. The founder of the Adventist movement, William Miller, had predicted that Christ would return to earth in 1844. The Adventists were forced to reassess their doctrine, for obvious reasons. Adventists like D.D. Palmer's father took the Bible literally and abstained from alcohol and tobacco. It's likely that, on occasion, the Saturday services of the small group of faithful in the Port Perry area would have been held at the Palmer's one-storey wooden frame home on Concession Road 7, as there was no Adventist church in the vicinity. Adventism was only one of dozens of religious movements that were bringing a strong sense of religious revival to North America in the nineteenth century. As we'll see, the sense of personal relationship with God and the spiritual conversion that were at the base of the revivalist movements would help lay the groundwork for chiropractic's birth.

Despite his father's deep religion, D.D. Palmer writes that his mother had the lion's share of unscientific thought in the family. "My mother was as full of superstition as an egg is full of meat, but my father was disposed to reason on the subjects pertaining to life," Palmer explains in a memoir he wrote in 1910.[3]

Thomas Palmer, D.D.'s father, was born in 1815, the youngest of four children. He was twelve years younger than his brother Henry, who became a shoemaker. Thomas followed in his older brother's footsteps — but, it appears, with much less success. In his personal journals, Palmer writes of his "father failing in business."[4] As a result, D.D., the eldest of six children, had to work to help support the family. He attended school until he was eleven and from then on appears to have been self-taught. Actually, Palmer's education is the subject of both speculation and legend in chiropractic circles. His younger brother T.J.'s autobiography tells the story of how he and D.D. were prodded by a "brutish taskmaster, one John Black" to tackle eighth-grade work when they were nine and eleven. They were then, according to the younger Palmer, "launched into the study of high school subjects that included the physical sciences."[5] Other sources suggest that D.D. Palmer got little formal schooling and was basically self-educated. He had no medical training. But census records indicate that a John Black did teach in a log school near the Palmers, so he may well have taught the two boys when he was in his late twenties.

Magnetic Healing on the Mississippi

After the end of the U.S. Civil War in 1865, Thomas Palmer moved his family to the coal mining town of What Cheer, Iowa, about 150 miles west of

Chicago. The elder Palmer probably hoped the post-war economy would offer him and his family better opportunities.

In 1871, D.D. Palmer married his first wife (of five), Abba Lord, and purchased ten acres of land near New Boston, Illinois. He kept his family fed by teaching in rural schools, raising bees, and growing fruit. The Mason jar having just been invented, Palmer made a decent living from selling preserves. He also cultivated a new variety of blackberry called Sweet Home, which canned well. Palmer marketed the bushes throughout the United States by mail order. He also developed a curious interest in goldfish, which he raised and sold. In 1874, Palmer married again, this time to a southern widow, Louvenia Landers. Little is known about what happened to his first wife, though she may have died in childbirth.[6]

By 1881, Palmer and his new wife had moved closer to his family in What Cheer and opened a grocery store, the ninth in what had become a prosperous small town. Palmer's business failed and he moved again, this time to Letts, Iowa, where he went back to teaching school. Three years later, Louvenia died. Palmer was left to care for an eleven-year-old from his second wife's previous marriage, two daughters, aged eight and six, and his first biological son, Bartlett Joshua Palmer. B.J. Palmer, as he is most often known, would grow up to become the great popularizer of chiropractic. The elder Palmer's relationship with his son would prove to be a hostile and difficult one, and the effects of it would shape much of what chiropractic has become. Six months after Louvenia's death, D.D. Palmer married again, this time to Martha Henning.

Around this time, spiritualism, theosophy, and magnetic healing began to fascinate Palmer. Spiritualists held that it was possible to talk to the dead through séances and other mystical means. Theosophists studied ancient and contemporary religions and sciences searching for synthesis. Magnetic healers believed they could treat a variety of ailments by diverting and clearing pathways for animal magnetism, which they believed flowed through the body like a liquid.

The most charismatic magnetic healer was Franz Anton Mesmer. In 1774, Mesmer, a German physician and a friend of Mozart, came to the conclusion that the universe was filled with increasingly refined fluids. The spaces between grains of sand, Mesmer wrote, could be filled with water; the spaces in water could be filled with air. The air itself (and everything else) was permeated by invisible ether. That ether, Mesmer said, was suffused with a perfectly refined substance, which, when present in a living being, he called animal magnetism. Using words Palmer would later re-employ, Mesmer wrote, "The animal body experiences the alternative effects of [animal magnetism], and is directly affected by its insinuation into the substance of the nerves."[7]

Mesmer thought this pervasive, subtle force (which no scientist had observed or measured) obeyed the laws of magnetism. For Mesmer, disease was the result of obstacles that blocked the flow of the universal fluid, or animal magnetism, in the body. The blockages impinged the contraction and dilation of blood vessels and so reduced the body's ability to conduct life. A body with animal magnetism ebbing and flowing easily within it would be free of disease. A skilled healer could clear blockages in this natural flow. That healer allowed the animal magnetism to heal the body naturally. Mesmer explains how he worked in his 1784 text, *Catechism on Animal Magnetism*.

> First of all, one must place oneself opposite the patient, back to the north, bringing one's feet against the invalid's; then lay two thumbs lightly on the nerve plexes which are located in the pit of the stomach, and the fingers on the hypochondria [region below the ribs]. From time to time it is good to run one's fingers over the ribs, principally towards the spleen, and to change the position of the thumbs. After having continued this exercise for about a quarter of an hour, one performs in a different manner, corresponding to the condition of the patient....It is always necessary that one hand is on one side, and the other hand is on the opposite side. If the sickness is general, the hands — made into a pyramid with the fingers — are passed over the whole body, starting at the head and then descending along the two shoulders down to the feet. After this one returns to the head: from the front and from the rear, then over the abdomen and over the back.

While Mesmer used actual magnets in some of his more public treatments, it's clear that he didn't consider them important or necessary. He believed that animal magnetism, being all-pervasive, could be controlled by a healer's will without touching a patient. He also believed it could be used as a medium for telepathy and precognition.[8]

Mesmer saw magnetism not just in human bodies but also in all animate and inanimate things. Early in his career, he related the ebbs and flows of animal magnetism in the body to the gravitational influence of the planets. So, for Mesmer, animal magnetism linked man to the universe. That belief tied him, philosophically, to a long line of vitalists (people who believe that life is driven by an invisible, spiritual force). Diverse healing systems, like acupuncture and, these days, therapeutic touch are all vitalist in nature.

Mesmer began his career as a magnetic healer in Vienna. With his charismatic and theatrical style and his hypnotic influence he was a sensation, especially with the female aristocracy. These rich women believed all manner of fashionable illnesses had been effectively treated by Mesmer's ministrations to their blocked and fragile animal magnetism. In fact, Mesmer was simply treating psychosomatic illnesses with sham treatments, which depended on the placebo effect and his natural showmanship and sex appeal. Viennese doctors quickly decried the flamboyant Mesmer as a fraud. In 1794, King Louis XVI appointed a commission (including Benjamin Franklin) to investigate Mesmer's techniques. The commissioners found no scientific support for the showman's methods, and his star began to wane in Europe.

In the America of the 1880s, though, magnetic healing was still a popular treatment for a host of illnesses. It became intermixed with the religious revivalism that was in the air, especially in rural areas of the country. Its key proponents in D.D. Palmer's part of the country were Paul Caster and his son. In the late 1880s, Palmer took courses from the Casters and became a doctor of magnetic healing.[9] In 1886, he opened his first office on Jefferson Street in Burlington, Iowa, a small town on the Mississippi River. He found himself in competition with doctors, homeopaths, purveyors of botanical cures, occultists, and the popular Casters. He didn't stay long, nor, it seems, did his third wife, Martha, who walked out on him. A year later, he opened up a new practice in Davenport, Iowa, a few miles north of Burlington. He took rooms in the Ryan Building and advertised himself as "D.D. Palmer, Cures Without Medicine." Palmer was in heavy debt when he opened the new business, but it soon became a moneymaker for him, thanks to word of mouth, testimonial advertising, and a 138-foot-long sign that could be seen by the passengers on board ships plying the Mississippi.

Palmer, much like Mesmer before him, treated a diseased organ by placing one hand under it and the other above it so that "magnetic radiation" could flow from hand to hand. But Palmer insisted that while other magnetic healers rubbed and slapped the entire body during a treatment, he isolated only the ailing organ and poured his magnetic healing energy directly into it. Palmer's clinic eventually filled forty rooms. Out-of-town patients could stay overnight, have meals, and take treatments in Palmer's drugless infirmary. Oddly, Palmer dedicated one room to his old passion, goldfish. He was adamantly opposed to drugs and surgery and took what would now be called a natural approach to healing, although in the late nineteenth century he was called a "drugless practitioner." In 1888, Palmer married Villa Amanda Thomas, his fourth wife. The new Mrs. Palmer took care of many of the clinic's administrative details but, ironically, had a drug addiction problem.[10] She died of a morphine overdose in 1904.

Heroic Medicine, Common Men, and Hellfire

To really appreciate Palmer's success and his relationship to the medicine of the doctors of the time, it's worthwhile pulling the lens back from his burgeoning clinic on the bank of the Mississippi and taking a wide-angle look at the state of medicine and the society of nineteenth-century America, especially after the Civil War.

It was a time of remarkable social, religious, and medical upheaval in the United States. American Protestant religions had already passed through two "Great Awakenings" of religious spirit and passion. While it was primarily Calvinists who drove the First Great Awakening from the northeastern United States, the Second Great Awakening, from about 1790 to 1830, was definitely a product of Southern Methodists and Baptists (who had learned some revival techniques earlier from Presbyterians). It was a time of fervent camp meetings, dramatic public response to the gospel, and "fire and brimstone" oratory that appealed more to the heart and the emotions than the intellect.[11] By the end of the Civil War, religious fervour had passed from the more established religions into the hands of newer movements like the Pentecostals, the Fundamentalists, the Holiness Movement, and the Adventists, like the Palmer family. These movements focused on the imminent arrival of Christ (who would establish a New Jerusalem in America), the need for a personal relationship with God, and the transcendent experience of giving yourself over to Jesus through a sudden spiritual epiphany.

The growth of these people's religions was fuelled by two social trends. The first was a late-blooming interest in European Romanticism throughout America during the middle of the nineteenth century. Writers like Thoreau, Whitman, Emerson, Hawthorne, and Melville captured the spirit of American Romanticism. This movement rejected science, intellectualism, and proscriptive religions like Calvinism. It celebrated the common man, simplicity, and harmony with nature. It considered Truth to be subjective, not tied to rigorous experiments and data. It also gave rise to "intentional communities," or communes, like the Shakers, who returned to simpler values in reaction to society's growing interest in progress, commerce, and industrialization.[12] The second social trend, closely linked to Romanticism, was the idealistic notion of democracy that grew out of War of Independence hero Andrew Jackson having been elected the seventh president of the United States in 1829. Jackson held himself up as the spokesman for the common man. Earlier presidents, like Jefferson, had been more intellectual and aristocratic than the self-made Jackson, who pushed for democratic reform throughout his two terms.

The blend of Jacksonian democracy, Romanticism, and Revivalism left late-nineteenth-century Americans suspicious of science, especially of intellectuals like doctors. What's more, the state of American medicine during and after the Civil War wouldn't have played in the doctors' favour.[13] At the beginning of the nineteenth century, American doctors were ruled by a belief that all disease resulted from overstimulation of nerves and blood. To deal with this, they used what were called "heroic" measures: bleeding patients, creating blisters, and administering purgatives and laxatives. Heroic medicine was often painful, traumatic, disfiguring, and useless. It was also, as can be imagined, very unpopular with patients. Up until the 1840s, the only anaesthetics were alcohol and opium, and surgeons often operated in the same soiled coats they wore to perform autopsies. But, encouraged by heroic medicine's leading American proponent, Benjamin Rush, American doctors continued using these dismal techniques.

For example, the treatment records of Dr. Samuel Overton,[14] a physician who practiced in Old Canton, Texas in the later part of the nineteenth century, demonstrate how long heroic medicine held sway. Even after 1850, Overton was still using cupping, a technique that involved applying small glass bowls containing a partial vacuum over lacerated skin to draw blood out of the body. He also used calomel (mercurous chloride), a powerful laxative with the nasty side effect of inducing tooth loss through the recession of often painful and bleeding gums. Overton frequently raised blisters on the surface of his patient's skin, using a variety of "counterirritant" compounds.

While doctors in France (and some progressive American doctors) were starting to stress data, analysis, and clinical examination, the "age of the common man" at play in America meant that doctors like Overton were more the norm. Nineteenth-century American surgery, especially during the Civil War, was torturous butchery. At the beginning of the Civil War, in 1861, an underprepared and understaffed Army Medical Department had to cope with rampant disease and infection at a time when the role of bacteria and viruses in infection and illness wasn't understood. For every solider who died in battle, two died from dysentery, diarrhea, typhoid, or malaria. A total of 560,000 soldiers from both sides succumbed to disease. An additional two hundred thousand died from battlefield injuries, often from post-operative infections. There was no antiseptic surgery at the time. Limb amputation without anaesthetic was a frequent solution to the massive wounds of battle. So, despite the tremendous advances medicine made as a result of the Civil War (hospital organization, research notes on disease and wound treatment), in its aftermath doctors were often viewed by the average American as a brutish elite too eager to bleed, burn, purge, or disfigure to no good effect.

Physicians' training at the time didn't improve their reputation. Early in the century, students had to buy tickets for lectures, were often illiterate, and had to bring their own cadavers for dissection if a school couldn't get enough. The students often hired illegal grave robbers to procure corpses for them. By 1875, there were seventy-three medical schools in the United States, but most were small, proprietary, and had few entrance requirements and no standard curriculum. Medical education in the nineteenth century was more a matter of apprenticeship than anything else.

By the middle of the nineteenth century, European physicians like Pasteur, Snow, and Lister had developed the concept of communicable diseases and bacteria, but the germ theory was not as contagious in America. It wasn't until 1880 that Dr. William Mayo first practiced antiseptic surgery in Rochester, Minnesota. Near the end of the century, when Palmer opened his magnetic healing clinic in Davenport, medical education was on the road to reform. In 1910, the wide-ranging Flexner Report (which examined American medical schools in detail) completely altered the state of medical education in America for the better. After the report, medicine in the United States made a remarkable climb out of the trenches of quackery and towards the modern high ground of evidence-based medicine rooted in solid science and serious education. But the poor education and carnage of the previous decades, mixed with Jacksonian democracy and religious revivalism, had created a fertile ground for common men who claimed to be able to heal without crude surgery, toxic drugs, or lethal infection. D.D. Palmer wasn't alone in trying to spread the word about painless, natural medicine in the 1880s. It was an age of quackery, patent medicine, and health crazes that were linked to moral purity and fundamentalist religion. Palmer fit right in.

The Golden Age of Quackery

At the beginning of the nineteenth century, Thomsonianism, driven by Samuel Thomson, held that all disease was caused by a clogged system that could be cleansed by vegetable tinctures. Electropathy, a close relative of mesmerism, came into vogue in the later part of the century. Its chief proponent, S.R. Wells, held that electricity applied topically to the body could adjust imbalances and could cure nervous disorders. All manner of electrical gadgets and items of clothing were sold — some with none-too-subtle sexual undertones. Hydrotherapists claimed that injecting patients with water, dousing them with cold water, or wrapping them in wet blankets or clothing could effect a variety of cures. It was also the era of traveling circuses, medicine shows, and acts like "Professor" Herbert L. Flint's traveling hypnosis show, in which B.J. Palmer, D.D.'s son, would become a stagehand.

Meanwhile, patent medicines like "Lydia Pinkham's Vegetable Compound" were taking the nation by storm. Their sales were fueled by outrageous ads in the rapidly growing number of American newspapers and by patent legislation that allowed makers to protect their products from imitations. Many of the patent medicines contained some vegetable extracts, but those harmless ingredients were mixed with unhealthy dollops of alcohol, sugar, opiates, and caffeine. According to an estimate by University of Toledo archivist Barbara Floyd, by 1859, quack medicines were generating $3.5 million in sales, an astounding amount that would skyrocket to $74.5 million in 1904.

The Crack Heard 'Round the World

So D.D. Palmer's Davenport clinic was just one of hundreds of different sorts of nonscientific solutions offered to suffering and enfeebled Americans. It's likely that, as successful as Palmer was with his infirmary on the lip of the Mississippi, he would have been an unremarkable footnote in the history of folk medicine if he hadn't run into a deaf black janitor who had the cleaning contract for the Ryan building, home of Palmer's clinic in Davenport. His adjustment of Harvey Lillard's spine was the crack heard around the world. Palmer describes the incident himself in *The Chiropractor's Adjuster*:

> One question was always uppermost in my mind in my search for the cause of disease. I desired to know why one person was ailing and his associate, eating at the same table, working in the same shop, at the same bench, was not. Why? What difference was there in the two persons that caused one to have pneumonia, catarrh, typhoid or rheumatism, while his partner, similarly situated, escaped. Why? The question had worried thousands for centuries and was answered in September 1895.
>
> Harvey Lillard, a janitor, in the Ryan Block, where I had my office, had been so deaf for 17 years that he could not hear the racket of a wagon on the street or the ticking of a watch. I made inquiry as to the cause of his deafness and was informed that when he was exerting himself in a cramped, stooped position, he felt something give way in his back and immediately became deaf. An examination showed a vertebra racked from its normal position. I reasoned that if that vertebra was replaced, the man's hearing should be restored. With this object in view, a half-hour's talk persuaded Mr. Lillard to allow me to replace it. I racked it into position by using the spinous process as a lever and soon the man could hear as before. There was nothing "accidental" about this, as it was accomplished with an object in view, and the result expected was obtained. There was

nothing "crude" about this adjustment; it was specific, so much so that no Chiropractor has equaled it.[15]

Palmer later treated another patient for "heart trouble." Again, he adjusted one of the patient's vertebrae and produced instant relief.

Then I began to reason if two diseases, so dissimilar as deafness and heart trouble, came from impingement, a pressure on nerves, were not other disease due to a similar cause? Thus the science (knowledge) and art (adjusting) of Chiropractic were formed at that time.[16]

Palmer believed he'd been given the "big idea" that explained the cause of 95 percent of all disease and disorders. Bones (not just the bones of the spine) out of place put pressure on blood vessels and nerves and thereby cause illness and weakness in the body. By manipulating the displaced bones, chiropractics (as Palmer called chiropractors at first) could offer therapeutic assistance. Palmer called the misalignments in the vertebrae "luxations" or displacements. He later came to call them "subluxations," as they were less than a full dislocation. The subluxation would become, literally and figuratively, the sore point of chiropractic for over a century.

The Lillard story is part of chiropractic legend. There are several variations of the tale. In one version, Palmer, in response to a joke Lillard is telling friends, hits him good-naturedly on the back with a book. Afterwards, the janitor notices a slight hearing improvement.[17] The date of the world's most famous chiropractic treatment is also in doubt, as is exactly which vertebra Palmer adjusted. The yarn is probably best considered chiropractic's creation myth rather than gospel truth.

Palmer was not the first (nor the last) folk healer to reduce all human maladies to a single simple cause. And some drugless practitioners were quick to point out that Palmer hadn't discovered anything at all. He'd just stolen their "big idea" and given it a new name. These were the osteopaths. Osteopaths believed that disease was the result of misalignments of the bones and organs. These alleged misalignments reduced blood flow and so brought on disease and disability. Andrew Still, the founder of osteopathy, explained the process in his 1899 book, *Philosophy of Osteopathy*:

The failure of free action of blood produces general debility, congestion, low types of fever, dropsy, constipation, tumefaction and on to the whole list of visceral diseases.[18]

The treatment Still prescribed was to carefully position a patient so that all bones met each other naturally and the pressure was relieved from vital blood vessels. Still makes it clear in his 1899 text that keeping the spine in alignment is a key treatment an osteopath can offer:

> Suppose a fall should jar the lumbar vertebra, and push it at some articulation, front, back, or laterally; say the lumbar, with one or two short ribs turned down against the lumbar nerves with a prolapsed and loosened diaphragm, pressing heavily on the abdominal aorta, vena cava, and thoracic duct; have you not found cause to stop or derange the circulation of blood in arteries, veins, lymphatics and all other organs below diaphragm? Then heart trouble would be the natural result. Fibroid tumors, painful monthlies, constipation, diabetes, dyspepsia or any trouble of the system that could come from bad blood would be natural results, because lymph is too old to be pure when it enters the lungs for purifying.[19]

Osteopathic principles were articulated by Still as early as 1874 and were familiar to Palmer. In fact, D.D. Palmer lived near Still and had, on more than one occasion, visited his home. The osteopaths felt they'd had the crown jewels stolen by a usurper. They had a point. It's difficult, reading Palmer's early writing, to find much of a difference between how he originally described chiropractic and what osteopaths practiced. Palmer, though, claimed his treatments could get the job done ten times quicker. Palmer also argued that while osteopaths focused on allowing a free flow of health, he worked on reducing the "friction and inflammation" he saw as the root of illness. Both schools of "healing without medicine" took a very mechanistic view of the body. As late as 1902, Palmer was writing:

> I look the human machine over and find what parts are out of place, why the blood does not circulate freely to all parts, why the nerves cry out with pain.[20]

Chiropractic historian Joseph Keating points out that this wording echoes Still's own writing on the mechanical metaphor and the body:

> The human body is a machine run by the unseen force called life, and that it may be run harmoniously it is necessary that there be liberty of blood, nerves and arteries from their generating point to their destination.[21]

Palmer Twists his Spine Theory

Palmer's theories of chiropractic changed dramatically over the next ten years, and they pulled further from osteopathy. At first, Palmer was extremely secretive about his chiropractic methods. He saw about one hundred patients a day, from 1:00 P.M. to 6:00 P.M. Each treatment took about thirty seconds, and Palmer wouldn't let any patient, or any observer, see him perform the manipulations. When he caught a customer trying to observe his technique in a mirror, he had it removed immediately. But through the encouragement of his son, B.J., and after a traffic accident that roused Palmer's fears of imminent death, he began to teach his chiropractic techniques to a select few in 1898. From historical accounts, it doesn't sound like the students got much of an education. Oakley Smith, an 1899 graduate, recalls his Palmer schooling this way:

> The first thing I learned was that there was no instruction to be given. There were no blackboards, no text books, no notes, not a single lecture. For six days I witnessed the giving of a number of treatments. That was the sum total of information that was transferred in exchange for tuition paid. The diagnosis as I witnessed it consisted of a quick gliding pressure from upper dorsal to middle lumbar to detect the position of posterior apical prominences. That was the sum total of examination that was given to any patient. The treatment consisted of giving a single forceful lunge on that prominent apex, using the flat of the hand as a contact. That was the sum total of the treatment. Nothing else was done. The patient's treatment for that day was finished. These treatments were given daily. There were no charts made, no histories taken, and no records made. After being permitted to watch this identical form of treatment on a number of patients for six days I was told that I knew all that was necessary for me to know, and that I should do the treating myself thereafter.[22]

Smith established his own school, the American School of Chiropractic, seven years after his short Palmer course. Palmer himself opened the Palmer School and Infirmary and, over the next few years, graduated a handful of students, including some doctors and osteopaths — and, in 1902, his son B.J.

From its very beginnings, chiropractic was plagued with the variations and divisiveness that continue to haunt it today. Many of D.D. Palmer's early graduates, like Smith, founded their own schools of chiropractic, each with his own unique interpretation of Palmer's original techniques and each with his own blending of chiropractic and other forms of therapy, including osteopathy. D.D. Palmer was dismissive of the rival schools. He called those who blended his technique with other therapies "mixers." Palmer was offering what he considered straight chiropractic. That "straight" vs. "mixer" battle lives on today in heated debates in the *Journal of the Canadian Chiropractic Association* and other chiropractic publications and advertisements. Straight chiropractors generally feel they need only to adjust subluxations to allow the body to heal itself. Mixers use other therapies and are more inclined than straight chiropractors to refer patients to medical doctors. But many mixers believe that the root cause of a depressed immune system is a misaligned spine. There is no scientific evidence to suggest this is true. In the United States, the straight/mixer debate is manifest in the two distinct chiropractic organizations that still exist. The American Chiropractic Association is a mixer group, while the International Chiropractic Association (started by B.J. Palmer) is more aligned with straight chiropractic. Numerous attempts to amalgamate the two organizations have been fruitless. In Canada, the Canadian Chiropractic Association is open to a broad definition of chiropractic and is more of a mixer organization.

Even as new variations of chiropractic rose around him, Palmer himself rewrote his theories on the fly — a right he felt only he had. In 1902, he and his wife abruptly moved to southern California, leaving his school and a mounting debt behind.[23] By 1903, Palmer became much more interested in nerves than blood. He developed the odd idea that the vibration of the nerves heated in the blood. The notion seems to have arisen from a clinic Palmer held in Santa Barbara, California in July of that year.[24] Palmer adjusted a patient's spine and noticed the dramatic changes in skin temperature his adjustments made.

Afterwards, he began to teach that nerve interference by displaced joints was the primary cause of disease. At the same time, Palmer wrote about chiropractic adjustments being more than therapeutic — they dealt with the root cause of the disease itself, not just the effects. "Therapeutical methods can only treat effects," Palmer wrote in 1904. "Causes cannot be treated; they must be made right by adjustment."[25] Palmer may have been responding to a 1903 charge against his son B.J. for practicing medicine without a certificate from the Board of Medical Examiners. If chiropractors weren't actually treating specific symptoms, but rather getting to the root cause of all disease, then, Palmer suggested, they weren't really providing therapeutic manipulations for specific ailments, they were offering "adjustments" that allowed the body to heal itself of all disorders naturally.

Ironically, an early student of Palmer's, Solon Langworthy, was also concentrating on the effect chiropractors could have on the nerves. As we'll see, it's Langworthy's writings about nerves, not D.D. Palmer's, that helped define the future direction of chiropractic. It was also during this period that Palmer began to distinguish between two kinds of nerves. The nerves that control the voluntary motions and actions of the body he labeled "educated" nerves. Those that took charge of the involuntary actions (digestion, etc.) he called "innate." With the use of those two words, Palmer had started chiropractic down an entirely new path. And Palmer's own life was about to take a dramatic turn.

D.D. Palmer returned to Davenport two years after his sudden departure to discover that in his absence his son, now twenty-three, had made the family business a success. But if he had left to avoid legal prosecution, he returned to find the same enemy had been waiting for him. In 1906, Palmer was convicted of practicing medicine without a license. He refused to pay the $350 fine attached to the sentence and was incarcerated for 23 days until his fifth wife, Mary Hudler, settled with the court.

Innate Takes Centre Stage

It was during his time in prison that Palmer began to conceive of "innate," not just as an adjective used to describe autonomic nerves, but as a separate, higher intelligence that controlled the function of the body and was a part of the Universal Intelligence. In his writings from this time, innate becomes capitalized and is often referred to as Innate Intelligence. In 1906, Palmer wrote that almost all bodily functions are managed by "Innate," except where the innate nerves are being "pinched and pressed upon, causing abnormal function."

So, ten years after his "discovery" of chiropractic, Palmer had already made significant refinements and shifts in his definition of his new form of treatment. What had started as a very mechanistic view of healing, much like osteopathy, had shifted dramatically to place more emphasis on the nerves and on a spiritual notion of a universal force flowing through the body. According to Palmer's 1906 thinking, if subluxations didn't block the flow, via the pinching or impingement of nerves, Innate would allow the body to heal itself through the application of Innate Intelligence, which was a fragment of a much greater Universal Intelligence. Unfortunately for Palmer, he was having more success with his theory than with his school or his son.

While in prison, D.D. Palmer transferred his assets to his son's wife, Mabel, to keep them safe from the law.[26] But after D.D.'s release from prison, B.J. refused to let him back into his own Ryan Street building. In an acrimonious dispute that had to be settled by an arbitrator, B.J. bought the school from his father. As well, Willard Carver, a lawyer who had unsuccessfully defended D.D. Palmer against practicing medicine without a license, became a chiropractor at a rival school and then went off and founded his own chiropractic school, teaching non-Palmer treatment methods. An even more deeply embittered and increasingly paranoid D.D. Palmer moved away from Davenport once again. While his early graduates and son opened successful and varied chiropractic schools and practices, the founder of chiropractic spent the next several years wandering in the chiropractic wilderness of Oklahoma and Oregon. He couldn't get along with a variety of chiropractic school partners and lashed out at B.J. and others he felt were not teaching or practicing true chiropractic. Meanwhile, he continued to rewrite his own theory.

By 1910, in fact, Palmer had completely revised his thinking about the pinching of nerves. Despite his earlier writings and teachings, he wrote in *The Chiropractor's Adjuster*:

> It has never been proven that subluxated vertebrae pinch, squeeze or compress nerves as they pass through the intervertebral foramina [the spaces between adjacent vertebrae].[27]

He now believed that a body's health depended on the state of its "tone." Tone was delivered to the body through the nerves and had its source in Innate Intelligence. If misaligned joints impinged on the nerves, there would be an increase or decrease of tension in the nerve. That "detuning" of the nerves would make it more or less able to transmit tone, and thus health, to the rest of the body. To Palmer, it was as if nerves were now like violin strings that needed to be maintained at the right tension so they could effectively resonate with the pitch of the Innate Intelligence that hummed like God's tuning fork. While the body could heal itself with Innate's help, only chiropractors could keep the nerves in tune.

Palmer believed that subluxations often caused an increase in nerve tension and so created too much nerve vibration. Using his 1903 theory that the nerves heated the blood, Palmer concluded that the increased vibration would create an excess heat that could cause inflammation and even kill tissues and stop organs from functioning. For Palmer, in 1910, bacteria, infections, and the body's natural defenses (white blood cells, etc.) had nothing to do with fever, swelling, or inflammation. It was all the result of nerves that had become too excited by bones that had minutely slipped from their ordained positions and relationships.

Palmer was certain that Innate Intelligence was a fraction of the Universal Intelligence that created and propelled the universe — God. For Palmer, Innate "never sleeps nor tires; recognizes neither darkness nor distance and is not subject to material laws or conditions." It was, in many ways, like the animal magnetism of Mesmer, but now Palmer had overlaid it with aspects of spiritualism and his deeply held religious convictions. He believed that the individual Innate that occupied every person's body came into existence before birth and survived the physical body's death. He also felt that Innate wished to communicate with chiropractors in order to allow them to help it heal the body naturally. In fact, Palmer came to believe that the secret of chiropractic was sent to him directly from God.

By 1910, D.D. Palmer had stepped away from whatever tenuous ties he had to what he considered science and had returned to the religious, spiritual, and vitalistic notions of his pre-chiropractic days. He effectively replaced the terminology of medicine ("therapy," "manipulation," and "diagnosis") with a new philosophical lexicon he felt reflected the more powerful, deeper nature of the assistance chiropractors gave the body and Innate. Chiropractors didn't treat symptoms and diseases, they simply listened to Innate and used their skilled hands to let it manifest itself in the body (his son B.J. would adopt this language for legal defence purposes). With Innate flowing freely, good health would follow. And Palmer felt he was the one and only person who could impart the true philosophy, science, and practical art of chiropractic. Why the change in theory, terminology, and attitude? It seems clear from his writing that Palmer was reacting to the success of his son's increasingly famous chiropractic school and to the other upstart chiropractors who were teaching and practicing variations on themes and theories that Palmer himself had advocated just a few years earlier. He was also reacting to the legal and medical professions, which he saw as plotting against chiropractors' ability to practice drugless medicine, and which had already had him thrown in jail once.

In a 1912 letter to a California chiropractor who wanted the state to license chiropractic, Palmer writes:

You ask, what I think will be the final outcome of our law getting. It will be that we will have to build a boat similar to Christian Science and hoist a religious flag. I have received chiropractic from the other world, similar as did Mrs. Eddy. No other one has laid claim to that, not even B.J. Exemption clauses instead of chiro laws by all means, and let that exemption be the right to practice our religion. But we must have a religious head, one who is the founder, as did Christ, Mohamed, Jo. Smith, Mrs. Eddy, Martin Luther and

others who have founded religions. I am the fountain head. I am the
founder of chiropractic in its science, in its art, in its philosophy and
in its religious phase. Now, if chiropractors desire to claim me as
their head, their leader, the way is clear. My writings have been
gradually steering in that direction until now it is time to assume
that we have the same right to as have Christian Scientists. Oregon
is free to Chiropractors. California gives Chiropractors only one
chance, that of practicing our religion. The protective policy of the
U.C.A. is O.K., but that of religion is far better. The latter can only
be assumed by having a leader, a head, a person who has received
chiropractic as a science, as an art, as a philosophy and as a religion.
Do you catch on?[28]

In fact, Palmer didn't go so far as advocating that chiropractic become a
religion, like other newcomers such as Christian Scientists, Mormons, and
Jehovah's Witnesses. He just wanted enough gospel armour to protect him
from the law. But just before his death in 1913, he was advocating that the
practice of chiropractic involved both "a moral obligation and a religious
duty" and that he was obeying God when he manipulated bones.

By correcting these displacements of osseous tissue, the tension
frame of the nervous system, I claim that I am rendering obedience,
adoration and honor to the All-Wise Spiritual Intelligence, as well
as a service to the segmented, individual portions thereof — a duty
I owe to both God and mankind. In accordance with this aim and
end, the Constitution of the United States and the statutes personal
of California confer upon me and all persons of chiropractic faith
the inalienable right to practice our religion without restraint or
hindrance.[29]

He had also come to believe chiropractic to be capable of miracles far
beyond simple symptom treatment.

[Chiropractic's] possibilities will become unlimited, when His laws
and our duties as a segmented, personified, portion thereof, are
scientifically understood. It will lessen disease, poverty and crime,
empty our jails, penitentiaries and insane asylums and assist us to
prepare for the existence beyond the transition called death.
It explains why all persons are not equal, mentally and physically;
or, if born alike, why some become superior or inferior to others
similarly situated, why certain individuals are not able to express

themselves as intelligently as others, why some persons are not mentally and physically alike at all times.[30]

He also believed that chiropractors had a religious duty to treat children, lest they remain infirm on Earth and in the afterlife.

> Many a child has been injured at birth by a vertebral displacement which caused an impingement upon one or more of the spinal nerves, as they emanate from the spinal canal, the fibers of which are distributed to certain organs. The result of this excessive tension is physical or mental debility, often both, which, from a lack of pathological knowledge, may be lifelong; the mental defect extending even into the next world. For we retain only that which has been acquired during this earthly, preparatory existence. By properly adjusting the neuroskeleton, these unfortunates may be enabled to acquire sufficient knowledge, rightfully due them, to become useful members of society and enjoy life in this world and the one to come. The chiropractor who can accomplish the above desirable results and refuses to do so, as a religious duty, should be compelled to perform it as a moral obligation.[31]

The Unscientific, Unsettled Legacy of Old Dad Chiro

In October 1913, D.D. Palmer died of typhoid fever at the age of sixty-eight. He had created chiropractic less than twenty years earlier. But in those two decades he had formulated theories and sparked controversies that would plague the profession for more than a century. Despite his rhetoric, his ideas contained little true philosophy and no science. He borrowed heavily from pre-scientific concepts like vitalism and spiritualism, stole techniques and concepts from mesmerism and osteopathy, and blended in religious overtones from revivalism and advertising techniques from patent medicine. He claimed his "big idea" was divinely inspired. It was certainly not based on any real science or scientific evidence, though it's clear that Palmer read widely about medicine and science. Near the end of his life, he wanted to move his theories beyond the realm of science and natural law. His ideas and his constant revisions both created chiropractic and laid the foundation for it to become a house divided. Tragically for D.D. Palmer, his later ideas were all but ignored by his ambitious and resentful son, B.J., who was about to hawk a watered-down chiropractic to a twentieth-century America like there was no tomorrow.

2

THE P.T BARNUM OF CHIROPRACTIC

How B.J. Palmer Sold, Simplified, and Nearly Destroyed Chiropractic

On the Web site www.chiropracticbooks.com, there's a whole section devoted to merchandise featuring the face of B.J. Palmer, the son of chiropractic's founder. You can buy B.J. Palmer sweatshirts, tapes, book bags, and even B.J. Palmer drinking glasses. You can also purchase a CD-ROM that contains all forty-one books B.J. Palmer wrote about chiropractic. Why does D.D. Palmer's son still have such a fervent fan club and an Old Fashioned glass with his face on it? It's because, much more than his father had done, B.J. Palmer made chiropractic the household word it is today. The younger Palmer marketed and sold the ideas of chiropractic like soap flakes. In fact, if it weren't for the driven, charismatic, and egomaniacal B.J., chiropractic would probably have faded and died in 1902, the year his father left a debt-ridden Palmer School behind him and opened a string of short-lived chiropractic colleges along the west coast of the United States. So perhaps it's fitting that today B.J. Palmer merchandise is being peddled on the Internet.

D.D. Palmer, B.J.'s father, was an inept businessman and, at best, a gifted amateur at advertising. For the most part, he simply aped the testimonial-driven sales methods patent medicine peddlers had perfected. B.J., on the other hand, was a promotions prodigy who cut his teeth working as a circus hand and a stagehand in a traveling hypnotist show. After his father's bitter departure, B.J., who had just turned twenty, took the most saleable parts of his father's ideas and unleashed an advertising campaign and a flurry of publications that made chiropractic seem like the perfect profession for the unskilled, unemployed, and unquestioning. He also sold it as the ideal treatment for just about anything ailing an American on the fresh edge of the twentieth century. The promotions for his school and for chiropractic treatments were equal parts cornball aphorisms, quackery, and "can-do" Americana, but they kept the failing Palmer school and infirmary afloat.

To his would-be students, he sold chiropractic as a modern, patriotic shortcut to easy street. In his 1906 book, *The Science of Chiropractic: Its Principles & Adjustments*, Palmer wrote:

> Are you looking for a profession? If so, choose one that is new, up-to-date, is remunerative from the start, practical in every way, progressive, fascinating, will make you prosperous while making others healthy and happy ... With a small outlay of cash and time you learn one hundred times more of the cause and its adjustment of disease than can be acquired in any medical college in a four-year course, or an osteopathic college in three years. ... The field of common labour is crowded. In Chiropractic there is an increasing demand for those who are qualified. Chiropractic is American. The cause of disease is comprehensible. Adjustments are readily learned and understood.[1]

In the same book, he told the general public that nerves pinched by misaligned vertebrae caused "100 per cent of all diseases."[2] The book contains a list of over one hundred disorders B.J. Palmer claimed chiropractic could cure. The catalogue included asthma, cancer, cataract, colic, epilepsy, hernia, insanity, spinal meningitis, smallpox, and urinary diseases. Palmer wrapped up the litany with these comforting words: "If your disease is not on this list, bear in mind that this chapter is not as large as a medical dictionary."[3]

He was also a prodigious writer of epigrams like:

> He that blowth not his own horn, for him shall no horn be blown.
> Early to bed, early to rise. Work like hell and advertise.
> The more you tell, the quicker you sell.
> Is life worth living? It depends on the liver.

His maxims revealed a strong belief in business, in advertising, and in the ability of the common man to pull himself up by his own bootstraps. They were featured prominently on the walls of the Palmer School of Chiropractic.

The Free-Thinking Father Figure

The epigrams (and a good deal else about B.J. Palmer) were inspired by an early twentieth-century literary figure, Elbert Hubbard, who appears to have become a father figure for the young man. Hubbard was an American publisher and writer and the founder of Roycroft, a handicraft community in East Aurora in New York State. Hubbard had been the head of sales and advertising for a soap company but quit in 1893 to start his own publishing enterprise, the Roycroft Press. He wore his hair long and flowing and affected poet blouses and a loose neck scarf. In 1895, the same year that chiropractic was born, Hubbard published the first issue of the avant-garde magazine *The Philistine*. His writings were strongly influenced by the American Romantics, such as Thoreau and Whitman, but they also have a strong Republican sensibility. Hubbard advocates hard work, duty, self-reliance, and faith in entrepreneurial capitalism. His 1899 essay, "A Message to Garcia," became an American business school classic. Hubbard was a charismatic figure whose writings attracted a community of free thinkers and craftsmen who produced a popular line of simple furniture. Hubbard himself was inspired by the artist's colony that William Morris (the English crafts-man, designer, and socialist) had built around his Kelmscott Press. Hubbard hosted annual conventions and went on the lecture circuit across America. By 1910, the Roycroft community had grown to over five hundred workers and artists. Hubbard wrote hundreds of pithy epigrams, the worst of which became inspirational business posters, *Reader's Digest* filler, and sermon fodder:

- The prophet without honor is the one who does not know how to advertise.
- Cheer up — there is always room at the bottom.
- Just please listen to my advice: Take nobody's.
- Education is a conquest, not a bequest — it cannot be given, it must be achieved.
- Quit blaming other people for your troubles — if you were big enough you wouldn't have any.
- The value of education lies not in its possession, but in the struggle to secure it.
- If you want others to think well of you, set them an example by thinking well of yourself.

They're all Hubbard's work. Hubbard had given a lecture at the Burton Opera House in Davenport, Iowa in 1906, though there is no evidence B.J. Palmer attended. However, in 1908, Hubbard visited Palmer at the Palmer

School of Chiropractic, and the two became friends. Hubbard and his wife died in 1915 when the ocean liner *Lusitania* was torpedoed by a German submarine off the coast of Ireland.

Photographs of B.J. Palmer from 1915 are a startling demonstration of the impact Hubbard had on him. Palmer sports the same flowing locks, poet's blouse, and loose tie as his friend and hero. But unlike Hubbard, Palmer wears a closely trimmed beard to mask his youth. Palmer also wrote and published a journal, *The Fountain Head News*, and, in 1915, launched the Palmer School of Chiropractic Printery. The print shop pumped out thousands of chiropractic books, pamphlets, advertisements, and newsletters, all of which advocated the miracles of chiropractic in B.J.'s hyperbolic and evangelical language. Palmer's message was always direct and positive: chiropractic worked. It was an idea he believed to his core. He was absolutely convinced that the fundamental principles of chiropractic were true, and he wanted everyone to know about them.

Palmer's understanding of the role of his school was equally clear-eyed. In a 1919 edition of *The Fountain Head News*, he wrote:

> Give me a simple mind that thinks along single tracts, give me 30 days to instruct him, and that individual can go forth on the highways and by ways and get more sick people well than the best, most complete, all around, unlimited medical education of any medical man who ever lived.[4]

Palmer also sold chiropractic merchandise, coordinated a series of chiropractic lyceums, and set out on speaking tours across America to pump up chiropractic. The tours often coincided with his testimony at fellow chiropractors' trials for practicing medicine without a license. Once again, B.J. was mirroring the actions of his free-thinking father figure.

Birth of a Salesman

Palmer's relationship with his real father, D.D. Palmer, was more complicated. D.D. Palmer had little time for his son, or any of his other children. When he did turn his attention to B.J., it was often to admonish or beat him. In his book *Fight To Climb*, B.J. has only black recollections of his home life:

> When each of our sisters reached eighteen, they were driven out of home and onto the streets of Davenport to make their living any way they could.
> [I was] forced to sleep in drygoods boxes in alleys, often when temperature was below zero.

All three of us got beatings with straps until we carried welts, for which father was often arrested and spent nights in jail.

Our older sister was badly injured and had been sickly all her life. Our younger sister had a severe abscess caused by beatings. [I] have a fractured vertebra and a bad curvature from same source.

None of this was because D.D. was naturally cruel or inhuman. He had a wife at the time (Villa Thomas) who was a dope fiend. She was a devil when without dope, and an angel when she had it. In those days dope was easy to get. She took it because of pain when she had her longstanding paralysis. To get rid of her scoldings against us, father would do what she told him to do. Father was so deeply involved and so busy with thinking and writings on Chiropractic, he hardly knew he had any children.[5]

Nor did B.J. have many kind words for his other stepmothers. His father had married three more times after the death of Louvenia Landers, his second wife and B.J.'s natural mother. In a 1906 letter, B.J. writes of his father's fifth and last wife, Mary, "Mrs. D.D. is one of the most unstable women I have met."[6]

The younger Palmer clearly respected his father's intellect and fortitude and had inherited his pigheadedness, obsessive need for control, and massive ego. Like his father, he frequently uses the royal "we" in his writings and clearly doesn't suffer fools, dissenters, or doctors gladly. Despite their similarities, D.D. Palmer seems to have had little time or affection for the often-troublesome son growing up in his distracted shadow.

B.J. Palmer only went as far as ninth grade in school; he refers to himself at that time as a "a mental derelict, a no-account kid bum."[7] In 1898, B.J. literally ran away and joined the circus. He was a hypnotic subject in "Professor" Herbert L. Flint's traveling hypnosis show. For three years, the younger Palmer toured the west, acting the part of a mesmerized audience member and letting the good professor smash a boulder on his chest as he lay ramrod straight across two chairs. It was in this act that B.J. Palmer got his first lessons in showmanship and bombastic salesmanship. Palmer also appears to have worked as a circus hand. He carried a love of the Big Top, the big show, and the tall tale all his life.

Palmer returned to Davenport in 1901 and graduated as a chiropractor under his father's instruction. A year later, he found himself in charge of the family's infirmary and school. It's not clear why D.D. Palmer left Davenport in 1902, although a student lawsuit and the threat of being arrested for practicing without a license hung over his head. But he did leave on short notice. Thanks to his natural talent for advertising and the financial aid and advice of local businessman Howard Nutting, B.J. clawed the school out of the $8,000 debt his father had left behind. In the next two years, Palmer pumped a substantial amount of Nutting's money into full-page newspaper ads and increased student enrolment dramatically. When his father returned to Davenport in 1904, the school was on much firmer financial footing. This was probably due in equal part to Nutting's financial coaching and B.J. Palmer's promotion. B.J. had a talent for spending money recklessly (especially on a variety of odd collections), as did his father, so it's unlikely that without a wise fiscal advisor he'd have made a go of the school after his father's abrupt departure.

By the time D.D. Palmer returned, the Palmer school had nine students and an active infirmary. Courses offered ranged in length from ten days for one hundred dollars to nine months for five hundred dollars.

Both the Palmers and their former students faced the constant threat of legal action for practicing medicine or osteopathy without a license. In 1906, D.D. Palmer spent time in jail for the crime. That conviction led to a final split between father and son, with D.D. leaving Davenport for the second time to head west. He sold his share of the chiropractic operation he founded to B.J.

How a Court Case Changed the Public Face of Chiropractic

It was the 1907 trial of Shegataro Morikubo that helped shape the scope of chiropractic practice. It also established B.J. Palmer as the legal angel of chiropractors everywhere.

Morikubo, a rarity as a non-white chiropractor — black students were not permitted to attend the Palmer school — had graduated in 1906 and had set up practice in La Crosse, Wisconsin. B.J. Palmer had established the Universal Chiropractors' Association (UCA) the previous year, mainly as a legal protective group for chiropractors. The Morikubo case was the first the fledgling organization dealt with. Palmer hired lawyer and Wisconsin state senator Tom Morris to defend Morikubo against charges of practicing medicine and osteopathy. In his successful defence, Morris got the prosecution to drop the charge of practicing medicine without a license. The lawyer was then left with the task of proving that Morikubo was not practicing osteopathy. Morris argued that chiropractors, unlike osteopaths, focused on the impingement of the nerves. Osteopaths, he pointed out, focused on the role of blockages of blood flow by all the joints of the body.

There are two interesting aspects to Morris's defence. First, in making his arguments, Morris relied heavily, not on the writings of the Palmers, but on those of Solon Langworthy, a Palmer graduate who had started his own school, the American School of Chiropractic, in Cedar Rapids, Iowa.

Morris's reliance on Langworthy's writings indicates that early on, chiropractic thought and teaching had extended beyond the Palmers' founding ideas. Langworthy's thinking on chiropractic was only one example of the divergent schools that would spring up then and continue to exist today.

Second, although Morris successfully argued that chiropractors focus on the nerves in their practice, that wasn't really true. Many graduates of the Palmer school in its earliest days still held to D.D. Palmer's original teachings that misalignments of the joints could cause impingements of the blood vessels and the nerves and so cause disease. So, while Morris painted a black and white picture to the court, with clear lines between osteopaths and chiropractors, the real-world practice of chiropractic was much more grey. Both Morris and B.J. Palmer seem to have been aware that they were glossing over the muddiness of the profession. Morris's defence was the first example of the chiropractic profession deliberately misleading legal and legislative bodies about the true nature of chiropractic. It would by no means be the last. Morris and Palmer also deliberately began adopting new terminology for the techniques of chiropractors to further distance themselves from other forms of treatment.

Writing in 1951, B.J. Palmer recalls the tactics of his early legal struggles:

> We are always mindful of those early days when UCA ... used various expedients to defeat medical court prosecutions. We legally squirmed this way and that, here and there. We did not diagnose, treat, or cure disease. We analyzed, adjusted cause, and Innate in patient cured [sic]. All were professional matters of fact in science, therefore justifiable in legal use to defeat medical trials and convictions.[8]

Many Canadian chiropractic organizations today use the same language and similar tactics.

"Get the Big Idea and all else will follow" was one of B.J. Palmer's favourite epigrams. In his ads, the subluxation is personified as a mischievous boy standing on a garden hose. "Get Off The Hose," B.J. exhorts. B.J. espoused Langworthy's ideas blended with those of his father — much to D.D. Palmer's disgust. In 1910, the elder Palmer wrote:

> Little did I think that B.J. Palmer, my only son, would prove to be the sneak thief who would try to appropriate the credit of originality and would desire to rob his father of the honor justly due him. Little did I think then that my only son would play the Judas, put me in prison, rob me financially and of credit justly due me.[9]

In the last years of his life, D.D. Palmer had turned his back on the notion of pinched nerves and had developed the theologically based theory of nerve "tone." But the reality is that the methods most chiropractors practice these days have more to do with the simplified, expedient version B.J. sold than the more complex notions that chiropractic's father came to believe in at the end of his life.

B.J. Palmer — Superstar

After 1907, B.J. Palmer championed what he called pure and straight chiropractic — the belief that diagnosis was unnecessary and that subluxations were the root of all "dis-ease." Palmer hurled invective equally at medical doctors and at those chiropractors who mixed chiropractic with other therapies like osteopathy or drug treatments. In fact, he went so far as to speak out against the licensing of chiropractic in states that were going to allow a scope of practice for chiropractors that he felt was too much like "mixed" chiropractic. He was also a vocal opponent of anything but the most basic of chiropractic educations. Palmer saw no need for chiropractors to learn anything about medicine, germs, immunization, or diagnosis. The reductionist B.J. Palmer was about to lead chiropractic into its golden age.

The Morikubo trial had turned B.J. into chiropractic's saviour, a role he played to the hilt. In an outrageous illustration that appeared on the lid of Chiropractic brand cigars (one of the many varieties of chiropractic merchandise B.J. peddled), Palmer is depicted as a brawny Christ astride the world. He keeps Death at bay with his right hand, while with his left he beckons to a sickly young woman helpless at his feet. His beatific head is surrounded by the concentric halos of the "philosophy, science and art" of chiropractic. Palmer would later state that Jesus healed by the laying on of hands and that "the first chiropractor was crucified." Clearly, in 1910, he saw himself as the first chiropractor's second coming.

Palmer was, by all accounts, astonishingly charismatic. He filled his students with an evangelical zeal for chiropractic. After hearing B.J., they were prepared to fight for chiropractic, go to jail for chiropractic, and preach the chiropractic gospel across America. Harry Runge, a 1912 Palmer School of Chiropractic graduate, described Palmer's power this way:

> B.J. had the students so they could hardly wait until they could get out into practice, to carry chiropractic to the world, and to get sick people well. He fills us with enthusiasm and self-confidence. We knew that we had the power to do these things right in the palms of

our hands. We were "miracle men" ... I wanted to be a pioneer, a leader, martyr if necessary.[10]

After his father's 1913 death, B.J. had complete influence on the Palmer School of Chiropractic. Enrolment, which had been climbing dramatically since 1904, rose from 462 students in 1916 to 2,776 in 1921.[11] That all-time high was a result of young men returning from the First World War with government funding for their educations.

Radio Station WOC — Chiropractic on the Air

The revenues from that spike in enrolments enabled Palmer to buy the most remarkable advertisement vehicle chiropractic had ever seen — radio station WOC. Palmer was an inveterate gadgeteer and early adopter of technology. He owned one of the first cars in Iowa and was fascinated by electricity. He purchased the one-hundred-watt station in 1922, after watching his son's experiments with a crystal radio. Because of its 130-foot antenna and its fortuitous location on the Mississippi, the small AM station had a remarkable reach. Palmer claimed listeners as far away as Aberdeen, Samoa, and the North Pole. The station's central location in North America meant it reached a good portion of the United States and parts of Canada. Palmer had purchased the station just as the radio habit caught fire. In 1921, there were few radio receivers in the United States, but by 1923, five hundred thousand sets had been sold.

B.J. made sure that the station's vast and growing audience got a daily dose of entertainment, news, and the latest word on the wonders of chiropractic. Several times a day, listeners got the clear message about the WOC wellspring:

WOC is coming to you from the Up-E-Nuf tower atop the Palmer School of Chiropractic, the Chiropractic Fountain Head, in Davenport, Iowa, where the west begins and in the state where the tall corn grows!

Often, on weekdays, listeners would hear a chiropractic lecture straight from Davenport. But many of the station's non-chiropractic features made it an American favourite and lifeline. The *Sandman Story Teller* was an enormously popular children's show. The station also created a cooking show, featured the PSC (Palmer School of Chiropractic) Orchestra and organ recitals, and delivered the weather, news, and sports of the day. In later years, WOC hired a young broadcaster named Ronald Reagan.[12] Using the Palmer

School of Chiropractic Printery, Palmer created a WOC station guide, calling cards, and pamphlets, which he encouraged chiropractors to leave out in their offices.

Palmer saw WOC as a never-ending advertisement for chiropractic. In 1924, he wrote:

> Anything that gets a listener-in to listening to WOC is getting 'Chiropractic' over more. It builds an interest that CAN BE turned into GOOD BUSINESS if you do your par. Are you?[13]

He also considered it a chiropractor's duty to support the station financially. In a 1923 letter to chiropractors, he wrote:

> WOC, however, has one BIG chore to perform that no other station has — educating the masses to Chiropractic. Chiropractic is a NEW SERVICE. It has been laughed at, scoffed at, ridiculed, and its followers called 'fakers' and 'grafters'. Chiropractic is less well known than any other commodity or service being broadcast by any station in America. People KNOW paper, automobiles, etc.
>
> The MISSION of WOC is to establish GOOD WILL FOR CHIROPRACTIC. Good will is cashable in business, in patients first and students later. WOC is educating millions daily, to a favorable mental receptivity to Chiropractic. For six months WOC has averaged 200 patients per month for chiropractors, according to our tabulation of your reports. This GOOD WILL is worth 200 patients per month NOW, with a steady growth month by month. The P.S.C. needs GOOD WILL as well as you. We are willing to carry our part of the load; but, as it NOW stands WE are carrying IT ALL. The P.S.C. must know very soon whether WOC quits or goes on.
>
> Are you willing to carry a share of the load for the upbuilding of that good will?"[14]

It's hard to overestimate the goodwill WOC really did generate. For all his faults, Palmer was a radio pioneer and a gifted broadcast marketer. In fact, his 1942 textbook, *Radio Salesmanship*, became a best-seller and a staple of North American broadcast schools.

B.J. Palmer had cornered the market on chiropractic education. In 1922, his school had twenty-three hundred students, from every state in the United States and twenty-four foreign countries.[15] He owned the chiropractic printing and merchandising business. WOC had no equal, and Palmer's face and voice were linked to chiropractic all over North America. His annual summer Lyceums filled Davenport and the circus tents set up on PSC property with nearly nine thousand chiropractors, who came from all over the world to hear the words of the master. Remarkably, though, according to chiropractic historian Cyrus Lerner, Palmer was not a rich man. In fact, Lerner argues that Palmer was in debt for several hundred thousand dollars, having squandered his money on collectibles and other personal indulgences. Lerner contrasted Palmer's financial condition with that of the attendees at the 1923 Lyceum: thousands of well-heeled chiropractors who had profited handsomely from their profession. Many were former patients, poor in health and pocketbook, who had improved their lot by adopting the profession that they believed had cured them. As Lerner puts it:

> They had become well, and they had become rich in their practice. [B.J. Palmer] had become poor and practically bankrupt in his work of teaching the philosophy of Chiropractic and wearing the mask of the Chiropractic genius. How did this affect him? Did it make him envious of them? It probably did, but what could he do about it? Absolutely nothing at the time.[16]

Palmer was also hounded and vexed by the "mixers," whom he saw as poisoning and polluting the profession. A year later, he would have a solution to both problems.

The Neurocalometer — B.J. Palmer Flies Too Close to the Sun

It was a sweltering Sunday morning in August 1924. B.J. Palmer once again presided over his annual Lyceum and homecoming in Davenport. He stepped dramatically into the D.D. Palmer Auditorium. The crowd had already participated in a triumphant parade through the city, seen demonstrations and chiropractic exhibitions in the circus tents on the PSC property, and met chiropractors from all over the world. Now the faithful were electric with anticipation. Palmer had promised them a revelation that would change chiropractic forever. The second-storey hall was packed. Palmer began a speech he called "The Hour Has Struck."

For the previous eighteen months, Palmer had been working to perfect a strange electrical device called the neurocalometer. Dossa Evins, a chiropractor and electrical engineer, approached Palmer with the invention at some point in 1923. The instrument had two narrowly spaced probes that could register a difference in temperature between them. In essence, it was a thermocouple (a device that measures differences in temperature) linked to a display. Evins believed the neurocalometer would let chiropractors easily locate subluxations, since it was thought that subluxations, causing an interruption in nerve impulse, would create a change in skin temperature. B.J. Palmer at first rejected the device out of hand. He later changed his mind and embraced the neurocalometer as a way to return chiropractic to its pure, straight roots and weed out the mixers. It was also a way for Palmer to make himself a very rich man.

In his speech to the Lyceum crowd, he explained the birth of the neurocalometer in almost biblical terms:

> ... we finally realized that we had in our profession the most valuable idea that has ever been given by man for man in the history of the world, the appalling immensity of the thing grew on us ...[17]

Palmer explained to the assembly that the neurocalometer could find major subluxations more effectively than even B.J. himself. It was so remarkable, he said, that even the untrained could use it to find subluxations. In later writing, Palmer called the neurocalometer:

> ... the most valuable invention of the age because it picks, proves and locates the cause of all dis-eases in the human race.[18]

The crowd was stunned. Some had heard of the neurocalometer already, as Palmer had been field-testing it. It was so well known in some circles that imitation neurocalometers were already on sale at the Lyceum, but few attendees were aware of Palmer's sweeping claims for the device. Their leader was essentially telling them that without the device they were washed up — they could be replaced by barbers or doctors who got their hands on neurocalometers. But the biggest shock was yet to come.

Palmer announced that the neurocalometer would only be available to "straight" chiropractors. But he had no intention of selling them the device. He would only lease it for ten years. He told the crowd that Sunday in August:

> The price until midnight September 14th remains the same. Beginning tomorrow morning at eight o'clock $100 cash and 13 payments of $50 each, each month, and when $500 has been paid you will be entitled to your technique and your Neurocalometer ... Those who pay the full cash of $500 in advance now get preferential position and delivery over all-time-payment contracts. The price after midnight of September 14th will rise to $2,200.[19]

In 1924, $2,200 could have bought a house. Palmer knew the leasing plan and the outrageous price of the device (which was manufactured for less than one hundred dollars) would cause a strong backlash. He'd already got a dose of it when he sold some field-test units. He told the crowd of his experience:

> I ran into many thousands of your human minds, with the multi-plicities of varying misunderstandings, where you did not have the vision, that could not see beyond your immediate today pocketbook — minds that were prompted by their prejudices, hasty judgments and unfair conclusions; minds that gossiped, minds that run to evil constructions.[20]

In fact, the attorneys of one chiropractor who attempted to sue Palmer over the neurocalometer deal had no misunderstanding at all:

> In all our experience as practicing attorneys, nothing more closely resembling a fraud and a swindle has ever been brought to our per-sonal attention than this proposition which your school is submit-ting to its graduates.[21]

Palmer claimed that the neurocalometer had been tested on a thousand patients, but according to chiropractic historian Joseph Keating Jr., the data, if it exists, has never been published. In fact, chiropractors had only Palmer's word that the neurocalometer was capable of the remarkable results he claimed. While it appears that the neurocalometer actually functioned as a thermocouple, there is no evidence that it could detect any subluxations. And there is no evidence that subluxations actually exist.

Despite the lack of evidence and the exorbitant leasing scheme, Palmer quickly sold a thousand neurocalometer leases at the Lyceum and a further thousand in the following year. The scheme made him a rich man, as he knew it would. Speaking about himself using the royal "we," he told the Lyceum crowd:

> You know we will make money on the Neurocalometer. I will be absolutely frank with you. We will make money on the Neurocalometer, but I promise you here and now to continue doing just what I have always done, to put every dollar we make on the Neurocalometer back into Chiropractic to feed the cow. Make me rich and Chiropractic profits. We will but make it all over into a bet-ter, bigger, busier Chiropractic and safer and sane chiropractors.[22]

In the *Fountain Head News*, Palmer was more direct about how the neurocalometer would create "safer and sane chiropractors."

> One of the designated intents and purposes of the Neurocalometer program IS THE ELIMINATON OF DIVERSITY AND THE ESTABLISHING OF ONE METHOD, in universal use in ALL offices that HAVE a Neurocalometer service to render …
>
> ChiropractORS are where they are purely because they cannot be trusted to preserve ChiropractIC in its purity for posterity … you place us in a necessary position or ruling adversely to any person using any other technique than that taught at the PSC.[23]

Palmer extended his disturbing quest for professional purity to chiropractors who were using knock-offs of the neurocalometers.

> We want the names and addresses of any and all Neurocalometer imitations. Get us the name of the instrument and the names and addresses of not less than two patients who have had them used on them. With this information we will be properly prepared to carry out a much desired program for you and much needed program for chiropractic.[24]

In fact, Palmer's dictator-like tactics and hard-sell techniques didn't cleanse the profession; they split it apart and effectively dethroned him as the unquestioned leader of chiropractic.

While Palmer loyalists bought into the neurocalometer deal, many more abandoned Palmer altogether. Even the loyal Lyceum crowd was shocked and splintered by their leader's astonishing speech. Palmer would never recover from the debacle. Four of his best instructors left to establish the Lincoln Chiropractic College; in 1925, stung by the negative reaction to his scheme, Palmer left the country on an extended world tour. The PSC's enrolment fell to four hundred after the introduction of the neurocalometer. The Depression left the school bankrupt and in the hands of the First National Bank of Davenport. Only the revenues from WOC saved the Palmer School of Chiropractic, and Palmer himself, from total financial collapse, despite earlier profits from the neurocalometer.

Keating writes that, despite the harsh lessons of the unpopular device, chiropractors continued to advertise and market in much the same way as Palmer had:

> Indeed, the profession, as a unified body politic, has never truly

renounced the marketing and advertising excesses modeled by B.J. and many clinical procedures and innovations since are noteworthy for the extraordinary and unsubstantiated claims which are made for them.[25]

In fact, Keating calls Palmer's introduction of the neurocalometer a "model of quackery."[26] That same quackery — the making of unsubstantiated claims — in chiropractic advertising is rampant on Canadian and American Web sites today.

Much like his father, B.J. would live the last part of his life a somewhat forgotten figure wearing a tarnished crown. He continued to try to reduce chiropractic to simple, non-scientific principles in an age when science demanded answers that neither he nor the profession that he marketed so effectively could provide. B.J. Palmer believed chiropractic worked, and he needed no more proof than what his hands could provide. His notion of research was simply to demonstrate what he already had no doubt about. He had attempted to build chiropractic up on printer's ink and testimonials alone, a habit that chiropractors still haven't shaken. He was an egotist and a liar. Even Keating, a chiropractic loyalist, makes no bones about this point.

B.J. taught his disciples that ends justified the means, and since his principles were true, his methods of putting them over were proper.[27]

As we'll see, his disciples are still very much alive in Canada.

3

SUBLUXATION: THE PHANTOM MENACE
How Chiropractic is Anti-scientific and Built on the Unproven Subluxation

Chiropractic's Big Idea is Also Its Big Problem

Here's the single most astonishing fact about chiropractors: they haven't proven that what most of them treat every day actually exists. All across Canada and the United States, chiropractors are charging millions of patients billions of dollars to locate and adjust "vertebral subluxations." Chiropractors think that there are disease-causing spinal misalignments that are amenable to adjustments. But the truth is D.D. Palmer more or less made the whole thing up.

What chiropractors have been doing for the last century is trying desperately to show *how* Palmer's subluxation could work, rather than investigating *whether* it exists. Of late, chiropractic leaders have been boasting of the profession's evidence-based direction and its commitment to research. But little, if any, of that research is directed at the key question for chiropractic. Two chiropractic researchers recently summed up the situation this way:

> In the long run, it makes little sense to us that a profession, especially one that promotes itself as "scientific," would continue to devote so much of its mental energy and resources aggressively involved in concocting theories to explain *how* a given therapy *might* have been responsible for any of a whole host of seemingly "miraculous"

clinical outcomes without first adequately demonstrating whether its therapies had anything whatsoever to do with them![1]

There is not a shred of scientific evidence to support the existence of chiropractic subluxations. It's as though hematologists hadn't really gotten around to demonstrating the reality of the red blood cell. Crazy as it seems, when chiropractors talk amongst themselves, they admit that they their entire profession is riding on a phantom.[2] Chiropractic historian Joseph Keating Jr. says:

> Chiropractors have always been ready to point out the shortcomings (real and imagined) in the theories and practice of medicine, but have been less inclined to focus their skepticism on the several common beliefs in chiropractic, most notably the hypothetical construct of subluxation-complex and the value of adjusting.[3]

Howard Vernon, a researcher at the Canadian Memorial Chiropractic College in Toronto, concludes a chapter in a chiropractic textbook by admitting that there is no scientific evidence that "links dysfunction in the spinal column with dysfunction in organ systems."[4]

When non-chiropractors investigate subluxations or manipulable lesions of the spine, their language gets even clearer. "Manipulable lesions may be a figment of the collective chiropractic and other physical therapy professions' imagination."[5]

Not surprisingly, when chiropractors go hunting for the phantom subluxations, they can't agree amongst themselves about where the lesions are hiding. Of course, in day-to-day practice, many chiropractors claim to be able to identify and treat subluxations — and they charge patients on that basis. But, when put to the test, they have consistently failed. In controlled conditions, chiropractors can't agree with one another about where the subluxations are, and they can't even repeat their own findings when asked to check the same patient more than once.[6, 7]

In 2000, a group of Danish researchers reviewed every available study on the validity and reliability of tests commonly used by chiropractors to detect subluxations and concluded:

> Thus far no manual or visual test has been identified that fulfills minimal criteria of consistent reliability and validity. Until such tests have been established, the presence of the manipulative lesion remains hypothetical.[8]

Keating, with his usual honesty, cuts to the chase:

We are not yet able to relate the palpable and manipulable lesion to subluxation theory, in part because we do not yet agree on how to find the spinal 'boo-boos.' The blackbox of the clinical subluxation has yet to be located, let alone pried open ... It may be that we find so little agreement among examiners in many reliability studies of subluxation-detection because subluxation is not a meaningful clinical entity.[9]

Translation? Chiropractors can't agree on where subluxations are because they're looking for something that might not even exist. And a simple study of human anatomy shows that in order for the basic theories of chiropractic to make any sense, your brain, spine, and nerves would have to function and fit together very differently from the way they actually do.

The Case Against Subluxations: The Body as Evidence

The vibrating nerves D.D. Palmer imagined at the end of his life, the pincer-like vertebrae advertised by B.J. Palmer, and the ear infections contemporary chiropractors claim to heal with a simple thrust all make no sense when you understand how the nervous system actually functions. And the venerable subluxation? A study of human anatomy suggests that even if it did exist, it would have no impact on disease or disorders. Let's dive deep inside the human body to find out why.

Your brain is about 3 pounds (1.4 kilograms) of gray-white jelly shaped like a giant walnut. At its base is a 17-inch (43-centimetre) "tail" of nerve fibre called the spinal column. This slightly flattened cylinder has the same jelly-like consistency as your brain and pours itself down your back inside your spine.[10] Actually, both the brain and the spinal column are almost floating. They're suspended in the skull and the spine by a liquid called cerebrospinal fluid. That cushioning juice is stored inside three layers of connective tissue — imagine tepid chicken broth in a thermal mug. Because of the buoyancy of the cerebrospinal fluid, your soggy, hefty brain has an apparent weight of only about fifty grams. That's good, because it puts less wear and tear on the blood vessels, nerves, and ligaments that attach themselves to it.

The spinal column contains millions of neurons — cells specially designed to send and receive electro-chemical impulses that let us do important things like see, digest food, run, and scratch where we itch. Under a microscope, neurons look like the roots of seedlings. They have thick central cell bodies and long, snaking arms called axons and dendrites. Nerve impulses travel along the length of an axon as migrating shifts in electrical charge. The fatter and more insulated an axon is, the faster the electrical charge can go. The top speed is about 120 metres per second. So, a sprinting nerve impulse could race from the toe to the brain of a tall man in about a sixtieth of a second.

A type of tissue called myelin insulates many axons, especially those close to the spinal column. Myelin is like the plastic covering on copper wire. It prevents the charge traveling through an axon from leaking into surrounding tissue and fluid. When the myelin sheath on the axon is damaged, the signals can fade or disappear. That's exactly what happens to people with multiple sclerosis. In MS, the myelin on important nerves gets inflamed or degenerates. As a result, the nerve impulses degrade, as does the sufferer's ability to see or move. Other, less insulating, materials like collagen protect the axons of non-myelinated neurons. In neurons with narrow axons, without myelin sheaths, nerve impulses can travel as slowly as eighteen metres per second.

Experiments have shown that if an axon is compressed at some point along its length, the speed of the charge traveling through it slows down at the compression point. But, just past the impingement, the charge rapidly accelerates to full speed. Imagine cars climbing back up to the speed limit after they pass an accident scene. That reality flies in the face of ideas promoted by both D.D. and B.J. Palmer, who believed that the signal or vibration in a pinched or impinged nerve would be weakened or degraded until the source of the pressure (a subluxation) was removed (by a chiropractic adjustment). B.J. Palmer characteristically reduced the idea to an erroneous but marketable metaphor — he portrayed nerve impulses as water in a garden hose and subluxations as a foot on the tubing. It turns out neurons are much more resilient than garden equipment.

At the end of the axons, the nerve impulse is relayed to the nearby dendrites of other neurons via an exchange of chemical ions (sodium and potassium are common couriers). It's as if the signals get out of their cars, kayak across a river, get into another car and keep on driving along a new highway. The exchange point is called a synapse. Of course, the interconnections between neurons are much more complex than even highway traffic. In the brain and spinal column, neurons are so dense it looks like the microscopic "seedlings" have been left too long in a tiny pot. The "root-bound" brain alone contains almost 100 billion neurons. Each of the body's neurons has only one axon, but multiple dendrites. Each dendrite can be over a metre in length, though many are far shorter. Each neuron can connect with thousands of others in a seemingly chaotic array of linkages that continue to be made after birth. As newborns, we have all the neurons we will ever have. But the dendritic connections between those neurons increase dramatically in the first two years of our lives. That's because we're exposed to new stimuli and are learning new skills at an astounding rate. Experiments have demonstrated that in cats, neural connections skyrocket after the eighth day of life — that's when kittens first open their eyes and start processing the world.

Many of the neurons and the connections between them are redundant. In fact, a good number of neurons making similar sorts of connections can get damaged before we notice any loss of muscle strength, sensation, or organ function. And even when neurons get damaged, the body can make new connections to nearby neurons that can fill in for the wounded ones. Of course, in cases of extreme trauma, such as a severed spinal cord, the damage is too severe for the body to route around.

Both Palmers imagined nerves as simple wires running from the spine to various muscles and organs in the body. In reality, however, the body's peripheral nerves are collectives of axons and dendrites snaking out from the spinal column to the general vicinity of various body parts. The signals they carry are much more diffuse and multi-pathed than the Palmers ever imagined or advertised. D.D. Palmer claimed to be able to trace specific nerves back to the source of irritation by using his hands on a patient's body. He also believed subluxations caused the nerves to heat up because of increased vibration. Palmer also held that normal nerve vibration was sufficiently energetic to warm the blood and the whole body. Nerves neither vibrate nor produce heat as they run their messages back and forth through the body. They are really just thin strands of carefully protected electrified jelly passing complex chemical notes to the other members of their collectives. The intricate choreography of elements, compounds, and charges that takes place each time a nerve impulse is triggered depends on processes, connections, and electrochemical dynamics that neither Palmer could or would have investigated. The Palmers' ideas are not brilliant, "ahead of their time" metaphors for these microbiological machinations; their concepts just make no sense in the stark reality of what really happens.

And while the Palmers were correct in believing that nerves exited the spinal column through spaces between the vertebrae, they got almost everything else about the process wrong — B.J. more so than D.D., as we'll see.

The Spine Doesn't Support Subluxations

The spine is a remarkable feat of natural selection and design. It's a stack of thirty-three bones held together by muscles, ligaments, suction, and the grace of gravity. The vertebrae, as the bones are called, have been organized into five groups. In our necks we have seven cervical vertebrae, and our upper back contains the twelve thoracic ones. In our lower back are the five lumbar vertebrae. These are followed by the five fused vertebrae known as the sacrum and the four fused vertebrae of the coccyx (a sort of bony vestigial tail). Vertebrae at different levels of our spine vary remarkably in appearance (though from above all look like the heads of exotic insects). Each contains a hole for the spinal column. The cervical vertebrae sport two additional holes for the vertebral arteries. A cushioning pad called the intervertebral disc is sandwiched between most vertebrae. It acts as both a shock absorber and a sort of ball bearing when we bend or twist. The disc is constructed much like a jelly doughnut. With age, wear, or trauma the soft "filling" of the disc can leak out and the disc can cave in, or prolapse. More on this unpleasant situation soon.

At this point, you might be thinking, if the vertebrae are stacked one atop the other like checkers, and there's a jelly doughnut stuck between them, how do nerves get from the spinal column to the rest of the body? Well, the vertebrae aren't flat. In fact, the surfaces between them are quite complex. While some parts of one vertebra fit snugly into the surfaces of its neighbours, there are also large vertical holes on either side. These holes are called foramina. Each foramen allows a peripheral nerve to exit from the spinal column. In fact, thirty-one pairs of nerves emerge along the length of the spine through the gaps between the vertebrae.

In the early twentieth century, B.J. Palmer taught that the misaligned (or subluxated) vertebrae above and below the spinal nerves could pinch them, causing disease and organ malfunction. Both parts of this theory are incorrect. Vertebrae almost never pinch nerves, and pinched nerves don't cause disease. Despite that, many chiropractors still offer it as an explanation for what they consider to be chiropractic's effectiveness.

The spaces between the vertebrae are actually almost three times bigger than the diameter of the spinal nerves that pass through them. The extra space is filled with blood vessels and protective fat. As D.D. Palmer himself discovered late in his career, the spaces actually increase in size when vertebrae are subjected to extreme movements. In *The Chiropractor* (published in 1914) he wrote:

> A displaced vertebra, one whose articular surfaces are separated, enlarges the foramina, there, [sic] does not occlude the opening, does not pinch, compress or squeeze the outgoing nerves as they pass through the intervertebral foramina.[11]

D.D. Palmer did conclude, however, that subluxations could occur because the spinal nerves could be stretched. Many contemporary chiropractors still use these two ideas to explain how chiropractic works.

However, in a dramatic experiment published in 1973, Yale University anatomist Edmund Crelin proved both Palmers dead wrong. In a test that reads like a cross between a *Popular Mechanics* article and a David Cronenberg film script, Crelin clamped a series of fresh human spines, with ligaments and spinal nerves intact, in a drill press. Using wires attached to an ohmmeter, he tested to see if the spinal nerves actually touched the edges of the foramina as he twisted and turned the spine with the controlled and measured force of the press. The results? Crelin couldn't stretch the spinal nerves or get the foramina to pinch or put pressure on them unless he exerted enough force to break the spine.

Chiropractic supporters, including the president of the American Chiropractic Association, argued that Crelin's experiment was irrelevant to chiropractic since it was carried out on dead spines. Crelin countered that, in fact, it was *less* likely for vertebrae in living spines to pinch, compress, or stretch spinal nerves, since live humans have reflex responses in the spinal muscles that would fight against any attempt to move the vertebrae dramatically.

It is occasionally possible for vertebrae to pinch or compress a spinal nerve. If an intervertebral disc ruptures, the vertebra above it can fall downwards. Or vertebrae can collapse due to osteoarthritis. Spinal tumours can also compress a spinal nerve. All of these examples, however, are extreme, and none is helped by chiropractic. In fact, chiropractic is contra-indicated in these situations. Accidents and other severe traumas can also put a joint out of alignment, but again, chiropractic is of little value in correcting the problem. The Palmers, and many chiropractors practicing today, argue that subluxations can be caused by the normal activities of daily living, stress, chemicals, and even the birth process. Even they admit that they have failed to produce any evidence that this is true.

But if vertebrae can't really go out of alignment, what's that snap or pop you hear when a chiropractor works on your back? That's the health care equivalent of a parlour trick. It's the same sound you get when you crack your knuckles. It's caused by gas rushing into a gap the chiropractic adjustment temporarily makes between one vertebra and another. It has no therapeutic value, but it sounds satisfying.

Let's suppose chiropractors could adjust misalignments in your spine. Could that really treat bed-wetting, ear infections, asthma, and other serious bodily disorders? Not at all. Here's why.

Autonomic Nervous System Not Sympathetic to Subluxation

The nerves that leave your spine have very little to do with how your organs function on a day-to-day basis. The spinal nerves, for the most part, control the function of your voluntary muscles and the sensitivity and health of your skin. Nerves that come from different parts of the spine rule the function of different parts of your skin and distinct muscles. Actually, it's a little more complex than that, because branches of one spinal nerve can braid together with branches from another to form plexuses that control movement in a specific region of the body, like the shoulders.

When a spinal nerve is damaged (perhaps due to a tumour's growth), that damage manifests itself in a muscle weakness or, in some cases, total paralysis in a part of the body. Shingles is a disease that attacks spinal nerves and results in a painful skin condition. Sciatica — pain in the buttock and the back of the thigh — is the result of pressure being put on the sciatic nerve by a prolapsed intervertebral disc in the lumbar area.

So, where are the nerves that control the organs of the body? They're all in our heads. In addition to the thirty-one pairs of spinal nerves, we have twelve nerves that are also part of the peripheral nervous system. They're called the cranial nerves. Most of them control important functions like our senses, speech, and information about the position of our head. But the tenth cranial nerve, called the vagus nerve, is different. It's connected to our major organs, such as the lungs, kidneys, and spleen. Like the rest of the cranial nerves, it does its job without ever passing through the spine. That's why, when someone's spinal cord is severed, the result is paralysis but not death from organ failure. This reality also makes D.D. Palmer's story of curing janitor Harvey Lillard of deafness quite curious. Palmer makes it clear that he adjusted Lillard's back (at the fourth thoracic vertebra). How could making an adjustment there make any difference to Lillard's hearing when the nerves to the ear are nowhere near the middle back? It couldn't. In his 1950 writings, B.J. Palmer makes a fascinating excuse for his father.

> Why did he "treat" Harvey's deafness IN THE NECK and SAY it was at the fourth dorsal? Answer is simple. Medical men said and emphasized it was dangerous to do anything IN THE NECK. To move those vertebrae was to cause fracture or dislocation and cause complete paralysis or immediate death by crushing spinal cord. Father absorbed this fear, notwithstanding evidence of having restored Harvey's hearing. Rather than have his students "treat" the neck and kill people, and kill off his Chiropractic idea, he shied all work away from neck and down lower on back where it was safer.[12]

While B.J.'s explanation should be sobering reading to chiropractors who continue to perform neck manipulations today, he is wrong in thinking that his father could have dealt with Lillard's deafness by adjusting a cervical vertebra. The cranial nerves don't pass through the upper part of the spine at all. The eighth cranial nerve, which supplies nerve impulses to the ear, remains tucked safely inside the skull, out of the way of chiropractors. Adjusting the neck could have no influence on it — or on hearing.

And despite B.J.'s explanation, his father later changed his mind about neck manipulation, especially of the atlas, the uppermost bone in the neck. In *The Chiropractor*, he writes, "Atlas luxations are the cause of a large percent of diseases, which may be relieved by adjusting the displaced atlas."[13]

In 1930, B.J. Palmer also showed affection for adjusting the neck. He advocated the "Hole-In-One" (HIO) technique. Palmer argued that chiropractors need only adjust the first two cervical vertebrae and all the others will fall in line like good soldiers. He based this on the readings of a bogus device, the neurocalometer,[14] which he co-developed and leased at an exorbitant fee to Palmer School of Chiropractic graduates. *(See "The P.T. Barnum of Chiropractic")*

In 1934, stung by medical critics who argued that it was anatomically impossible for normal vertebrae to pinch nerves, B.J. Palmer traveled to Germany to try to obtain what chiropractors call the "wet specimen"[15] — a set of upper cervical vertebrae that were fixed and purged of tissue almost immediately after the death of their donor. It does not prove subluxations occur. In fact, by this point in his career, with anatomical evidence weighing against him, Palmer began to argue that subluxations actually take place in the spinal cord itself and not in the nerves. Again, there is no evidence that this is true.

The Hole-In-One technique is still used by many chiropractors in Canada and is one reason there are about fifty million neck manipulations performed in this country each year, even though the vast majority of Canadian patients see chiropractors for low-back pain.

Let's recap. The peripheral nerves that emerge from the spine deal only with the voluntary muscles and skin. The peripheral nerves that control the senses (apart from skin sensitivity) and the major organs are either tucked inside the skull or bypass the spine completely on their way to the organs of the body. So even if it were possible for vertebrae to pinch, compress, or impinge on nerves (which it's not, unless there's decay, tumour, or trauma), the nerves they'd compress don't feed vital organs. If chiropractors could remove the subluxations (which they can't), they'd only be freeing up nerve impulses to the skin and muscles.

But the peripheral nerves aren't the only type we have. Another set of nerves makes up what's called our autonomic nervous system. These are the nerves that control the bodily functions we don't have to think about, such as digestion, sweating, panic reactions, and blinking. There are two types of autonomic nerves: sympathetic and parasympathetic. The sympathetic ones control our sudden reactions to stress (rapid heartbeat, hormone secretion, pupil dilation, etc.). The parasympathetic nerves are more involved in the day-to-day operations of the body and innervate many of the smooth muscles that line the bowel and blood vessels.

When you spring bolt upright in bed at 3:00 A.M. as a phone call shatters the silence, your body's fear reactions are controlled by your sympathetic nerves. In those moments of blissful sleep before the phone rang, your body was running on autopilot, and your parasympathetic nerves, which maintain and restore energy and automatic functions, were at work.

In his writing, it seems clear that D.D. Palmer was unaware of the parasympathetic nerves. B.J. Palmer was aware of the sympathetic nerves, but, according to his father, chose to ignore them completely, deducing, with no proof, that the daily unconscious maintenance of the body was driven by "Direct Mental Impulse."[16]

Most of the sympathetic nerves begin in the mid-back area of the spine. The starting points of the parasympathetic nerves are in the brain stem above the spine and in the lower part of the spine, called the sacrum, which is made up of fused vertebrae that can't be adjusted by chiropractors.

As well, there's no proof that the autonomic nervous system plays much of a role, if any, in organ disease. In fact a 1997 study published in the *Journal of Manipulative Physiotherapy* concluded that there was not:

> ... the slightest bit of clinical evidence of which we are aware that patients with broken necks or broken backs, or patients with entire hips or shoulders blown apart by shotgun blasts, or even patients with mechanical neck or low back dysfunction subsequently go on to develop higher incidences of any segmentally or regionally related internal organ disease.[17]

So, even if chiropractic adjustments did have any impact on the autonomic nervous system, they wouldn't have any impact on organ disorders. Despite common sense and this anatomical evidence, in 1994, the American Chiropractic Association assisted in the publishing of a text about chiropractic health care careers. The book contains a schematic from *Gray's Anatomy* of the sympathetic nervous system and its association with the viscera. The caption in the chiropractic text reads:

> The illustration helps to show that every vital organ in the body is connected with and controlled by nerves from the spinal cord and

brain. Through this knowledge, one can more fully understand why chiropractic treatments can relieve so many human ailments.[18]

The illustration supports no such claim.

And, as we've seen, the subluxation as described by B.J. Palmer, D.D. Palmer, and many chiropractors today is an anatomical impossibility. In the last couple of decades, some chiropractors have looked for more complicated neurological and dynamic definitions of a subluxation. Some theorized that a subluxation was a limited range of motion in all or part of the spine. According to some chiropractic theorists, that abnormal range of motion caused nerve pressure. Others said it produced nerve "interference." Still others said it caused nerve compression. But in general, the idea was that through a complicated neurophysiological feedback process called subluxation complex, the subluxations caused all sorts of bodily problems.

The subluxation complex is based on the idea that there is an intricate cross-communication between the central and autonomic nervous systems. However, no adequate mechanism that clearly explains the process has been created or proven by chiropractors. And since they made it up, and are the only ones who believe it, it's up to them to prove it. The subluxation complex ideas hinge on the autonomic nervous system's ability to create disease. But, as two Palmer College of Chiropractic — West researchers point out:

> Although there is certainly no question that somatic pain has the propensity to elicit a number of global and/or regionally related somato-visceral reflex responses, the collective scientific evidence to date (along with a bit of common sense) provides little support, if any, for the notion that these autonomic responses are capable of initiating processes of frank disease.[19]

Current definitions for this sort of subluxation are anything but elegant. Here's one drafted in 1996 by the Association of Chiropractic Colleges in the United States:

> A subluxation is a complex of functional and/or structural and/or pathological articular changes that compromise neural integrity and may influence organ system function and general health. A subluxation is evaluated, diagnosed and managed through the use of chiropractic procedures based on the best available rational and empirical evidence.

That definition, though, is just theoretical. Dr. Howard Vernon, an instructor and researcher at the Canadian Memorial Chiropractic College (CMCC), sums up the current state of affairs this way, in the textbook *Foundations of Chiropractic — Subluxations*:

> The profession, it seems, is either still 'fixated on' or feels more satisfied with its conceptual models and its elaborate speculative pictures than with pursuits of more basic scientists, who seek to depict or study subluxation as it really occurs.[20]

In the text, Vernon details eighteen studies that attempted to create and test the effects of subluxations in animals. He concluded that there have been no sustained lines of investigation in the studies, no replications, and no clinical implications. That is to say, there has been no real proof, the blame for which Vernon lays squarely on the shoulders of chiropractic.

Another textbook that is required reading at the CMCC, *The Chiropractic Theories*, calls the subluxation a manipulable lesion. The book, written in 1994, asks these questions:

> Is there a manipulable lesion? Indeed, is there a specific, identifiable lesion that responds favourably to spinal manipulation or to chiropractic manipulation therapy ... Or, are there physiological and clinical effects of [chiropractic manipulation therapy] that can be reliably and reproducibly measured whether or not a lesion is detected? ... Tireless efforts to quantify and qualify the [subluxation] and to find a suitable outcome measure or measures capable of predicting manipulative effectiveness have met with mixed and often disappointing results.[21]

In other words, chiropractors have failed to prove the existence of the subluxation and have failed to prove that the chiropractic adjustment has any effect on visceral disease. The subluxation, no matter how contemporary chiropractors define it, is unproven. And it's clear from even a basic understanding of anatomy and neurology that the simplistic notions about subluxations and the spine and nerves that both Palmers advocated, and which are still used by many chiropractors today, simply don't make sense.

So, while chiropractors believe their unique adjustments can treat much of what ails us, there's no evidence in the body, nor any body of evidence, to indicate that it's true.

Subluxation, Common Sense, and Science

You don't need to be an anatomist to see the silliness of chiropractic's subluxation. Common sense tells you the idea isn't very practical.

The human skeleton is meant to support and protect the organs of the body. There isn't any evolutionary advantage for vertebrae to be so sensitive that a slight misalignment could result in serious organ dysfunction, like kidney failure or heart problems. That's especially true if those misalignments can be caused, as many chiropractors believe, by stress or the simple activities of daily living. If our early ancestors could have been felled by a few bumps to their spines, the world today would probably be ruled by cockroaches, not humans. And if all health flowed from the spine, quadriplegics would experience total organ shutdown and death. But they don't.

As well, it is a little too convenient that for chiropractors, the body has the innate ability to heal itself, but that gift doesn't extend to the backbone. For many chiropractors, it takes God to heal the body, but chiropractic to heal the spine.

In 1995, two chiropractic researchers, Donald Nansel and Mark Szlazak, posed a lot of good, common-sense, scientific questions that the chiropractic profession should have been asking for decades. The answers they provided exposed the fundamental fallacies of subluxation-based chiropractic. Nansel and Szlazak rightly ask, if subluxation theory is correct, then shouldn't people with low-back pain be riddled with diseases in organs that are fed by the nerves coming off the lumbar spine? Surely, cases of people suffering from this phenomenon would have shown up in the medical literature by now. But, as Nansel and Szlazak point out, they haven't.

> There is not the slightest suggestion that patients suffering from severe primary mechanical low back pain, for instance, are more prone to develop higher incidences of prostate or testicular carcinoma, colitis, ovarian cysts, endometriosis, pancreatitis, appendicitis, diabetes melitis, or any other category of regionally or segmentally related organ disease. Indeed, in and of itself, the rather conspicuous absence of even one such obvious epidemiological somato-visceral disease correlate seems to cast serious doubt as to the existence of a clinically significant regionally or segmentally related "somato-visceral disease" mechanism.[22]

In other words, if subluxations were real, low-back-pain sufferers should be the sickest people on earth. And low-back pain would be an obvious predictor for a whole host of lower abdominal diseases. But neither is true.

Why Science Doesn't Matter

For many chiropractors, it is a given that there is a subluxation, and that adjusting it makes people healthier. Many chiropractors don't think science, or scientific evidence, is necessary for their belief. For these chiropractors, proof comes from a higher source.

As remarkable as it seems, according to a 1997 study by Leslie Biggs, a sociologist at the University of Saskatchewan, about 22 percent of Canadian chiropractors subscribe to the Palmers' teachings. Those teachings include the idea of the chiropractic subluxation and Innate Intelligence. Keating describes Palmer's understanding of Innate as being a fraction of Universal Intelligence, or God, which controls all biological functions in the body by flowing through the nervous system. Palmer believed Innate was part of an intelligence that filled the universe, was eternal, and bonded with the body at birth. He even came to believe that Innate communicated with chiropractors, guiding their adjustments. As we've seen, these ideas, which have more to do with spiritualism than science, were strongly influenced by Palmer's religious upbringing and interest in vitalism and animal magnetism. A significant percentage of Canadian and American chiropractors still think Innate exists and is fundamental to chiropractic.

Chiropractor Lon Morgan described chiropractic's Innate Intelligence problem in a controversial 1998 journal article:

> Some chiropractors feel that holding to, even reviving, Innate philosophy is essential to chiropractic's survival. They view Innate as the fundamental identifying principle of chiropractic, that which separates us from medicine. Innate thus serves as a guide to keep us from suffering the perceived fate of the osteopaths. To tamper with this bedrock legacy from the Palmers runs the risk of fracturing the very foundation of chiropractic.[23]

Like a terrible family secret blurted at a dinner party, Morgan's article pulled into the spotlight an embarrassing fact about the profession. It is still hopelessly tangled up in pseudo-scientific nonsense. Morgan courageously confronted the profession's fundamental conflict and discussed a problem that never makes it into chiropractic media releases and glossy brochures. He wrote:

> The severe divisiveness of Innate within chiropractic has been profound. By instilling in [chiropractors] the notion that nothing else is needed, the concept of Innate discourages thoughtful analysis,

serious scholarship, and research. It further impedes our professional development and societal acceptance.

Other penalties include isolation from the scientific community and a loss of critical thinking ability by our practitioners. Many chiropractors are quite ignorant of developments in other health care fields, which could have a significant impact on how we might approach clinical practice. This lack of awareness leads to a false sense of security that nothing else is required. As a result chiropractors remain professionally isolated and permanently confined to treating less than 10 % of the general population.

Innate Intelligence clearly has it origins in borrowed mystical and occult practices of a bygone era. It remains untestable and unverifiable and has an unacceptably high penalty benefit ratio for the profession. The chiropractic concept of Innate Intelligence is an anachronistic hold-over from a time when insufficient scientific understanding existed to explain human physiological processes. It is clearly religious in nature and must be considered harmful to normal scientific activity.[24]

Morgan is not the only chiropractic commentator who has criticized the profession for adhering to Innate. Keating has also exposed Innate for the divisive nonsense it is:

…we surely stick out like a sore thumb among professions which claim to be scientifically based by our unrelenting commitment to vitalism. So long as we propound the "One cause, one cure" rhetoric of Innate, we should expect to be met by ridicule from the wider health science community. Chiropractors can't have it both ways. Our theories cannot be both dogmatically held vitalistic constructs and be scientific at the same time.[25]

Although both Keating and Morgan state what appears to be obvious and reasonable, their articles unleashed a blizzard of adversarial and outraged letters from chiropractors that went on for months and filled pages in the *Journal of the Canadian Chiropractic Association*. While the profession tells governments, universities, and the general public that it is based soundly in science, some of its members beg to differ. One letter-writer proudly embraced Innate:

It is true that the concept of Innate Intelligence separates us from medicine, but we are a very separate and distinct profession that no one else can duplicate. Our philosophy is that 1. the body is a self-healing organism, 2. that the Master control of the body is the Nervous System, 3. that interference of Innate through the interference of the Nervous System results in Dis-ease. And 4. that chiropractic eliminates that interference.[26]

Chiropractor Michele Whitney, who at the time was the chair of the Chiropractic Awareness Council of Canada, wrote:

The chiropractic profession was founded on very specific principles. These principles are here to stay whether you like it or not. Call me an "innatist," a "subluxationist," a "fundamentalist." Bring on the CHIROPRACTIC INQUISITION!"[27]

But the most vehement reaction came from chiropractors who believed in Innate, not just because it originated from the profession's founding fathers, but because they saw what they believed was irrefutable proof in their offices every day. In their letters, they reveal the startling scope of diseases that Innate-embracing chiropractors proudly tackle.

Perhaps Dr. Morgan would like to come and spend a few days in my clinic where we see patients with all sorts of visceral conditions that have responded to chiropractic care. Where we see how our scientifically-applied correction of the subluxations allows the body to heal dysfunctional bronchial passages where asthma has been present for years. Where we have seen GI [gastro-intestinal] dysfunction of 20 years change in a matter of months so that meds are no longer needed. Where we see heart arrythmias settle down and blood pressure drop over thirty points systolic, and stay that way on six-month follow-up. Where we see little children with epileptic seizures stop having them. Where we see a little boy who was told he would be blind by the time he was eight years old absolutely amaze the doctors at the University of Ottawa with his retina regeneration.[28]

When Keating wrote a skeptical article about chiropractic "philosophy" and Innate, he too was attacked by chiropractors who believed the only proof they needed was in their own two hands:

I realize that Keating has never experienced the sound of clean inhalations of an "asthmatic" child after an adjustment. I realize that he has never seen the child with an "ear infection" immediately stop crying after an adjustment. I also realize that he has never met the eyes of a desperate patient asking the chiropractor to just try and do something and then both the patient and chiropractor receiving results beyond expectation or scientific understanding.[29]

As well as anger, what the letters revealed was an astounding ignorance of the basics of scientific evidence and the process of evaluating the efficacy of any health care intervention. It's unwise to rely only on your own clinical experience to figure out if a treatment works for diseases and disorders that often go away on their own, like colic or headache, or have symptoms that come and go, like MS and asthma. It is too easy in these cases for practitioners to trick themselves and their patients. The placebo effect, the natural remission of some diseases, and dozens of other factors, including the practitioner's belief in the treatment, can confound even the most well-meaning health care provider. But many chiropractors' belief in Innate seems to blind them to this simple truth. This led Nansel and Szlazak to chastise the profession in an articulate and honest letter in the *Journal of Manipulative and Physiological Therapeutics.*

We must admit that we have grown increasingly weary of dealing with those in the chiropractic profession who persist in their use of the case study as a means of convincing patients and chiropractic students of the "effectiveness" of the "chiropractic adjustment" for just about everything from psoriasis to colon cancer. Simply put, the first tenet of the scientific method dictates that in the face of any positive clinical outcome, the *most* that can be concluded is that the therapy in question did not *totally prevent* the patient's recovery, although one should also consider the possibility that the therapeutic intervention might actually have slowed down or interfered with the recovery.[30]

They go on to point out something that should have been clear to the profession decades ago. If chiropractors are going to take credit for every good result that comes after an adjustment, then they need to take responsibility for every negative outcome as well. They write:

...both ethical as well as intellectual balance would require that an equivalent amount of mental energy be devoted to the generation of theories that, for instance, might explain how a given cervical adjustment might have *caused* the asthma attack that occurred a few minutes later, the heart attack that occurred later that morning, the bacterial pneumonia that developed that evening, the appendicitis that flared up the following week or the gastric tumor discovered a month later. After all, are not such occurrences also part of the chiropractic clinical experience?[31]

Of course, Nansel and Szlarzak believe treating subluxations doesn't affect health one way or the other.

Chiropractic and Anti-science

Nansel and Szarazak simply bring science to bear on chiropractic, something most chiropractors have little time for. This manifests itself in three ways.

First, many chiropractors distrust the medical science establishment, with which they have been at loggerheads for decades. Scientific medicine has rightly questioned the beliefs of chiropractors and derided their unproven techniques and their unquestioning acceptance of received wisdom. The challenge by medicine has not been just an academic one, but has, on many occasions, found physicians and chiropractors pitted against one another in courts of law. It's important to understand that many chiropractors don't consider scientific evidence as valuable as their own personal clinical experiences. In fact, argues Keating, many chiropractors, having rejected science, are left with no yardstick by which to measure evidence.

> As the history of chiropractic reveals, unjustified claims-making has a long tradition, and may be so ubiquitous as to be invisible to many [chiropractors]. An important component of the problem as I see it, is that many (perhaps a majority) do not adhere to a scientific epistemology, and therefore accept very weak information as scientific "proof" or substantiation. If we are unable to recognize unjustified, unsubstantiated claims for the value of chiropractic care then we will not be able to guide, let alone police ourselves.[32]

Second, and perhaps more important, many chiropractors feel they have no need for science. Like D.D. and B.J. Palmer, many chiropractors retain a deep disdain for scientific evidence, convinced that perceived success is somehow above or beyond science. This attitude, which chiropractic historians say pervades the profession, is the main reason that chiropractors have not created a significant body of meaningful research into the fundamental questions of chiropractic, let alone created anything of value outside the profession. Chiropractor Joseph Donahue is remarkably candid about this issue, admitting what scientists have been saying about chiropractic for years:

> What better proof can you have of this problem than our scientific stagnation? For example, one cannot name one unique, well-accepted scientific achievement of chiropractic. Our meager scientific output should make it obvious, profession-wide, that we have been on the wrong philosophical track.[33]

It's that attitude, not their professed lack of funds, that has inhibited serious research by chiropractic. While it's true that chiropractic organizations don't have access to the same funding pools as mainstream medicine, some of the experiments that could prove or disprove some chiropractic tenets aren't hard or expensive to do. For example, some chiropractors claim the birth process causes subluxations in newborns. So, put fifty babies in room, half born by Caesarean section, half by vaginal birth, and ask ten chiropractors to independently sort them out. How much could that cost?

Third, many chiropractors fear scientific investigation and evaluation of chiropractic beliefs and treatment because the ideas of Innate and subluxations broaden the parameters of the profession beyond simple spinal manipulative therapy. If those beliefs wither under the glare of scientific scrutiny, chiropractors have little left. No one recognizes this more than working chiropractors themselves. Despite the repeated claims by the chiropractic leadership that the profession is increasingly embracing science, many front-line chiropractors don't want to hear the brutal truth that science is delivering about their profession and don't want to abandon their unscientific underpinnings.

Chiropractor Tom Preston, from North Bay, Ontario, couldn't be clearer:

> Without our philosophy of vitalism and the intrinsic abilities of the body to heal itself we are just an overpriced physiotherapy department that would fast become redundant. With more and more MDs, physiotherapists, massage therapists, and yes, the lay public as well, learning to manipulate, our profession would be lost in the maze of healthcare providers and become defunct in 25 years. How do I know this? There are chiropractors going bankrupt all over North America. It has been my experience that these usually aren't the philosophically sound vitalistic chiropractors but usually the ones who try to duplicate the services of the physiotherapist.[34]

None of this would surprise University of Saskatchewan sociologist Leslie Biggs. In 1997, she surveyed Canadians chiropractors about their attitudes on chiropractic philosophy and scope of practice. She found a profession deeply divided. Only 18.6 percent of the chiropractors surveyed believed that chiropractic should be limited to the treatment of musculoskeletal disorders, the only part of the practice that is supported to some extent by scientific evidence. Biggs found that 22 percent were "empiricists," practitioners who believed that chiropractic was an alternative form of care, subscribed to the philosophies of chiropractic founders D.D. Palmer and B.J. Palmer, and supported a broad scope of practice, using chiropractic to treat problems beyond simple musculoskeletal issues.[35] The rest, about 60 percent, fell somewhere between these two poles and were described as moderates. But even among the moderates, there was a marked disdain for the evidence-based practice that the CCA says it supports. Biggs's survey found that 74 percent of chiropractors surveyed do not accept that controlled trials — the highest standard of scientific evidence — are the best way to validate chiropractic methods. More than half (51.3 percent) believed that personal clinical experience was the best way to validate chiropractic. Only 8.4 percent of the chiropractors surveyed agreed with controlled trials.

As for the notion put forward by chiropractic officials that modern chiropractors are science-based health professionals, Biggs found little evidence to support it. A majority of chiropractors surveyed, almost 60 percent, "believe that there is evidence for the treatment of non-muskuloskeletal problems with chiropractic methods (a contentious issue within chiropractic)." A full 47.1 percent claimed, "chiropractic science has proven that chiropractic is valid for non-musculoskeletal problems."[36]

All of this was published in 1997, informing the chiropractic leadership that a majority of the profession rejected the idea of evidence-based chiropractic and believed chiropractic was effective for non-musculoskeletal problems and that more than one-fifth of chiropractors subscribed to the outdated, pseudo- and anti-scientific views of the profession's founders, D.D. and B.J. Palmer.

Craig Nelson harvests the fruit of that kind of fuzzy thinking. Nelson is an associate professor of chiropractic at Northwestern College of Chiropractic in Bloomington, Minnesota. For fun, he collected examples of what he called "chiro-babble" — egregious statements and studies from chiropractic journals and magazines. But by 1993, Nelson had stopped laughing. He found three articles that went beyond the pale. One suggested using Innate Intelligence to beat slot machines; another said x-ray analysis could indicate latent homicidal tendencies, and the third chiropractic article said AIDS was non-infectious and could not be transmitted sexually. Nelson found these non-scientific, nonsensical ideas were "sickening, irresponsible and pathetic."

In a letter to the *Journal of Manipulative and Physiological Therapeutics*, he wrote:

> There is only one possible defense that one can offer for these outrages. That is, that they are aberrant and not representative of the profession. I am no longer certain this is true. There seems to be a whole new generation of chiropractors raised on New Age mush, whose wit has been dulled by century-old dogma, and whose intellectual role model is a television evangelist. At the very least this faction represents a large, vocal and influential minority in chiropractic ... My sense of amusement with all of this has vanished primarily because of a growing awareness that: a) the number of chiropractors who are animated by 19th century pseudo-science seems to be growing rather than shrinking, and b) these chiropractors will abandon their philosophy when hell freezes over.
>
> This letter is written to suggest that a profession that tolerates, through its silence or inaction, this sort of irresponsibility deserves whatever it gets.[37]

In the end, chiropractic is left with two things: Innate, which is untestable, and the subluxation, which has not been proven to exist. In the face of that, many chiropractors simply fall back on their belief that what they do is effective, proclaiming the mantra "Chiropractic works!"

In 1989, Keating warned the profession that that stance was facile and wouldn't carry the profession into the twenty-first century.

> Those chiropractors who "already know chiropractic works" because God has revealed this, or because D.D. or B.J said so, or because "it just makes sense," or because personal experience or anecdote has confirmed it, are unlikely to conduct nor critically evaluate much clinical research, since they have their answers before the research questions are asked. Yet, these anti-scientific ways of "knowing" are still actively propagated at several chiropractic colleges and seminars throughout the profession.[38]

That warning of more than a decade ago has gone largely unheeded. Early in 2002, the Ontario Chiropractic Association unveiled a new television advertising campaign. Its tagline?

"Chiropractic Works."

4

THE NOT-SO-WELL-ADJUSTED CHILD
Many Chiropractors Treat Infants and Children,
and Most of What They Do is Questionable

Judy Matthews⁺ has just been given a complete checkup in the offices of a Burlington, Ontario chiropractor who treats children. Judy is an active, healthy eleven-year-old girl who likes to play baseball and soccer. She has no major health problems.

But the news from the chiropractor is not good. In fact, it's frightening. The chiropractor performed a series of tests, including measuring her shoulder height, leg length, and pelvis height, and examining her spine. He also used a machine to check her "nerve flow" and took an x-ray of her spine. After examining the results, he delivered the verdict: early osteo-arthritis, mild scoliosis or curvature of the spine, pronounced asymmetry, and multiple subluxations that were causing what could become serious health problems. "It is not advanced," said the chiropractor. "But it has got to be handled. All the symptoms she is experiencing now are the result of subluxations she has in her spine since, probably, birth." The chiropractor, like many who treat children for common disorders, believes just being born can result in disease-inducing spinal misalignments.

The treatment? The chiropractor emphasized that Judy needed immediate chiropractic care — adjustments six days a week for two weeks, then three times a week for six weeks, then more tests, then adjustments two times a week, and then, once her condition improved, about once a week. The approximate cost of this course of therapy, not counting additional tests and x-rays? Approximately five thousand dollars. Under Ontario health insurance

---

⁺ *Not her real name.*

(OHIP), about half of the cost of chiropractic visits is covered — up to an annual cap. In this case, most of the cost would have to be paid by the child's parents. All of this is disturbing and confusing for Judy's mother, because Judy is perfectly healthy.

In fact, Judy was part of a test of pediatric chiropractic we performed in February 2001 for the Canadian Web site canoe.ca (www.canoe.ca). Judy was the niece of a fellow reporter. It was a simple test. The chiropractors were told Judy was generally in good health, but suffered a few earaches, some mild headaches, and a few allergy symptoms. Her mom said she was worried about the possibility of asthma. She had heard from neighbours that chiropractic care could be beneficial for children and wanted the chiropractor to check her over. Our colleague, her uncle, accompanied Judy to each of the chiropractor's offices. After visits to five chiropractors, we had Judy checked out by an expert pediatrician, Dr. John Wedge.

Dr. Wedge is chief of surgery for Toronto's Hospital for Sick Children and an experienced pediatric orthopedic surgeon. He met Judy and her mother in the Orthopedic Clinic at Sick Kids. He examined the young girl's shoulders and her hips, measured her legs, and checked her spine.

"This is a perfectly healthy girl," said Dr. Wedge.

We asked if she needed immediate and ongoing treatment.

"No. She just needs lots of good exercise, a good stretching program that would be good for everyone," he said.

That wasn't the consensus of five chiropractors in the Greater Toronto Area who advertised or marketed themselves as treating children. Four disagreed profoundly with Dr. Wedge's assessment. In fact, the four chiropractors found numerous "serious" problems with Judy's spine — specifically, subluxations that needed chiropractic treatment.

Each chiropractor we visited found different subluxations and came to different conclusions about what was wrong with Judy, but four out of the five agreed on one thing: she needed chiropractic adjustments to get healthy. Only one chiropractor who examined her said she was fine and recommended no chiropractic manipulation. The other four put her through a barrage of tests and found imbalances, partially locked vertebrae, asymmetry, uneven weight distribution, and a spinal column riddled from top to bottom with subluxations. They found subluxations in the upper, middle, and lower spine, but not necessarily in the same vertebrae.

They used a wide variety of methods and tests for locating the subluxations, including palpating the spine, taking a thermographic scan (looking for heat differences), and using surface electromyography (SEMG). Thermographic scanning and SEMG are unproven diagnostic tools. Spinal palpation has not been shown to be reliable in isolating subluxations, which themselves are theoretical.

Three chiropractors recommended x-rays. Our colleague in every instance declined x-rays to protect Judy from unnecessary radiation, but in one case, Judy's mother was called directly by the chiropractic office, and she gave permission over the phone.

The chiropractors said Judy had, among other things, one shoulder lower than the other, one leg longer than the other, one hip higher than the other, one ear lower than the other, something called "anterior head carriage," scoliosis, or curvature of the spine, early osteo-arthritis, and numerous sub-luxations, all of which, according the chiropractors, could cause earaches, headaches, allergies, asthma, arthritis, learning problems, and more serious problems later in life, including digestive and reproductive problems, the chiropractors said. Four out of five chiropractors recommended chiropractic adjustments, either by hand or with a small pogo-stick-like tool called the Activator. So, is Judy ill, and does she need ongoing treatment and tests at great cost to the taxpayer and her parents?

No, said Dr. Wedge. First, osteo-arthritis is the arthritis of aging, the result of injury and daily wear and tear on joints. It is almost never seen in children. "For someone to have idiopathic osteo-arthritis at this age, I've never seen it," said Dr. Wedge. "Never heard of it." He found no neck problems, no lower back problems, no evidence of scoliosis — a real and sometimes serious curvature of the spine — and he detected no appreciable difference in shoulder and hip height, and even if he had, some degree of asymmetry in people is perfectly normal. Minor differences in leg length are pervasive in the population, and in the vast majority of cases cause no ill effects.

"Everyone is asymmetrical, it's part of the human condition. There is a whole industry based on this asymmetry and it's called tailoring," he said. "And yet, you have another whole industry based on this variation and it's called chiropractic."

Chiropractors Also Claim to Treat Ear Infections

Are the chiropractors we called a minority? Apparently not, according to a telephone survey we undertook as part of the same canoe.ca investigation. This time, we had a fellow reporter, Natasha Marko, telephone fifty chiropractic offices randomly selected from the Toronto phone book. We made no attempt to include chiropractors who claimed to treat children. These were just ordinary chiropractors, selected by chance.

Marko posed as a young mother with a two-year-old child prone to chronic ear infections. She asked if the chiropractor treated young children and whether they would be able to help with ear infections. When possible, the chiropractors were also asked to explain how chiropractic manipulation would be able to help with the infections.

Of the fifty chiropractic offices contacted, forty-five said they treated young children, and thirty-six said they could help with ear infections.

The survey is important because chiropractic treatment of childhood infections, such as otitis media (ear infections), and conditions, such as asthma, colic, attention deficit disorder, and a host of other childhood disorders, has been a flashpoint of controversy in the medical community and within chiropractic itself. Critics say that there is no scientific evidence that chiropractic manipulation is of any benefit to these conditions. In addition, the claim by chiropractors that subluxations may be involved in illness and disease in children is unproven.

But despite a lack of mechanism, chiropractors claim they know their manipulations work because they have seen successful cases in their practices. "We definitely have had wonderful results with kids that I've seen in the past with chronic ear infections," said a west-end Toronto chiropractor interviewed during the survey.

Pediatricians say there is no scientific proof that chiropractic is beneficial for childhood illnesses, and in some cases, it may even be dangerous. Dr. Paul Munk, a pediatrician and former president of the Canadian Paediatric Society, notes that although 86 percent of episodes of acute otitis media heal themselves, those that do not can lead to serious illness. "However, how do you know if a particular child is one of the 14 percent who would respond to antibiotics and thereby avoid developing mastoiditis, cerebral abscesses and meningitis along with permanent hearing deficit and learning problems — all of which used to happen to a small percentage of acute otitis media sufferers prior to the advent of antibiotics?" asked Munk. Currently, these complications are seen very rarely because of the use of antibiotics.

The chiropractic community itself is divided over what conditions their techniques are capable of tackling. A small minority of chiropractors limit their practice to musculoskeletal conditions, but most chiropractors treat a wider range of problems. Chiropractors subscribing to subluxation theory believe that virtually nothing is beyond their scope because the body can heal itself, provided the spine is free of subluxations, which they remove with spinal manipulation. As one east end Toronto chiropractor surveyed said, "What we do is see if there is something the child has that would respond to adjustments or if there is what we call a subluxation, so we'd know that we could tap into the nervous system and make the correction."

Chiropractors have been unable to prove through research that spinal manipulations have an effect on specific childhood conditions such as ear infections. So where, exactly, do chiropractors get the idea they can treat childhood disorders like earaches?

When we interviewed Jean Moss, the president of the Canadian Memorial Chiropractic College, she sidestepped the issue of whether her college teaches that chiropractic can treat middle ear infection. She said the usefulness of chiropractic treatment for ear infections depends on whether the infection is acute or chronic. Children can experience chronic ear pain, which she claimed is more often associated with the small muscles surrounding the upper cervical area and down in the muscles of the jaw. "Sometimes reducing those musculoskeletal symptoms helps the patient feel better. It doesn't cure the infection. That does need antibiotics, but it does help and it does seem to assist with the process and reduce the level of pain." However, she admitted that there is no strong evidence to support claims that chiropractic can help with the symptoms of ear infections. "No there's not. There is anecdotal clinical evidence from people in their practices. There are some case reports, which is the lowest level of research," she said. But the pediatric chiropractic textbook Moss's school offers for sale in its bookstore and makes available to its students in its library says nothing about adjustments treating only "ear pain." In fact, in one example of a patient with otitis media with effusion (ear infection), the text says all symptoms cleared up after neck adjustment.

> The patient was adjusted at C3 in the seated position. He received six adjustments over a 4-week period and had a complete resolution of symptomatology. The patient cooperated easily and fully during the adjustment procedure and appeared to enjoy the process.[1]

And, unlike Moss, other chiropractors and chiropractic professional organizations seem unequivocal in their view of the benefits of chiropractic manipulation for childhood problems like ear infections. The Web site for the Chiropractic Life Centre in Kingston, Ontario told this story to visitors in June 2002:

> A young boy came in yesterday with a heart-breaking history of ear infections, subsequent hearing loss, speech problems, many rounds of antibiotics and forthcoming tympanostomy surgery (tubes in the ears). This issue of Lifeline is dedicated to all children with ear infections so that their parents learn that there is an alternative available to stop their child's needless suffering. If there is any child you know who can benefit by reading this newsletter, please forward this information to their parents.
>
> As you well know, Chiropractic care does not cure any disease.

> The purpose of a Chiropractic adjustment is to allow the innate intelligence of the body to work at one hundred percent of its potential without interference. This enables every cell in the body to work in harmony, whether that cell resides in the leg, the stomach, the hand or the ear.[2]

The Centre's rhetoric echoes not only B.J. Palmer's unscientific philosophy but also his careful and deliberate use of words to avoid legal problems. The site goes on to explain exactly how chiropractic adjustments can deal with ear infections:

> The Eustachian tube functions via the contraction of a small muscle called the tensor veli palatini, which is controlled by nerves that emanate off the spine from C1 to C4. These small nerves come together into the superior cervical ganglion, which provides nerve supply to the tensor veli palatini.[3]

In fact, the normal function of the tensor veli palatini is controlled by cranial nerves, none of which pass through any vertebrae in the neck. But the lack of mechanism doesn't stop even provincial chiropractic organizations from making unfounded claims.

The Ontario Chiropractic Association lists "recurring ear infections" in one of its pamphlets as one of the "common health conditions of infants and children that may respond to chiropractic care." Those are fighting words for pediatricians who don't believe chiropractors can treat or diagnose ear problems. "They're claiming they can treat an infection with spinal manipulation. It's anatomically and scientifically impossible," said Montreal pediatric practitioner Dr. Murray Katz.

William Jarvis, a retired professor at Loma Linda University in California and author of many books and articles on chiropractic, agrees with Katz. "What they say makes no sense," says Jarvis, co-editor of the *Journal for the Scientific Evaluation of Alternative Medicine*. "It only makes sense in the chiropractic paradigm of life force — that somehow the subluxation creates a chain of events that leads somehow back to the ear." And pediatrician Paul Munk doesn't know how chiropractors would know how to examine a child's ear. "What training does a chiropractor get in ear examination by someone knowledgeable in that art?" he asked. "You could also look into my ears with an otoscope and probably not be aware of what the normal anatomy and physiology of that region is — thus this would be a useless exercise."

Dr. Linda Spigelblatt, a Montreal pediatrician and a director in Quebec of the Canadian Paediatric Society, agrees. "To my knowledge, they are not taught how to look in the ear by ear, nose and throat specialists. Ear examinations are notoriously difficult," she said. "Studies have shown that ears are very difficult to evaluate. And so for a doctor with many years of training, it is difficult to evaluate the ear. For a chiropractor, who has had basically no equivalent training, I am not even sure how they would evaluate the ear."

But Ear Infections are Just the Start

Many Canadian chiropractors are claiming positive results not just with ear infections but with other childhood disorders, including asthma, colic, bed-wetting, colitis, and sometimes just about anything under the sun. The Chiropractic Life Centre's site, for example, tells users:

> It is our vision and mission for everyone on earth to be under regular Chiropractic care. As Chiropractors, we do not heal or treat specific diseases. We locate subluxations, provide adjustments to the spine to relieve nerve pressure, and this in turn makes the body a more effective self-healing organism. It does not matter what the medical diagnosis is. We, as Chiropractors, seek to improve health regardless of the patients' condition. ... So who needs Chiropractic? In the words of Dr. Sid Williams, founder and president of Life University, "Chiropractic should be universally utilized as a major tool for disease prevention, extending longevity, improving the health of children, of working adults, of athletes, and of aging people alike."[4]

Later on the same page, the centre lists sixty-six different disorders it believes are treatable by chiropractic. They include:

Hearing problems	Croup
Sinus problems	Asthma
Common cold	Bronchitis
Allergies	Jaundice
Runny nose	Constipation
Sore throat	Diarrhea
Tonsilitis	Bladder problems
Cough	Bed-wetting.

These are all common childhood disorders, and it's clear from the Centre's site that children are welcome at the clinic. The site has been making these claims online for over two years.

But the Centre's not alone, and the Web's not the only outlet for pediatric chiropractic messages. In a recent issue of *Alive* magazine, a Burlington, Ontario chiropractor writes:

> The major cause of most [subluxations] is actually the process of being brought into the world — birth. For an infant, it can be very stressful. Subluxations associated with birth trauma can cause hyperactivity, lowered resistance, ear infections, asthma and bed-wetting, as well as signs of "central motor impairment ... If allowed to remain, subluxations are the starting point of nerve system and body malfunction."

And a Waterloo, Ontario chiropractor writes on his site:

> Our children (Adam, 7 1/2 years old, and Mitchell, 6 years old) have no need for any medication or drugs. They do not take Tylenol, aspirin, cough syrup, antibiotics, or any other pills or potions you can think of. Chiropractic, and a healthy lifestyle, have made their bodies and immune systems strong. Our oldest son, Adam, has **never** taken antibiotics in his life!
>
> Chiropractic has great success with asthma, ear infections, and aches and pains, when these are caused by nerve interference. The above mentioned conditions and many others are most commonly the result of nerve interference (SUBLUXATIONS).
>
> Allow your children to reach a new level of health. Have their nerve interference (SUBLUXATIONS) removed from their spines, allowing their inborn (**innate**) intelligence to regulate and control their body. This is how nature intended it to be![5]

Some chiropractors even go beyond visceral disease. At the Web site for the Sudbury, Ontario chiropractor, visitors are told that even learning disabilities, seizures, and autism can be treated by chiropractic. The site offers parents these encouraging words:

Wellness for Children
Our techniques produce extraordinary results!
ADD — ADHD — Allergies — Autism — Asthma — Dyslexia — Learning Disabilities — PDD — Seizures and more ...

Cranial Adjustments for Children
Since 1985, we have examined many learning disability related patients. In every single one of these cases there was a structural mis-

alignment in the skull. It is essential when treating children with learning difficulties, that cranial adjusting be included in the treatment protocol.[6]

This chiropractor uses "cranial adjustments," in which the bones of the skull are supposedly manipulated. There is no evidence such treatment has any effect on health or disease. The site has been making these claims for more than two years.

The site's statements baffle Dr. Joe Byrne, chief of psychology at IWK Grace Health Centre in Halifax. "I know of no clear scientific evidence, using accepted scientific methods, that supports the claims that these chiropractic techniques have demonstrable positive and enduring effects on the core symptoms of ADHD [Attention Deficit Hyperactivity Disorder] or LD [Learning Disorder]," he said. Dr. Byrne, a pediatric psychologist, is a recognized expert in the field and has done extensive research into the diagnosis and treatment of ADHD and LD. Byrne reviewed the claims made by chiropractors and searched for relevant studies involving chiropractic treatment. He said there are "remarkably very, very few studies available," and those are seriously flawed by deficient research design. Byrne concluded, "These few studies yield results that cannot, in my opinion, be interpreted to scientifically support the proposed methods of intervention."

It's not just individual chiropractors who believe chiropractic can cure all manner of childhood illnesses. The Ontario Chiropractic Association pamphlet mentioned above also states:

When should you first take your child to a chiropractor? As soon as possible after birth. Chiropractic care at an early stage could prevent many common childhood illnesses from developing.[7]

In June 2001, *Canadian Chiropractor* magazine devoted almost its entire issue to pediatric chiropractic. It contained articles on how chiropractic could help with ear infections and scoliosis.

But are these just rogue chiropractors and fringe organizations? Hardly. The Ontario Chiropractic Association represents 83 percent of all the province's chiropractors. According to a 1999 survey of twelve hundred Canadian chiropractors published in the *Journal of the Canadian Chiropractic Association*, 84.5 percent said they treated children under two years old. On average, about 92 percent of the chiropractors who filled out the survey's questionnaire said they treated patients under eighteen.[8] What did they treat them for? Here's a list from the study:[9]

Condition	Percent
Musculoskeletal	96.8
Headache	89.5
Muscular (sprains/strains)	89.1
Articular/joint conditions	82.9
Gait/posture	77.6
Asthma	60.5
Otitis media (earache)	51.8
Colic	46.1
Menstrual complaints	44.8
Immune system	43.4
Gastrointestinal	37.2
Hyperactivity	34.2
Enuresis (bed-wetting)	31.3

According to the survey, the top three reasons for treatment in patients under the age of two were prevention (31.3 percent), colic (16.1 percent), and otitis media (16.1 percent). In children up to eleven years of age, the top was prevention. There is no scientific evidence that chiropractic manipulations prevent any childhood disorder.

The study concludes by pointing out, "the results of this study show that almost all Canadian chiropractors were involved in the treatment of patients under the age of 18."[10] It also states:

> The occurrence of musculoskeletal conditions in this study appears to be somewhat less predominant than in studies relating to adult patients. This may mean that patients under the age of 18 are more likely to present with non-musculoskeletal conditions.[11]

In other words, parents are bringing their children to chiropractors for conditions (like ear infections, hyperactivity, colic, asthma, and bed-wetting) that aren't related to the musculoskeletal system, the nervous system, or joints, and many chiropractors are treating them.

That's certainly the message you get if you visit the Web site of the Chiropractic Awareness Council. The CAC is a Canadian organization of chiropractors dedicated to "promoting public awareness of Chiropractic life principles by promoting awareness of the devastating effects of the Vertebral Subluxation Complex on the expression of Human Potential."[12] It is difficult to enumerate the false claims made by the CAC because virtually every statement they make in relation to chiropractic and health is unsubstantiated and unsupported. For example, on their page about babies, the site reads:

The birth process is considered one of the most traumatic events of our lives on our spine and nervous system.

Irritation to the spine and nervous system can be traced to a variety of different ailments in infants such as allergic reactions, colic, unexplained crying, difficulty breathing, poor appetite.

Spinal check-ups should be made at these key moments in a baby's development:

- after birth process (as soon as possible)
- when the baby starts to sit up
- when the baby starts to crawl
- when the baby starts to stand
- when the baby starts to walk

Then they add a warning: "Failure to visit the chiropractors following these important stages of spinal development can lead to scoliosis, a weakened immune system, 'growing pains,' motor impairment, ear, nose, and throat infections, frequent colds and hyperactivity."[13]

None of these statements is true.

But Are They Really Treating Anything?

Some chiropractors are careful to say they don't treat any specific conditions. They claim they just let the body heal itself naturally by removing subluxations. The chiropractors we visited during the canoe.ca survey stated, often more than once, that they do not "treat" any specific condition such as ear infections. As one chiropractor we took eleven-year-old Judy Matthews to said, "Just so you know, we don't treat ear infections. We don't treat anything, because your body can heal itself provided there's proper nerve endings in the brain getting into the body." Another said, "Now, one thing I want to emphasize is that this is not a treatment for asthma or headaches or whatever. This is to make her body work normally so she doesn't have any of that stuff.... In medical terms everything is geared towards a treatment for something. I don't treat a darn thing." This issue of whether chiropractors "treat" illness or disease is a crucial one. For pediatrician Dr. Munk, this position explains their approach to specific complaints. He said:

... Four out of five chiropractors did not even look into the ears to make this diagnosis. By assessing the vertebrae and nerves only, they are trying to evaluate the child's problems with their eyes shut and their hands tied behind their back.

Dr. Charles DuVall, an Ohio-based chiropractor and outspoken critic of the profession, is more direct about the issue: "The chiropractors, no matter what you tell them, say 'it is a subluxation and we have to adjust your spine.' It all comes back to this: If all you have is a hammer everything looks like a nail."

Dr. Katz agrees. "It's said that chiropractic is a treatment in search of a disease. So, if you have a five-year-old child with ear infections, I look in the ear. They look in the neck." Even if the idea of nerve interference had merit, the nerve for the ear does not pass through the neck, explains Katz. "It's a scam."

The chiropractic approach also raises serious questions for Dr. Spigelblatt. "You can basically then say if it doesn't work, well, I never said it was going to work because I never said I was going to treat you. It strikes me as a way of non-committing yourself to any harm or good," said Dr. Spigelblatt. "Basically, they are saying they will re-adjust the spine so that the body heals itself and if the body doesn't heal itself, then it almost implies there is something wrong with self."

Professor Jarvis said, "In three decades I would say it is pretty much the same old story. They try to kind of weasel around that idea that we don't diagnose disease, we analyze the spine and correct spinal problems and of course, all good things follow."

The "we don't treat anything" model also flies in the face of attempts chiropractors have made to show their therapy does help specific conditions such as asthma or colic. As Dr. Spigelblatt notes, "In the studies that are done, they do treat specific conditions. There have been studies published by chiropractors on enuresis [bed-wetting], on ear infections, on asthma, and low back pain."

In reality, chiropractors seem to want it both ways: they want to be able to treat all childhood illnesses with chiropractic manipulation, but they want the freedom of not being responsible for the outcome of specific problems.

The Proof Isn't Out There

But whether or not chiropractors say they're treating the spine or treating specific childhood disorders, there's no proof they're doing any good what-soever, and chiropractors' own studies demonstrate that. A 1995 study of the evidence for the efficacy of pediatric chiropractic, done by chiropractor Allan Gotlib, came to this conclusion:

> The biomedical information available through literature based retrieval with respect to pediatric health conditions and manipulation

as a therapeutic intervention is scattered, fragmented, lacks sufficient methodological rigour and remains primarily at the empirical
or anecdotal level. Health care practitioners utilizing manipulation
with therapeutic intent have some distance to go in substantiating
on a scientific basis the successful outcomes realized on a daily
empirical basis in the clinical environment. In comparison to other
professions, chiropractic appears to have taken an initial leading role
in reporting manipulative therapy as a therapeutic intervention with
respect to certain pediatric conditions.[14]

Translation? Chiropractors who treat children only think it works, and no
other health professionals agree with them. They have no real evidence.

A 1998 study of the effect of chiropractic manipulation on childhood
asthma published in the *New England Journal of Medicine* came to this
conclusion:

In children with mild or moderate asthma, the addition of chiropractic
spinal manipulation to usual medical care provided no benefit.[15]

In 1999, a randomized controlled trial compared drug therapy with spinal
manipulation for the treatment of colic and found some improvement with
manipulation.[16] However, according to the Canadian Paediatric Society:

... despite adhering to a sound methodology, the two study groups
could not be compared because treatment was not blind, and the
chiropractor-treated group had more interactions between chiropractors and the parents and baby during the treatment sessions.[17]

In 2001, a Norwegian research team carried out a double-blind clinical
trial in which eighty-six infants with colic received either chiropractic spinal
manipulation or a placebo. Both groups showed a slight improvement.
The researchers concluded that chiropractic manipulation is no more
effective than placebo for treating infantile colic.[18] Colic, while disturbing for
parents, is a self-limiting disorder — it often clears up on its own.

There is no good scientific evidence that chiropractic adjustments can
treat any childhood disorder — including low-back pain. That's something
even some chiropractors admit. In an October 2001 review of unsubstantiated
claims in chiropractic brochures, chiropractic researchers write:

Currently available experimental data do not justify any claims for
the value of chiropractic care in populations of children ... The

symptom-producing effects, if any, of spinal subluxations have not
been scientifically established.[19]

Because of this lack of evidence, in 1994, the chairmen of Departments
of Pediatrics and Pediatric Hospitals in Canada released a statement about
pediatric chiropractic. They wrote, in part:

> Chiropractic spinal adjustment is NOT required as preventative
> therapy to maintain a child's health … There is no scientific evidence
> whatsoever that the so-called chiropractic spinal adjustment
> results in any correction of the child's spine. These adjustments are
> ineffective and useless.[20]

The Alberta Society of Radiologists also weighed in on the debate when
their members voted unanimously to refuse to take x-rays for chiropractors
of patients in the pediatric age group.

In May 2001, Dr. Wedge and three other prominent physicians at
Toronto's Sick Kids hospital joined the fray. They called for the Ontario
Ministry of Health to put an end to the chiropractic treatment of children in
the province. In a May 11 letter, the doctors wrote that they find it "ethically
unacceptable" that chiropractors claim they can deal with learning disabilities,
ear infections, scoliosis, asthma, bed-wetting, colic, "and many other childhood afflictions." The letter is signed by Dr. Wedge, the hospital's surgeon-
in-chief, Dr. Hugh O'Brodovich, the chief of pediatrics and pediatricians, Dr.
Ross Barlow, and Dr. Michael Levis. It was sent to Mary Beth Valentine, a
program policy director with the Ministry of Health, and to Tony Clement,
the province's health minister. "Our goal is the mandated cessation of
pediatric chiropractic, period," said Dr. Levis told us in an interview after the
letter had been sent. In their letter, the four also stated that the College of
Chiropractic of Ontario "seems either unable or unwilling to enforce and
ensure a strict adherence to its legally mandated scope of practice." They
called on the ministry to step in to "expeditiously rectify this situation which
has the potential to adversely affect the health of the children of Ontario."

The CCO questioned the physicians about why they sent the letter to the
ministry and the media but not to the CCO. It challenged the doctors to
provide names of chiropractors and details of any concerns the doctors had
about the chiropractors' treatment of children. The CCO warned them it
would not let the matter drop, and if the doctors could not provide specific
examples of infractions, it demanded a written apology and retraction.

In March 2002, The Canadian Paediatric Society issued a strong warning
about chiropractors who use spinal adjustments on young children to treat

colic, bed-wetting, ear infections, and asthma. The society raised concerns about the use of chiropractic care for ailments it feels have nothing to do with musculoskeletal complaints. It said there was no scientific evidence to support chiropractic adjustments in children for back pain, let alone asthma or colic.

Beyond the Scope of Practice

As the Canadian Paediatric Society pointed out in its statement, besides lacking evidence, the chiropractic treatment of children for ear infections, asthma, autism, and other disorders goes well beyond chiropractors' licensed scope of practice in all provinces. Chiropractors are only meant to treat and diagnose ailments associated with the functions of the spine and their effects on the nervous system or with the structure and function of joints. For example, here's part of the Chiropractic Act that governs Ontario chiropractors:

> Chiropractic Act, 1991
> CHAPTER 21
> 3. The practice of chiropractic is the assessment of conditions related to the spine, nervous system and joints and the diagnosis, prevention and treatment primarily by adjustment, of,
>   a) dysfunctions or disorders arising from the structures or functions of the spine and the effects of those dysfunctions or disorders on the nervous system; and
>   b) dysfunctions or disorders arising from the structures or functions of the joints. 1991, c. 21, s. 3.
> 4. In the course of engaging in the practice of chiropractic, a member is authorized, subject to the terms, conditions and limitations imposed on his or her certificate of registration, to perform the following:
> 1. Communicating a diagnosis identifying, as the cause of a person's symptoms,
>   i. a disorder arising from the structures or functions of the spine and their effects on the nervous system, or
>   ii. a disorder arising from the structures or functions of the joints of the extremities.
> 2. Moving the joints of the spine beyond a person's usual physiological range of motion using a fast, low amplitude thrust.
> 3. Putting a finger beyond the anal verge for the purpose of manipulating the tailbone. 1991, c. 21, s. 4

Most people reading that portion of the act would not imagine it covered autism, bed-wetting, colic, or asthma. But for chiropractors who believe that the all human disorders arise from subluxations, almost every childhood ailment is fair game. That attitude proved disastrous for eleven-year-old James Turner.

The Tumour That Didn't Have to Leave a Boy Paralyzed

James is the son of Canadian stock car racer Alan Turner. Turner is suing Barrie chiropractor Gary Dyck for $2.75 million. He claims Dyck paralyzed his son by adjusting his neck and back. In July 2001, Turner filed a statement of claim with the Ontario Superior Court of Justice in Hamilton, Ontario. The following allegations were made in the document and have not been proven in a court of law.

According to the statement of claim, Turner's son developed chest pains while swimming and was taken to the office of the Barrie chiropractor on July 24, 2000. Dyck adjusted James's neck and back without obtaining x-rays, conducting a proper investigation, or making a diagnosis, alleges the statement of claim. The next day James felt worse, but he was taken back to Dyck's office for a second appointment, where his spine was again allegedly manipulated without x-rays, examination, or diagnosis.

After the second treatment, James's condition deteriorated rapidly. He was rushed to The Royal Victoria Hospital in Barrie, "where he was in great distress, having lost the use of his legs and bladder function," claims the statement. He was then taken by emergency ambulance to The Hospital for Sick Children in Toronto, where he received an MRI (magnetic resonance imaging) and neurosurgery.

Sick Kid's doctors discovered James had a benign tumour (known as a ganglioglioma) on his spinal cord. This type of tumour is non-cancerous and slow growing. With proper detection and medical treatment, about 75 percent of afflicted children escape paralysis if the spinal cord is undamaged at the time of diagnosis. However, doctors at Sick Kids found that there was swelling in both the tumour and spinal cord, which caused James to become permanently paralyzed. Further examination confirmed that the tumour had been damaged and had bled, according to the statement of claim. "The damage to the spinal cord was preventable and was caused by the negligence of [Dyck]," the statement alleges.

As a result of Dyck's treatment, the family states that James now suffers paraplegia (loss of the use of his legs), pain along the right side of his neck, weakness in the left hand, and poor bowel and bladder control. James will require ongoing home assistance, rehabilitation, and treatment, according to the statement of claim.

In his statement of defence, Dyck agreed that he treated the Turner boy in July 2001, but that he only did so after obtaining a patient history from both the boy and his grandmother, completing a physical examination and making an appropriate diagnosis. The statement notes that Turner's spinal tumour was a rare condition ant that its presence could not reasonably have been known or discovered by Dyck in the circumstances. He notes that neither the boy's family doctor nor the physicians at the Royal Victoria Hospital found the tumour. It was only at Sick Kids, after substantial neurological examination and testing and an MRI scan, that doctors became aware of the tumour on James' spine, according to the statement.

More importantly, the statement of defense maintains that the chiropractic adjustments to Turner's thoracic and cervical spine were performed properly and gently and had nothing to do with damage to the tumour. "The adjustments to the thoracic spine, in particular, were performed without rotation, twisting or substantial pressure and did not result in damage to the pre-existing spinal tumour and its clinical manifestations and were not affected by the adjustments or any other chiropractic treatment provided to James Turner by Dr. Dyck," reads the statement. The statement also claims that the damage to the tumour may ahve been caused by sports-related injuries. Like the allegations in the statement of claim, none of the statements in Dyck's defence document have been proven in a court of law.

Anti-immunization Still Lives

Some chiropractors are so sure of chiropractic's power that they think it can keep their young patients' immune systems so strong that they don't need to be vaccinated.

When meningitis hit the community of Kitchener-Waterloo, Ontario in 1994, it hit hard. When it was over, two teenagers were dead and two others were left as amputees. In the midst of the outbreak, public officials worked tirelessly to vaccinate children against the disease and to keep the public informed. But one health professional in the Kitchener area took a very different stand. Chiropractor Jeff Winchester picketed one of the temporary vaccination clinics set up at a local high school. To drive home his point, Winchester carried a sign that read, "Meningitis shot is not mandatory." When interviewed by the local newspaper, the Kitchener-Waterloo *Record*, Winchester said, "I think all inoculations are dangerous because they mess with the body's natural immune system." One year later, Winchester wrote a letter to the editor of the same newspaper regarding inoculation against chicken pox. He wrote:

As humans, we have an innate (God-given) healing ability. We are born with self-healing, self-regulating bodies. The concept of inoculating children with formaldehyde, mercury, acetone, rabbit brain tissue, etc., seems to be a stupid choice.[21]

Another Waterloo area chiropractor, James Gregg, supported Winchester. During the meningitis outbreak he told the Kitchener-Waterloo *Record* that some people are at high risk for meningitis but that "a mass vaccination program isn't needed."

And the Kitchener-Waterloo chiropractors aren't alone. Bob Pike runs the Pike Chiropractic Healing Centre in Keswick, Ontario. Two years ago, Pike ran a series of ads about immunization in a local newspaper, the *Georgian Advocate*. One ad informs readers that vaccination is "breaking the chain of natural passive immunity" so that mothers are no longer able to pass antibodies to their babies in their milk. Another ad argues it is an "abuse of rights" for a medical officer of health to remove unvaccinated pupils from a school in the event of an outbreak of an infectious disease. "Threatening the unvaccinated with expulsion is, in my opinion, a tactic calculated to manipulate parents into a choice based on fear instead of freedom," Pike writes.

Dr. Patricia Marchuk, a family physician practicing in the same community as Pike, points out that unimmunized children are asked to stay home during an infectious outbreak for their own health. "An infectious disease can break out in a school because no vaccine is 100 percent effective," she explained. "Unimmunized children are asked to stay home because we know that are very vulnerable," she said. "It's for their own protection, not persecution." Dr. Marchuk has also attended "vaccine awareness evenings" run by chiropractor Katrina Kulhay. The sessions are held at the Kulhay Wellness Centre in downtown Toronto and are often attended by young mothers. Kulhay promoted the evenings with ads that encouraged parents to:

- Be informed … if you plan to vaccinate your child and/or receive a flu shot
- Learn what vaccinations **really** contain
- Don't be misinformed … it is **not** mandatory to school vaccinate your child
- Know the possible serious immediate and long-term health side-effects.[22]

At the sessions, Kulhay has shown a video called *Vaccination — The Hidden Truth*, about the dangers of vaccinations. Interview subjects in the video state that vaccines cause the diseases they're supposed to cure. One speaker, Greg Beattie, states, "They don't tell us that if your child misses the whooping cough vaccine it is less likely to develop asthma." The interview subjects in the video also say that vaccines cause sudden infant death syndrome (SIDS), cancer, attention deficit disorder, and multiple sclerosis. The video states that vaccines contain animal proteins that stay in human DNA for generations. None of those statements is true.

After the video was screened, Kulhay spoke to the crowd about vaccination. Attendees can also collect information sheets about the dangers of vaccination. One, titled *The Dark Side of Flu Shots,* states that animal DNA can be passed to humans through vaccination and points out that "natural health advocates" consider the use of a high-protein, sugar-free diet; full-spectrum lighting; and supplementation with zinc, vitamin C, echinacea, and sublingual oil of oregano drops as an alternative to a flu vaccine.

In a recent interview with us, Kulhay said her awareness evenings are just about giving her patients choices about immunization. But Dr. Marchuk, the Keswick-area family physician, was appalled by the awareness evening. "I felt so terrible for all those people. If I didn't know what I knew, I would have been horrified by the video," she said, "and the young mums were. Young parents are so vulnerable to this of thing, because they want to do everything right."

Kulhay is not the only chiropractor raising concern about vaccination. A Burlington, Ontario chiropractor tells visitors to his Web site:

> DPT and Tetanus Vaccinations double the prevalence of asthma and allergy Symptoms! This confirms our fears that vaccinations do have their price.

At the Web site of a Stirling, Ontario chiropractor, visitors can find this anti-immunization material:

> There are very few good studies demonstrating the effectiveness of vaccines in humans ... The associated risks for injecting a vaccine into a child are much greater than most realize. There is substantial evidence that vaccines contribute to an increase in the incidence of Sudden Infant Death Syndrome (SIDS). This is often not reported as such and many parents are never even told that the vaccine their child received may have been the reason why their baby died.
>
> Some other short term and long term health problems associated with vaccinations are the following: anaphylactics [sic], allergies, asthma, arthritis, colitis, mental retardation, seizure disorders, the spread of HIV, and certain forms of cancer. There have never been any long term studies conducted that would show the

long term safety of these injections....

There are also unplanned substances that have been found in vaccines. Both animal RNA and DNA have been found. These substances have the potential of making genetic alterations to the person it is injected into. This means the damage that occurs might present itself in future generations.[23]

None of those statements is true.

All these chiropractors openly demonstrate their negative opinions of immunization, despite a policy issued by the College of Chiropractors of Ontario (CCO) that makes it clear that chiropractors should be familiar with scientific research on immunization and should state its benefits. Here's a portion of that policy:

> 1. Members who disseminate information about immunization to patients or to members of the public have an obligation to inform themselves about immunization, including scientific research.
> 2. In disseminating information about immunization to patients or to members of the public, members shall:
> a) advise that immunization is not within the scope of practice of chiropractic nor do chiropractors have the legislative authority to immunize patients;
> b) outline, within the member's knowledge and expertise, the effects, benefits, risks and side-effects of immunization, versus no immunization for: individual patients and the public at large; and
> c) advise that the *Immunization of School Pupils Act* provides for circumstances in which school pupils may be exempted from immunization.[24]

The CCO policy is by no means an endorsement of immunization and, in fact, section C of the policy gives support to chiropractors who counsel their patients against school immunization programs. The Canadian Chiropractic Association's official position is more direct in its support of vaccination. Its April 2002 policy on immunization reads:

> The CCA accepts vaccination as a cost-effective and clinically efficient public health preventative procedure for certain viral and microbial diseases, as demonstrated by the scientific community.[25]

But much of the material mentioned above, which clearly ignores the CCA and CCO policies, has been on chiropractic Web sites for more than two years. It's easy for any patient, journalist, or chiropractic official to find. And a survey we did of many other chiropractic Web sites in Canada found no material of any kind supporting vaccination. It appears that both the CCO and the CCA have done a pitiful job of enforcing their own policies. It's also interesting to note that in 1999, one of the anti-immunization chiropractors was appointed to the CCO's Fitness to Practice Committee despite the CCO having been fully aware that he not only practiced pediatric chiropractic but had participated in the "ChiroPediatric World Tour," an event that advocated treating children with chiropractic for a wide assortment of childhood disorders and that was critical of vaccination.

The chiropractic policies do raise an important question though. Why would chiropractors, who are legislated to treat musculoskeletal conditions, have any opinion about immunization at all? What does that have to do with the spine? Absolutely nothing, unless you subscribe to the unproven and unscientific idea that subluxations can cause disease and depress the immune system.

The fact that national and provincial bodies need to have an express policy about immunization indicates that it is a serious problem within chiropractic. It's a little like an auto mechanic's association having a policy about its members commenting on aviation safety. The problem is, anti-immunization is central to chiropractic philosophy. We've already seen that a basic tenet of chiropractic is that a body free of spinal subluxations is capable of maintaining its own health. As a natural extension of this unfounded belief, a significant portion of the chiropractic community agrees that, at best, immunization is unnecessary, and, at worst, it pollutes the bodies of otherwise healthy children.

Chiropractic opposition of immunization can be traced to its founder. In 1889, six years before he "discovered" chiropractic, D.D. Palmer wrote, "Vaccination is a medical delusion."[26] One of his early advertisements is headlined, "Vaccination is a Medical Delusion of the Nineteenth Century." Palmer also wrote that:

> Hundreds of scientists are devoting their lives to the study of bacteriology, germ investigation, a microscopical branch of biology, in order to determine their relationship to health and disease, not realizing that life action is due to the combination of intelligence and matter, spirit manifestation through material.[27]

In 1906, his son B.J. Palmer, added:

> The idea of poisoning healthy people with vaccine virus … is irrational. People make a great ado if exposed to a contagious

disease, but they submit to being inoculated with rotten pus, which if it takes, is warranted to give them a disease.[28]

In fact, B.J. didn't believe in contagion at all.

Chiropractors have found in every disease that is supposed to be contagious, a cause in the spine. In the spinal column we will find a subluxation that corresponds to every type of disease. If we had one hundred cases of small-pox, I can prove to you where, in one, you will find a subluxation and you will find the same conditions in the other ninety-nine. I adjust one and return his functions to normal.... There is no contagious disease.... There is no infection... There is a cause internal to man that makes his body in a certain spot, more or less a breeding ground [for microbes]. It is a place where they can multiply, propagate, and then because they become so many they are classed as a cause.[29]

He even felt that chiropractic adjustments could reverse the damage he felt vaccination did:

Vaccine virus, or other poisons which create disease conditions will not permanently affect the patient when the Chiropractor keeps the vertebra in proper position. We have checked the fun of doctors and saved children from being poisoned, by adjusting the vertebra that the pus poisoning was displacing.[30]

Those century-old attitudes continue to inform many chiropractors' views on vaccination. Chiropractor Lon Morgan wrote about chiropractic opposition to immunization in a 1997 article in the *Journal of the Canadian Chiropractic Association*. In it, he laments the position taken by his colleagues and confirms the results of our chiropractic Web site survey. He writes:

Chiropractic's anti-immunization attitude has been based, not on an objective evaluation of scientific evidence, but on a visceral rejection of anything associated with medicine. ... Despite an ever-increasing amount of scientific data supportive of immunization ... many conservative chiropractors are still oblivious to the public health significance of this information. Some continue to publish articles filled with selective and outdated statistics ... and there is still a significant number of chiropractors who do not accept or are not aware of scientific evidence supporting the role of immunization.[31]

Morgan's thoughtful and frank article sparked five pages of letters, the majority of which passionately disagreed with him. A Hagersville, Ontario chiropractor wrote:

> Chiropractic's anti-immunization attitude is not based on a reject of everything medical, rather on the basic principles of the profession. The human body is a "self regulating" and "self healing" mechanism and needs no outside influences to function properly. This is Chiropractic Philosophy.[32]

That sentiment was shared by another chiropractor from Cambridge, Ontario:

> I am definitely anti-vaccination. I don't believe they are effective and in fact know that they damage the health of not only the individuals that receive the vaccinations but also future generations as well.[33]

Morgan had some supporters as well, including a Toronto-based chiropractic instructor:

> I have been teaching part-time at the CMCC and I have noticed among some students and faculty a tendency to lean toward the chirovangelists in our midst who are trying to undermine evidence-based chiropractic, using the arguments of a betrayal of chiropractic philosophy. (Of course they have no understanding of the word "philosophy" and should rather use the word "dogma"). I am afraid this scholarly review of the scientific literature will fail to convince them as they believe they are the only holders of the "chiropractic truth." Moreover, these believers adhere to a conspiracy theory, unfortunately common among some of our American compatriots. But in this case it is not their government being taken over by the U.N., but the evil drug companies, with their lackeys in the medical field, who are conspiring to kill us with their drugs and vaccines.[34]

Jean Moss, the president of the CMCC, says that the college is not anti-immunization and doesn't teach against vaccination. However, a June 2002 study of the attitudes of CMCC students about vaccination published in the *Canadian Medical Association Journal* (*CMAJ*) drew some fascinating conclusions.[35] The study shows that only 40 percent of fourth-year students at CMCC agreed with vaccination. The study also uncovered that only 38 percent of fourth-year CMCC students said yes to the question "Would you want your children to be vaccinated against infectious disease with any currently recommended vaccine?" But the most disturbing study result is this: The longer students are at CMCC, the less likely they are to support vaccination. The researchers suggest that while the CMCC is presenting immunization neutrally in its core course material, students are picking up the anti-immunization attitude from guest speakers, student club presentations, and other informal routes. It's curious, though, that a college that prides itself on being "science based" will not only send potentially 40 percent of its graduates into the world with an anti-immunization stance, but also allow that attitude to blossom while the students are within its walls.

Immunization, despite chiropractors' claims to the contrary, is perhaps one of the single most researched beneficial public health procedures in history. Its safety and efficacy are grounded in solid science and research, a reality CMCC should embrace while inoculating its students against nonsense. A commentary in the same issue of *CMAJ* raises this alarm:

> The greatest concern about the negative attitudes toward vaccination of some of the CMCC students is that, in light of the growing prevalence of chiropractic care in Canada and elsewhere, there is a risk that these attitudes will be passed on to patients.[36]

Why this prevalence of anti-vaccination thought at the CMCC, and why does it get worse the longer students study there? Perhaps it has something to do with the "chiro evangelists" mentioned in the Toronto chiropractor's letter to the editor. Or perhaps it's the anti-vaccination materials available at the college. *Pediatric Chiropractic*, a textbook available at the college, questions "universal immunization in developed countries." It also features a twenty-page chapter that focuses almost exclusively on vaccine failures, side effects, and adverse reactions to popular vaccines for measles, mumps, rubella, polio, influenza, and diphtheria/pertussis/tetanus (Dpt). In general, the chapter takes a skeptical view of vaccination. The authors of the text conclude the chapter by stating that "our emphasis on presenting the adverse consequences of certain vaccines is healthy and it may allow parents to make more informed choices." Visitors to the CMCC's bookstore have also been able to purchase the book *A Shot in the Dark — Why the P in the Dpt Vaccination May Be Hazardous to Your Child's Health*. The book, which is also available in other popular bookstores, paints a horrific picture of the impact of the whooping cough (pertussis) vaccine.

Perhaps the study's results aren't so surprising. Perhaps, too, it shouldn't come as a shock that many anti-immunization chiropractors are CMCC graduates.

Playing the Freedom of Choice Card

When challenged, chiropractors like Kulhay and Winchester, echoing the *Pediatric Chiropractic* authors, claim they are simply educating the public, allowing them to make more informed decisions about immunization and allowing them to exercise their free choice. But for many chiropractors, a call for free choice is simply code for espousing anti-immunization. For example, Winchester says he wants people to make responsible decisions about getting immunized. "My opinion on immunization is very clear," says Winchester. "It's a freedom of choice issue. The law in Ontario is very clear also that no inoculation is mandatory and everyone has the right to choose what goes in their body and, unfortunately, I hear too many times that people are told that it's mandatory, that you have to get a shot to go to school. It's a whole series of lies and basically I get sick of hearing that after a while."

But the information chiropractors like Winchester disseminate is often grossly unbalanced and usually focuses exclusively on negative side effects. Winchester argues that the medical community provides only positive information about immunization and that he just lets people know they have a choice. "In a medical doctor's office you're never given a choice. You're never told that you have an option," he says. "So in our office if anyone asks, or if we get talking about it, [patients] are told they have an option. We don't tell people what to do. And you know I'm tired of the medical community saying things like that. I'm also tired of the medical community saying 'Chiropractors say that if you get your backs adjusted then that replaces immunization.' It does not. They're two separate issues." Winchester has made his choice. He's chosen not to vaccinate his son.

But Do They Have a Reason to be Alarmed?

Do the chiropractors have a legitimate concern about vaccination? Not at all. Years of medical research shows that vaccines are effective and that the risks associated with them are extremely small compared with the risks associated with contracting a vaccine-preventable disease.

"Vaccination is a much safer way to acquire immunity than experiencing the diseases," said Dr. Ron Gold, an infection control expert, retired pediatrician, and author of *Your Child's Best Shot*, an immunization guide for parents published by the Canadian Paediatric Society. Dr. Gold says the evidence for the safety and efficacy of vaccines is enormous. There are there are three major types of evidence that support the use of vaccines:

Randomized placebo controlled trials in which participants are divided into groups and receive either the vaccine or a placebo. The groups are then followed over time to compare their rates of disease. Such studies have been carried out with killed and live polio vaccine, pertussis vaccine, diphtheria toxoid, Haemophilus b vaccine, pneumococcal vaccine, meningococcal vaccine, measles, mumps, and rubella vaccine.

Epidemiological evidence that shows a specific disease declines after the introduction of an effective vaccine program. Strong data exists for all vaccines, says Gold.

Epidemiological evidence that shows a disease reappears after vaccination programs are discontinued or when the proportion of children vaccinated decreases. This type of evidence is illustrated by past pertussis outbreaks in the United Kingdom, Sweden, Japan, and all of the countries of the former USSR when vaccination use decreased or stopped. An epidemic of diptheria also occurred in the former USSR when vaccination programs were interrupted.

But arguing with chiropractors who are against immunization is nearly useless, says Dr. Gold. "It's just as it is with many alternative medicine believers, because it's a belief system," the infection expert explains. "Whether it's fundamentalist Christianity or something else, it is difficult to have a rational argument based on the science. There is no scientific nor rational basis for [their] irrational belief."

Practice Building

There's another reason, besides belief, that chiropractors are adjusting children for a variety of disorders. There's good money in it. Many chiropractors use pediatric chiropractic as a "practice builder," a way to get more patients on to the adjustment tables more often. Currently, in Canada, there's about one chiropractor for every six thousand Canadians, a ratio that's becoming less favourable to chiropractors as more graduates begin practicing before existing chiropractors retire. About 10 percent of Canadians use chiropractic, a number that hasn't been keeping pace with the rise in the chiropractor-to-patient ratio. That means that new chiropractors, who on average only clear about $45,000 per year, are going to be scrambling for customers and income. A 1999 survey of pediatric chiropractic indicates where these numbers lead:

Chiropractors treating patients under the age of 18 were significantly younger and more likely to have received formal or informal training specific to treatment of patients under the age of 18 than those not treating these patients. The differences between chiropractors in different age and training groups were greatest for the youngest age categories.[37]

Translation? Fresh, cash-strapped chiropractors are struggling for patients, so they are treating more young children and taking training courses to learn how to do it. Often those courses and training are sold with emphasis on both skills and practice building.

The textbook *Pediatric Chiropractic* makes this clear. The description on the back cover reads:

> See how **Pediatric Chiropractic** can help expand your practice and offer innovative care to the next generation.[38]

But in the world of practice building, that's soft sell. At The Future Perfect Web site, chiropractors are told that pediatric chiropractic will help them "Grow Your Practice Like You Never Have Before." The site goes on, "We are committed to sharing with you the essentials, secrets and Future Perfect pediatric practice management procedures of ultra successful practitioners."[39]

But the hardest sell of all is reserved for children's parents. In *At Your Own Risk,* author Ralph Lee Smith tells the story of his 1969 attendance at a three-day chiropractic practice building seminar by Share International, the sales arm of the Parker School of Professional Success. At the seminar, attendees were given the *Textbook of Office Procedure and Practice Building for the Chiropractic Profession.* Smith explains:

> "To get new names [of potential patients] from non-responding patients," says the text, "say, 'if other illnesses in your family are worrying you, it will slow down your response [to chiropractic]. How is everyone in your family?' Patients and others should be told to 'Remind your friends that chiropractic is good for practically *all* diseases.'"[40]

Remarkably, the scare and guilt tactics Smith writes about haven't disappeared in the intervening thirty-three years. If anything, they've become more aggressive.

The Art of Management Inc. is a Toronto-based practice building company. Here's some of what the company suggests to chiropractors keen on attracting more children to their clinics:

Approach teams such as little league soccer, contact sports, school teams, etc. where kids get knocked around.

When you do your initial intake or patient history form, ask the patient if they have children. Later, when the patient is doing well physically, have your [chiropractic assistant] sit down with the patient for a 10 minute consult regarding their children and THEIR physical conditions. Educate the parent on why it is vital for children to be treated NOW. Make appointments.

Have a package of information on Chiropractic and Children. This should contain data on sports injuries, colic, scoliosis, headaches, earaches, etc.

Parents tend to be oblivious to the amount of knocking-around kids experience in a day. Suggest they follow their kid around for a day and catalogue these bumps so they can see why a kid needs adjustments now to prevent chronic problems from developing.[41]

The Art of Management site also offers practice-building tips from a successful Burlington, Ontario chiropractor. Here's the advice he offers other would-be pediatric chiropractors:

First of all, there is no magic formula for this. The starting point is that YOU need to understand fully the concept of subluxation and the devastating effects that can have on health and that chiropractic is a life saving procedure. Your passion for chiropractic will exude and infect your patients. If you have a "back pain, headache, relief care" kind of chiropractic practice, you're not going to have a successful pediatrics practice.

You need to have a lot of informational resources (research articles, scientific journals, and newspaper clippings, etc.) in the practice to help parents feel comfortable about bringing their children in. There is often an attitude of "you're not seeing my kid unless you have proven yourself to me first." They have to understand well what chiropractic is before they'll bring in their kids.

Tell patients, "You're here getting a pain fixed that your child may be at home developing." Get them to bring their children in now.[42]

The chiropractor's advice is not only in direct contravention of CCO policies, it's also blatant quackery, and it encourages chiropractors to treat outside their scope of practice. There is no evidence that subluxations have "devastating effects" on health, nor is there evidence that chiropractic has saved lives. The tips also raise another important question: if he's encouraging other pediatric chiropractors not to have just a "'back pain, headache, relief care' kind of chiropractic practice" what, exactly, are such clinics billing provincial health insurance plans for when they treat children?

But most disturbing is the unnecessary fear and guilt these tactics instill in parents. "You're here getting a pain fixed that your child may be at home developing," the chiropractor tells patients. There's no proof that's true at all. Those tactics only get worse when a parent meets with some pediatric chiropractors face to face.

During our test with eleven-year-old Judy, we paid a visit to a Burlington clinic. Here's what the chiropractor told Judy's uncle about the results of the tests on his niece. Keep in mind that Judy is a perfectly healthy little girl with no spinal problems.

> **Chiropractor:** When she was little, I believe something might have happened to her, and I am thinking of two things — either falling off like the monkey bars, or a staircase, I'm kind of siding toward actually her being delivered, you know what I mean?
>
> **Reporter:** When she was born?
>
> **Chiropractor:** Yeah. The surgeon or somebody grabbing her head, twisting it one way or the other. A lot of stress created. I would estimate probably 85 to 95 percent of all the problems I see in adults start from the process of delivery if you can believe it. Certainly in all the kids that I see — asthma, headaches, scoliosis, Crohn's Disease, and all these weird, bizarre things that people have later on in life, they start when they're little. ... You know that weakness she had? In her right arm? And she's right handed?
>
> **Reporter:** Oh yeah.
>
> **Chiropractor:** That's a big, huge malfunction. Weakness in the fingers, right side and she's right handed. Okay. We should have picked this up in the left if anything, but not on the right. And it's quite prevalent. So that's the malfunction. Things are working ... but they're not working to the degree they actually and she's only ten ... Now, if something in the body is not functioning normally, it causes other malfunctions to occur. If something in the body is not functioning normally and it's allowed to remain, in time does it get better or worse?
>
> **Reporter:** If you don't treat it?
>
> **Chiropractor:** Yes.
>
> **Reporter:** It gets worse.
>
> **Chiropractor:** Yeah. And at some point it starts to break down, get

cyclical, next it's a disease. This is a funny word, this word scares people. But this word came from this word (Dis-ease)

Reporter: Dis and ease.

Chiropractor: Yes, in other words, something is just not at ease. Medicine has taken the hyphen out to shorten it — disease. Now the reason I am going through this is that the disease that she is kind of easing into is the very, very, very early stages of arthritis starting. Now, it is not advanced.[43]

Thankfully, the chiropractor's diagnosis of Judy is completely useless and wrong. We contacted Bob Wheeler about the claims made about pediatric chiropractic on his company's Web site. He said he was simply relaying information that was passed on to him by memebers of the chiropractic community. He would not comment on the medical concerns about pediatric chiropractic.

The site also provides comments about an Oakville, Ontario chiropractor who treats children:

[The chiropractor's] practice's open-plan concept really works for her because people can see kids getting adjusted and they often ask her about it. Whenever patients mention that their children have an ailment that chiropractic can treat and prevent, she suggests that the parent bring them in for a free initial exam.

[The chiropractor] also conducts a Healthcare Workshop that all new patients attend. As part of the overall chiropractic education, she introduces a few cases relating to children. Afterwards, patients ask her questions about their nieces, grandchildren, or their own kids.

Talking to PTA groups is a successful action for [the chiropractor]. She gears the information towards general health for the main part but mentions kids issues and concerns more towards the end.[44]

We also paid a visit to an Oakville pediatric chiropractor with Judy. Here's the advice she gave Judy's uncle on the phone after performing a "thermography scan" of Judy's back. Thermography, as used by chiropractors, has not been proven to provide any useful information about health.

Chiropractor: Okay. I can tell you that her scan is horrible. Her thermography scan is terrible. From the top of her neck all the way down to the upper part of her low back is showing nerve interference. That's a huge area in someone her age. Now, I haven't seen her x-rays obviously because I don't think you've had them done yet, is that correct.

Reporter: Well, that's the other thing, her mother doesn't want to have x-rays.

Chiropractor: Okay, her mum would need to speak to me then. But I really think that it's necessary, especially seeing what I'm seeing on the scan and what I saw in the exam. We also see a bit of restriction of range of motion in her neck, which is very unusual to see in a child. And a lot of postural changes. A head tilt. A high shoulder on the left. A high pelvis on the left. She also has anterior head carriage, which means her head sticks forward over her shoulders which means there is tremendous amount of pull and stretch on the spinal chord which is not a very healthy position for the neck at all.

And she also has significant weight discrepancy, meaning that she was leaning more to the left than to the right. And in her case, she's got about a nine pound difference — one side versus the other — which is a significant amount — especially again in a child. You don't expect this much showing up in a child.

Now, things like ear infections, headaches, asthma, all that tends to occur from that top part of the spine where she's showing the majority of the irritation.

So, what we're seeing symptomatically and what we're seeing in the exam and the test results definitely point to these things originating or coming from problems with the nervous system.

Reporter: What were you hoping the x-ray would show you?

Chiropractor: The x-ray will tell me what phase of degeneration her spine is in, how far advanced this condition is. What kind of changes we're seeing in the spine itself. And it also helps to rule out any congenital abnormalities, things she was born with, any abnormal bones or formation of bones, or curvatures, it just gives us a little bit more detailed information.

Reporter: So what do you think would happen if we didn't treat these things?

Chiropractor: Generally, what we tend to find is they will get worse as time goes on. Now, I can't say that 100 percent for sure, but that's what we have tended to see in the past. And, I mean she is already showing symptoms, so I don't think it is a wise idea to leave it.

Reporter: What type of treatment do you recommend coming out of this?

Chiropractor: Chiropractic care, obviously. I'm not exactly sure what you mean? Frequency, length of time... that kind of thing?

Reporter: Yeah.

Chiropractor: For that I need to see her first. I want to adjust her first.

See how she responds to the adjustment and then I can give you a better indication. That's what we go over in the next couple of visits. The next visit back we go through how to read a thermography scan, phases of degeneration, what you would see in x-rays, how to interpret an x-ray, just information about chiropractic, how problems can develop, and then the time after that I go through frequency, length of time, cost, payment options, all that sort of thing...[45]

Again, there was nothing wrong with Judy, who was given a clean bill of health by Dr. Wedge, an experienced pediatric orthopedic surgeon.

Other chiropractors in other provinces use similar practice-building techniques. Sharon Mathiason, whose daughter Laurie died of a chiropractic-induced stroke, has been a vocal opponent of "Spinal Health Care Week" in Saskatatoon schools. During these events, chiropractors have offered a five-week lesson plan for teachers, who were encouraged to invite chiropractors into the class. And until Mathiason complained to the Ministry of Education, chiropractic organizations sponsored chiropractic-branded contests aimed at kids. "It was just a practice building tool for chiropractor," said Mathiason. "It was nothing more than blatant conversion. We could just as easily have a John Deere tractor week. It would make as much sense."

Chiropractors also make use of a children's colouring book featuring a bulldog named Oliver, chiropractor-friendly stickers, and posters of cuddly bears getting their spines adjusted. The stickers have been available at the CMCC bookstore.

The Art of Management site suggests chiropractors interested in building their pediatric practices make sure such material is easily available to parents who visit:

> Educate patients well on kids and chiropractic. Parents often need to hear the message many times. Have brochures on chiropractic for children, such as the ones put out by Koren Publications or the Peter Pan Potential in California.[46]

Peter Pan Potential is a pediatric chiropractic promotion firm founded in 1989 by Claudia Anrig,[47] the co-author of *Pediatric Chiropractic*. Koren Publications, based in Philadelphia, publishes a variety of pediatric chiropractic brochures and advertises itself as having the "premier collection of chiropractic products, practice building tools and childhood vaccination resources." The publications are laced with quack claims and scare tactics aimed at parents. The Koren site contains this advice in a patient newsletter:

Not only is their effectiveness in question but there is growing evidence that vaccinations cause autism, allergies, learning disorders, ADD & ADHD, asthma, diabetes, dyslexia, hearing problems, vision problems, digestive disorders, stuttering and developmental delays.[48]

Koren pamphlets, which are available in many Canadian chiropractors' offices, celebrate pediatric chiropractic as being effective for bed-wetting, emphysema, asthma, shaken baby syndrome, and the imagined birth trauma. A Koren brochure states:

> With the birth process becoming more and more an intervening procedure ... the chiropractic adjustment becomes even more important to the child's future.[49]

Like almost all statements about pediatric chiropractic, this one is frightening, and frighteningly wrong.

Government is Paying for It

Whether chiropractors are drumming up new business, treating healthy children, adjusting pregnant mothers, dealing with autism and learning disabilities, or manipulating children with earaches, provincial health insurance plans are helping to pay for it. In total, across the five provinces where chiropractic is partially paid for by government health insurance, the treatment of children costs an estimated $15 million per year, according to provincial statistics. And parents paid that much and more out of their own pockets, because chiropractors can charge above insurance rates for their services. In all, pediatric chiropractic in Canada costs at least $40 million a year.

To appreciate the concern about chiropractors treating children, consider this. Chiropractors in British Columbia treated 1,279 individual babies under 12 months of age in 1998–99. They billed the provincial government's health plan for 3,717 services to those babies, which cost taxpayers in that province more than $45,000. But what were those babies being treated for? "I don't know," a spokesperson for the B.C. Ministry of Health told us. "That's a good question."

In Ontario in 2000–2001, the Ontario Health Insurance Plan (OHIP) paid out $10 million for the chiropractic treatment of patients nineteen and younger. Nearly $6 million of that was spent on children under the age of fifteen and $1.4 million on children four and younger.

It's the same in other provinces. In 1999, in Saskatchewan, chiropractors performed 1,218 services on children under 12 months of age. In

2000, the Saskatchewan government paid out $412,325 for chiropractic treatment of children under 14 years of age. In 1998, in Manitoba, chiropractors performed services on 4,493 infants in the same age group. And again, provincial health officials did not know what chiropractors were seeing those babies for. But in April, 2002, the Manitoba government took another look at the situation and cancelled insurance coverage for chiropractic treatment of children under nineteen years of age. The Manitoba Chiropractors' Association, with the help of the U.S.-based International Chiropractic Association (ICA), rallied chiropractors and their patients. They sent thousands of letters demanding coverage be reinstated and in July the government reversed its decision. Across the board, provincial insurers who pay for pediatric chiropractic don't really know what they're paying for. That's because chiropractors don't have to indicate what disorder they're treating when they adjust children. So a chiropractor could treat a child for asthma, ear infections, or autism and bill the government for the "adjustment" he made to the child's spine. And while provincial government officials have no idea what chiropractors are treating children for, pediatricians, and even some chiropractors, say they don't know what possible effect the adjustments could have on children anyway.

Retired chiropractor and author Samuel Homola has limited his forty-three-year chiropractic career to the treatment of musculoskeletal problems. "As far as I am concerned there isn't anything they could be treating them for that would be reasonable and logical," he said. "I certainly wouldn't recommend that anybody take a child that young to a chiropractor. ... There is no reason at all for a chiropractor to treat a baby that young. To me it's just horrendous that there would be that many chiropractors treating that many babies under 12 months of age," said Homola. "It's an absolute waste of insurance money to pay a chiropractor to treat a baby ... They are not pediatricians, they have no business diagnosing the conditions, much less treating them."

In Saskatchewan, the number of treatments in that age group has gone up, on average, 33 percent per year since 1996, even though the number of infants in the province hasn't increased. Pat Toth, the assistant director of Compensation and Professional Review for Saskatchewan Health, says he really doesn't know what chiropractors are treating in children that young, and he doesn't know why there was such an increase in chiropractic treatments in infants in his province. "It sounds to me like that's something that there should be a concern about."

Toth sits on a Joint Chiropractic Professional Review committee in Saskatchewan. That committee reviews billings by chiropractors, but Toth says its deliberations are private.

As we've seen, some of those billings are for treatments for childhood disorders like ear infections, bed-wetting, colic, asthma, and even attention deficit disorder and learning disabilities. And prominent medical associations, like the Canadian Paediatric Society, say that chiropractic adjustments are useless for these conditions in children.

Chiropractors are licensed health care professionals in Canada. That means they are self-regulated, administering their own discipline and overseeing how their members practice and bill. In provinces where health insurance plans cover part of the cost of chiropractic treatments, the scope of practice covers only disorders arising from the structures or functions of the spine and their effects on the nervous system. The intention of provincial health care payments is to reimburse chiropractors only for treatments that lie within the profession's scope of practice. But chiropractors bill for services within only a few broad categories: initial visit, subsequent visit, or emergency visit, and x-rays. The billing forms indicate that a chiropractic service has been rendered, but does not in most cases specify what that service was intended to remedy. "That's the responsibility of the college," said Nadine Criddle, a British Columbia Ministry of Health spokesperson, referring to the regulatory body that oversees chiropractors in B.C. She said the province's medical service plan (MSP) simply administers the payments.

It appears that the provincial chiropractic regulatory bodies are not acting as effective watchdogs over the profession's treatment of infants and children. "The primary function of the regulatory bodies is to protect the public, not the profession," said Dr. Murray Katz. "The claims that are being made are obviously questionable and should be investigated at the initiative of the college without necessarily any individual complaints from patients."

And the chiropractic profession itself appears to be divided on the issue of pediatric chiropractic. Not all chiropractors treat infants and children. Studies indicate that there is a tiny minority of chiropractors who practice science-based chiropractic, which focuses solely on musculoskeletal conditions. "We exist almost as 2 separate professions — those that follow the mantra/religion of the subluxation and all of its ills (which of course require extensive chiropractic intervention), others who prefer to limit ourselves to musculoskeletal complaints and treatments," says Dr. Mark Bodnar, a chiropractor in Bedford, Nova Scotia. "Personally, I feel strongly that if chiropractic would give up on these outdated (and in many cases inappropriate) treatment/philosophical attitudes we would open ourselves to significant referrals and public acceptance doing what we do best (and what very few other professions have proven effective at) — musculoskeletal complaints."

Chiropractic organizations in Canada suggest that chiropractors are just treating children for musculoskeletal complaints. On its Web site, The Canadian Chiropractic Association, the professional association representing chiropractors across the country, writes:

> Chiropractic treatment is based on the basic biological and physio-logical sciences which apply equally to children as they do to the adults. Chiropractic treatment is as beneficial to children as it is to adults, and children should be seen by chiropractors when appropri-ate. The scientific literature is now demonstrating that low back pain is a very prevalent condition amongst school children.[50]

The site does not mention the chiropractic treatment of childhood illnesses. Marlene Paulin, a spokesperson for the Ontario Chiropractic Association explained that chiropractors treat children and adults primarily for musculoskeletal disorders. These organizations are simply ignoring dozens of other Canadian chiropractic Web sites and chiropractic studies that demonstrate that that's just not the case. All sorts of childhood illnesses are being treated by chiropractors — a fact that officials in both organizations are certainly aware of, and are certainly misrepresenting. They present chiropractors as back doctors for babies, which is not the way pediatric chiropractors portray themselves at all.

Retired chiropractor Samuel Homola says that treating children like tiny adults doesn't make sense. "A small child and a young baby don't have the musculoskeletal problems that an adult has," said Homola. "I don't know of any musculoskeletal problems that they could treat babies for. And how would they even determine that they had a problem?"

Dr. Stephen Barrett, retired psychiatrist, author of many books on health fraud, and founder of the quackwatch.com Web site, says it is a waste of public funds to pay for chiropractors treating infants and children. "They are not only wasting money, but I think it is mentally harmful to a child to grow up thinking that having your spine examined is a normal part of life and that there is something wrong with you that the chiropractor needs to fix once a week or once a month."

It's clear that a significant portion of chiropractors are treating often per-fectly healthy children and letting the government pick up part of the tab. That's wasted money, because there is no childhood disorder that chiroprac-tic has been proven to be able to treat. All pediatric chiropractors do when they adjust children's spines is confuse children, frighten parents, bill patients, and bilk the government as they build their practices on the backs of kids.

5

NECK MANIPULATION AND STROKE
"But Mom, She is *a Doctor"*

Early on a warm summer evening, twenty-year-old Laurie Mathiason slipped and fell down a stairway at the A&W where she worked in Saskatoon, Saskatchewan. It was July 23, 1997. She told her boyfriend, Doyle, that she had hurt her back, and he suggested she try his chiropractor. Laurie agreed.

Over the next months, the chiropractor adjusted the vertebrae of Laurie's back, including those in her upper neck. In 21 separate visits, the chiropractor manipulated Laurie's vertebrae 189 times. Though Laurie's initial complaint was low-back pain, the chiropractor, on each visit, manipulated her neck.

On February 3, 1998, Laurie went in for her usual visit to the chiropractor. As she lay on the examining table face up, her chiropractor rapidly twisted her neck left and right. Laurie felt pain directly after the adjustment and a short time later was unable to turn her neck. That night, at the A&W, she walked into tables and dropped ashtrays and burgers. Her friends recall telling her repeatedly that she was a klutz. Her mother, Sharon, told her she should go to a doctor. "But mom," Laurie replied, "she [the chiropractor] *is* a doctor."

The next afternoon her neck was stiff and painful, and she booked another chiropractic appointment in the hope of getting some relief. The chiropractor's office was in a shopping mall where her mother worked part time at a nearby health food store. Just before 2:00 P.M., Laurie dropped by her mother's store with Doyle to say hello. Accompanied by Doyle, she went to her appointment, and there the chiropractor manipulated her neck once again. This time, Laurie immediately began to cry. Her left eye rolled up into her head, her right eye roamed randomly, and she went into convulsions. Doyle tore through the mall to get Laurie's mother. He told Sharon that something had happened at the chiropractor's office and that she'd better come quick. They ran through the mall together, and when Sharon dashed into the room, she found her daughter foaming at the mouth. Laurie had turned blue. "She didn't know me. I was calling to her, I was saying, 'Mummy's here, Mummy's here,'" Sharon recalled.

Laurie went into a coma. At the Royal University Hospital in Saskatoon, doctors did all they could to help her, but she never regained consciousness. Three days later, Laurie Jean Mathiason died. Neurologists at the hospital told Laurie's parents that their young, healthy daughter had died as a result of a massive stroke. Her tragic death touched off a firestorm of controversy about the relationship between chiropractic neck manipulation and stroke that continues today. But to understand both the debate and what happened to Laurie that day on the chiropractor's table, you need to have a clear picture of the complex and delicate relationship between the spine and blood vessels in the human neck and brain.

Vertebral Arteries and the Brain

Your brain is the most demanding organ in the body. It constitutes about two percent of your body weight, but it needs twenty percent of the body's oxygen supply and requires a steady supply of glucose. And, although it is a marvel of engineering, the brain is fussy. If you shut off the flow of blood to the brain for ten seconds, you lose consciousness. After twenty seconds, electrical activity in the brain ceases and it loses the ability to communicate with the parts of the body it controls. Cut the supply off for more than twenty seconds, and parts of the brain go dead. Sometimes that can lead to paralysis or an inability to speak, walk, or remember. Sometimes it means death.

The body is well equipped by nature to deliver oxygen and nutrients to the brain. Inside your neck you have two sets of arteries that bring blood to the head. In the front of the neck are the carotid arteries. They're the ones that doctors put their fingers on to check for a pulse. They supply blood to the front part of the brain. In the back, travelling up the spine and into the neck and brain, are another set of blood vessels called the vertebral arteries.

Your head is supported by the top section of your spine, seven vertebrae known as the cervical vertebrae. They are numbered, from the top of your skull to the bottom of your neck, as C1 to C7. On each side of the cervical vertebrae, holes penetrate the bony structures. Your vertebral arteries resemble thin strands of cooked spaghetti. They enter the neck at the bottom, at about C6, and snake up either side of your neck, threading themselves through the bony rings in the vertebrae like fishing line through the eyes of a rod. They are tethered to the vertebrae of the neck, and they are the only arteries in the body so intimately linked to bone. These hollow, muscular arteries carry oxygen- and nutrient-rich blood fresh from the heart up to the brain. The carotid arteries in front take a fairly direct route into the brain, but the vertebral arteries are different. As they emerge from the top vertebrae, these arteries both take a torturous hairpin turn, travelling horizontally before disappearing into the base of the skull through an opening known as the foramen magnum, which is Latin for "big hole." Inside the skull, just below the brain, the two vertebral arteries join to form vertebral basilar artery.

Though this design is meant to protect the delicate blood vessels, the bony gauntlet the vertebral arteries run ironically makes them more vulnerable to damage. Because they are bound inside holes on either side of the cervical vertebrae, the vertebral arteries turn when the neck turns. That extra loop where the arteries wind their way around the top cervical vertebra, also known as the axis, gives the blood vessels a bit of play when the head itself rotates from side to side. Though flexible, the arteries can only give so much. If they are pulled too hard or too far, they can stretch and tear. This is particularly true of arteries affected by atherosclerosis — commonly called "hardening of the arteries" — a disease of the blood vessels in which the artery walls can be made brittle by a buildup of waxy plaque. People have very infrequently damaged their vertebral arteries doing mundane and seemingly harmless activities such as coughing, sneezing, swinging a golf club, looking up at the sky, playing volleyball, or painting a ceiling. Doctors even coined a term, the "beauty-parlour stroke," for what sometimes happened to women getting their hair washed in the standard hairdresser's sink.

If the head is rotated or stretched beyond its normal range of motion (about fifty degrees), especially if it occurs suddenly, the thin lining of the vertebral arteries, called the intima, can tear. This is called a vertebral dissection, and it can happen in a couple of ways, both bad news for the brain.

In one scenario, a flap like a piece of loose wallpaper can form on the intima. Blood eddies and slows as it tries to make its way around the flap, but when blood slows, it also thickens. As it thickens, a clot can form around the flap. Tiny bits of that clot, called emboli, can break off and lodge themselves higher up in the smaller vessels that grow like dense roots around the brain. Those emboli can cut off blood flow, and thus cut off brain function. Later, the clot itself can break away just like a scab and lodge itself in an artery, interrupting blood flow and suffocating a piece of vital brain tissue in the process.

In the other scenario, the gap in the inner lining of the artery can act as a new pathway for the arterial blood rushing by. High-pressure blood that enters the tear flows into the muscular layer of the artery, called the media, swelling it so much that it can narrow the actual artery and decrease or completely cut off blood flow in the artery. In either case, a stroke can result.

Dissections can occur in other arteries too. The carotids, for example, are large arteries that run up the front of the neck surrounded by soft tissue. They can also be dissected by sudden neck trauma, though this has been only rarely associated with neck manipulation.

The Mathiason Inquest

Because Laurie Mathiason was so young and died in unusual circumstances, the coroner called an inquest into her death. An inquest is an official investigation designed to find out exactly where, when, and how someone died and to determine if there is any way to prevent similar deaths in the future. In September 1998, a four-day inquest was held into Laurie's death.

The six-person inquest jury heard testimony from more than a dozen medical and chiropractic experts. In the end, they were told that Laurie's vertebral artery was most likely ruptured by neck manipulation during the February 3 visit to her chiropractor. The chiropractic adjustment the next day probably dislodged a blood clot in the artery. That clot then traveled along the artery into her brain, where it had fatal consequences. The coroner's jury determined the cause of Mathiason's death was "traumatic rupture of the left vertebral artery."

The jury heard testimony from medical experts that the damage to Laurie's artery was directly related to the chiropractic manipulation of her neck. As the coroner, Dr. John Nyssen, said at the inquest, "So at this point, the public knows that Laurie died of a ruptured vertebral artery, which occurred in association with a chiropractic manipulation of the neck."[1] What seemed perfectly clear at the inquest would become the subject of debate in the months and years after it, a debate created by chiropractors.

At the conclusion of the inquest, the jury presented its recommendations, designed to prevent similar deaths in the future. Each and every one of the jury recommendations concerned chiropractic neck manipulation. They recommended that the Ministries of Health in Canada provide funding immediately to implement studies to:

a. determine the incidence of strokes associated with cervical spine manipulations.

b. determine the benefits and harmful effects that are associated with single and multiple cervical manipulations.

c. pursue the development of effective screening tests that will identify patients who are at high risk of complications when receiving cervical spinal manipulations.

They also called on the government to "develop a prototype patient and family medical history form which elicits pertinent health data prior to Chiropractic treatment" and to work with "Chiropractic Associations to ensure that the contents of the consent for treatment form be discussed by the Chiropractor and the patient at the initial visit." They called for screening tests to be made mandatory before chiropractors performed neck manipulation, and they asked that all health care experts work together to "maximize benefits and minimize risks inherent in cervical spinal manipulation treatments."

Finally, and perhaps most importantly, they called for full disclosure to ensure the safety of the public. The jury recommended that the government collaborate with chiropractic associations to "ensure that literature indicating the risk of strokes and other inherent risks associated with Chiropractic treatment, be visible and available in the reception area of every Chiropractic clinic."

When the inquest closed, chiropractic spokesmen in Saskatchewan appeared to accept the inquest's outcome and the recommendations of the jury. "I don't think there are any unreasonable recommendations within that group," Alexander Grier, president of the Chiropractors' Association of Saskatchewan told a reporter at the *Star Phoenix*, the daily newspaper in Saskatoon. It didn't take long for the backpedalling to begin.[2]

Misinformation Campaign

For Laurie's mother, sitting through the four days of the inquest into her daughter's death was one of the toughest challenges she had faced in her life. But Sharon Mathiason took some small solace in the fact that the findings of the inquest were unequivocally clear and in her hope that the recommendations might help some other young woman or man avoid Laurie's fate. It was only a matter of days before those hopes were shattered, and in the ensuing weeks and months, Sharon would experience a new pain — the maddening frustration of hearing her daughter's death diminished and denied.

Only two days after the inquest wrapped up, Sharon listened as CBC Radio's Mary Lou Finlay interviewed Paul Carey, the president of the Canadian Chiropractic Protective Association. At first, Carey conceded the most obvious point, saying that the death was "associated" with chiropractic, but then quickly backed away from even that. "The jury members did not make a direct relationship to the chiropractic adjustment. They did not say that that had caused [the stroke]. It may have, but they could not make that leap, because there was some evidence that it may have pre-existed the visit to the chiropractor. The chiropractor may have caused the clot to move or, uh, just been an unfortunate participant at the time." Later in the interview he again stated that chiropractic may have been involved but "we're not even sure if that was the real cause."[3]

In the next months, official chiropractic statements, press releases, and newsletters would continue to twist the facts of Laurie's death and misrepresent the outcome of the inquest. For example, the Canadian Chiropractic Association (CCA) issued a news release on October 6, 1998, that stated, "The jury did not make a finding that chiropractic treatment was the cause of this tragedy."[4] In an information sheet to Canadian chiropractors, the CCA made a similar statement: "It is notable that the jury listed the cause of death as a tear in the vertebral artery and not a cervical manipulation."[5]

In the months following the inquest, chiropractors continued to maintain that Mathiason's death was not related to chiropractic manipulation. In the November 2, 1998 issue of the newspaper *Dynamic Chiropractic*, the headline on the Mathiason story was "Chiropractic Acquitted in Canada — Patient's Death after Manipulation Not Attributed to DC."[6] In a November 1, 1998 newsletter to patients, the Circle Centre Chiropractic Clinic in Saskatoon repeated several misrepresentations. First, the newsletter writers took a broadside at the media: "Instead of informing the public of the basic facts surrounding this case and the relative safety of neck adjustments, the media chose to sensationalize and essentially misinform." And finally, they repeated and strengthened what was rapidly becoming the accepted version of the inquest in chiropractic circles: "The jury of the inquest in their official report did not find fault nor make recommendations against chiropractic or the chiropractor."[7]

Of course, as the officials in the chiropractic community were well aware, inquests are not mandated or even allowed to find fault, nor are they allowed to ascribe personal or individual blame.

Sharon Mathiason tracked these misleading statements, and more than a year after the inquest, the same kinds of fudging and blurring of the facts of Laurie's death continued. In a letter to the editor in the *Hamilton Spectator*, a chiropractor warned, "Let's be careful not to pass judgment too quickly. An inquest into the death of a Saskatchewan woman last year did *not* conclude that her death was caused by a chiropractic adjustment."[8]

The same claim was made in an advertisement taken out by more than a dozen chiropractors in Burlington, Ontario. The headline on the March 5,

2000 advertisement in the Burlington *Post* was, "The Truth about Chiropractic and Neck Adjustment," and it read, in part:

> Regarding the Saskatchewan inquest of 1998, the jury concluded that the patient died due to a tear in the vertebral artery; it **did not** conclude that she died as a result of a chiropractic neck adjustment. The Coroner's inquest did not say the chiropractic adjustment caused the stroke. It could have been other activities of daily living."[9]

When Sharon Mathiason saw this ad, she was astonished that the findings of the inquest could be so completely misconstrued by the chiropractors. The statements in the ad were not just partially inaccurate, they were a contradiction of what actually came out of the inquest process. In fact, the pathologist who testified at the inquest, Dr. Robert Macaulay, told the jury that Laurie's death was due with "99 percent certainty to the neck manipulation." There was no evidence or testimony that Laurie died as a result of her regular daily activities.

Perhaps even more ironic has been the way that the chiropractors have dealt with the jury's recommendation that they inform the public about the risks associated with chiropractic treatment. In Saskatchewan, the provincial chiropractors' association used the directive to produce a series of brochures promoting chiropractic and selling its safety. The title of one brochure was "Why Chiropractic is a safe health choice."

When Sharon Mathiason reads these denials, misleading statements, and outright falsehoods about her daughter's death, she says she is "absolutely flabbergasted."

"It is a deceit," she said. "I say that what chiropractors are doing is waging a coordinated, intentional campaign of fraud and deceit on the Canadian public. This does not allow anyone who is contemplating going to a chiropractor to have a full and accurate truth about Laurie's death. People are not being properly informed of the risk of chiropractic."

The Mathiason family agreed to a settlement with the chiropractors in February 2001, and as part of the terms of the agreement, the chiropractor did not accept responsibility for Laurie's death. As well, the agreement prohibits Sharon from disclosing the amount of the settlement. Nevertheless, she has continued to speak out in general terms about the dangers of neck manipulation and to vigilantly criticize misleading and inaccurate statements sent out by the profession. She is an avid letter writer, and her "corrections" of chiropractic misstatements often appear in leading newspapers. She was also an outspoken critic of Saskatchewan chiropractors' campaign to introduce chiropractic to school-aged children each year during Spinal Health Week in the province. Mathiason said the Chiropractors Association of Saskatchewan provided an information package about the spine to schools across the province. The material, including a poster and activity sheets, is aimed at Grade 5 students. Mathiason sent letters criticizing the campaign to the department of education, to the ministry of health, and to her provincial government representative. In the letter, she named the chiropractor who performed the neck manipulation on her daughter that caused the fatal stroke.

She received a letter from lawyers demanding an apology and a retraction. Mathiason said she cannot afford fights with lawyers. Now a widow (her husband died suddenly in the spring of 2001 of a heart attack at the age of fifty-seven), she lives modestly on a tight budget. As well, she has had to suffer through the losses of her sister to cancer and, more recently, of a nephew to a brain tumour. She said she is less able — both emotionally and financially — to wage a public battle against chiropractors, their marketing tactics, and their misrepresentation of her daughter's death. But she will continue to lobby against upper neck manipulation. "It's a procedure that has to stop."

Neck Manipulation, Strokes, and Deaths

Almost no one denies that neck manipulation, delivered by chiropractors or anyone else, has the potential to do harm. Reports of complications following chiropractic neck manipulation date back to 1925, with the case of a patient suffering a dislocated atlas (the top vertebra of the spine). The first documented case of stroke following a neck manipulation was a 1947 published report of two patients who became unconscious during chiropractic adjustment and died in less than twenty-four hours.[10]

Since then, there have been numerous case reports of neurological complications following chiropractic neck manipulation, the most common being posterior circulation stroke related to vertebral artery dissection. Most chiropractors acknowledge in their own writings that neck manipulation, particularly adjustment of the upper neck, carries with it the danger of damaging the arteries in the neck, either the carotids that run up the front of the neck or the vertebral arteries that run up the back.

In his book *Current Concepts in Vertebrobasilar Complicatons following Spinal Manipulation*, chiropractor Allan Terrett opens his first chapter with a strong statement to his fellow chiropractors: "It has to be accepted that VBS [vertebrobasilar stroke] following SMT [spinal manipulative therapy] does occur."[11] He states the seemingly obvious because, despite the substantial evidence accumulated over more than fifty years concerning neck adjustment and stroke, some chiropractors continue to deny the connection.

Terrett himself refers to articles published in the chiropractic literature calling the causal link between chiropractic neck adjustments and stroke "junk science" and laments that these statements do not help the profession in "accepting the problem, addressing the problem, or searching for solutions to the problem."[12] His advice appears to be having little impact in some quarters. As recently as 2002, the World Chiropractic Alliance took the official position that "the only reasonable conclusion which can be drawn is that chiropractic adjustments do not pose any significant risk of stroke and are remarkably safe."[13]

Setting aside the "stroke denier" contingent in chiropractic, the real debate around neck adjustment and stroke focuses on numbers. How often does a chiropractic neck adjustment damage the vertebral or carotid arteries? How many people suffer neurological complications following a neck adjustment? And, finally, how many patients who have their necks adjusted by chiropractors suffer strokes? In other words, what is the incidence of harm from chiropractic neck manipulation? This is a key point, because all interventions, even the taking of an aspirin for headache, carry risk. If the risk is low and the benefit substantial, then the intervention is considered a good one. If the risk is high or the possible outcome catastrophic, and the benefit is dubious, then the medication or therapy doesn't make much sense. The debate about chiropractic neck manipulation hinges on these precise points.

How often do chiropractors cause neurological damage by manipulating people's necks? The answer depends on who you ask and how you look at the numbers.

In their public statements and materials intended for patient consumption, chiropractors put the risk of suffering a stroke after neck manipulation at between one in a million and one in two or three million. They sometimes suggest to patients that the risk of one in a million is about equal to your chances of being hit by lightning.

The numbers becomes even smaller if you base the estimate on reported legal and insurance claims. Using this technique, a 1995 American study, which only counted *paid out* claims, arrived at a number of twenty cerebrovascular accidents a year. The authors estimated that the insured chiropractors performed about forty-three million cervical manipulations a year, producing a harm rate of about one stroke per two million cervical manipulations.[14]

In Canada, using a similar model, Paul Carey, president of the Canadian Chiropractic Protective Fund, which insures the vast majority of chiropractors in Canada, ran the numbers. He used provincial government health insurance plan records to estimate that chiropractors performed more than one hundred million manipulations over five years (1986–1990). Carey noted that this number is likely low because figures for the four eastern provinces were not available and services provided outside the health insurance plans were not counted. He estimated that about half of the manipulations, or fifty million, were cervical. During that time period, 13 cases of CVA were documented, resulting in an incidence rate of 1 for every 3.8 million manipulations. In Quebec over the same five-year period, only one case of CVA was reported, creating an incidence rate of one accident per fourteen million manipulations. Excluding Quebec, Carey estimated the rate at about one per three million, leaving him to wonder if "previous estimates have been overstated."[15]

A similar and more recent review, which examined the malpractice data from the Canadian Chiropractic Protective Association, was conducted by Scott Haldeman and Paul Carey. The authors looked at all claims of stroke over a ten-year period (1988–1997). They found forty-three cases of neurological symptoms following cervical manipulation. Of those, twenty were deemed minor, with the remaining twenty-three diagnosed as stroke by a neurologist. The authors then estimated the number of neck manipulations performed by chiropractors in Canada over that time period. Extrapolating from survey data, they estimated that chiropractors covered by the CCPA performed 134.5 million cervical manipulations over a ten-year period. Using these numbers, they estimate the rate of stroke after neck manipulation to be 1 in 5.85 million. This, say the authors, is "significantly less than estimates of 1 in 500,000 to 1 in a million cervical manipulations of earlier studies.[16]

Almost nobody outside of chiropractic accepts these numbers. Researchers and physicians say it is ridiculous and misleading to estimate incidents of serious injury based on insurance claims alone. Those claims, they say, cover only a fraction of the incidents that actually occur.

In smaller countries, where it was possible to actually track treatments against injuries, the numbers look different. In Denmark, researchers looked at cervical spine adjustments and found that the incidence of CVA was 1 in every 120,000 cervical treatment sessions, tracked over a ten-year period from 1978 to 1988.[17] In the same study, they found the manipulation of the upper neck about four times more commonly associated with injury than that of the lower neck. Some studies put the incidence rate of neurological complications as high as one in forty thousand[18] cervical adjustments, and even one in twenty thousand,[19] but chiropractors nevertheless argue that the treatment is one of the safest interventions in health care.

When The RAND Corporation did a review of all the literature on neck manipulation and mobilization, they found the procedure to have a very low risk rate. They calculated the risk for complications arising from cervical manipulation was 1.46 per 1 million manipulations.[20] The RAND authors assumed that one in ten negative outcomes was reported in the literature, and using that methodology, they found the rate of serious complications from cervical spine manipulation to be 6.39 per 10 million manipulations and the rate of deaths to be 2.68 per 10 million manipulations. The authors of the RAND study and the authors of other studies comparing the risks of complications from neck manipulation with the use of non-steroidal anti-inflammatory drugs (NSAIDs) found both to be small, with neck manipulation significantly smaller — one hundred times smaller in one study.[21]

At the conclusion of his book-length treatise on neck manipulation and injury, Terrett couldn't be more clear: "On analysis, SMT as delivered by chiropractors is one of the most conservative, least invasive and safest of procedures in the provision of health care services."[22]

Diane Rodrigue

Try telling that to Diane Rodrigue. Today, laboriously using a voice machine to help her speak, the forty-four-year-old quadriplegic will tell anyone who will listen to never, ever let a chiropractor do a neck adjustment. In May 2002, Rodrigue appeared on national television in a CTV documentary to warn Canadians against chiropractic neck manipulation. The fact that she is alive and spreading her message is something of a miracle in itself.

In the winter of 1994, Diane Rodrigue lay in the intensive care ward of the Sudbury General Hospital attached to a ventilator. She was thirty-six years old. She couldn't breathe, couldn't move, and couldn't talk. But she could listen. She could listen as doctor after doctor told her she had been paralyzed by a stroke she suffered after a chiropractic neck manipulation. They said she would never get better and would probably succumb to pneumonia. According to Rodrigue, the physicians asked her if she wanted the ventilator turned off so she could die.

Rodrigue chose to live, and a month later, when she stopped taking morphine and could think clearly, decided to sue her chiropractor for five million dollars. She discussed the suit with her lawyer via her mother, who read her lips. Rodrigue and the chiropractor settled out of court for one million dollars.

In 1993, Diane Rodrigue was the office manager for the Temiskaming District Ministry of Housing, overseeing a staff of four. The ministry's office was in the same building as chiropractor Kristin Shepherd. Rodrigue was suffering from headaches, and some of the other women in her office had been visiting Dr. Shepherd. "They came back saying it had done them a world of good," said Rodrigue. So she decided to try it.

On her first visit, Shepherd talked to her about chiropractic medicine and explained that subluxations, or problems with the alignment of her spine, could cause health problems. She sent Rodrigue for neck and full-spine x-rays. On the next visit, according to Rodrigue, Dr. Shepherd told her that vertebrae in her spine were out of alignment and that this was causing her headaches. She then adjusted Rodrigue's hip, back, and finally her neck, rotating it sideways.

After a couple of weeks of treatment, Rodrigue said she realized her headaches and neck pain got worse after each adjustment, not better. Three weeks after her first adjustment the pain got so bad she vomited. The next morning, she called her chiropractor at home. "I was really frightened," Rodrigue recalls. That day Shepherd met with Rodrigue and agreed that she shouldn't get any neck manipulations. "She wrote in red letters on my chart 'No neck manipulation, slight traction only' and put red stars beside the words," said Rodrigue. She continued to go for treatment, getting just traction, or a slight pulling on the neck, from her chiropractor.

Dr. Shepherd, now practicing in New Liskeard, Ontario, says she only recalls Rodrigue getting her neck adjusted beyond light traction once during her visits to her, although she says she also adjusted her hip and back. She says that the level of traction applied to Rodrigue's neck would have been very slight. "I don't know how to describe it, would be enough to move a Kleenex across a desk. It was so light," she explains. Rodrigue is unclear about exactly how many times her neck was manipulated during her visits. Dr. Shepherd recalls noting the warning on Rodrigue's chart.

In January 1994, Rodrigue went for her last session with the chiropractor, a review and final assessment. That assessment was done by Dr. Michael Nenonen. He had been filling in for Dr. Shepherd for a week. Nenonen had previously treated Rodrigue on two occasions.

During the last assessment session, Rodrigue says Nenonen suggested that he give her an adjustment. Rodrigue agreed. According to Rodrigue, Nenonen adjusted first her hip, then her back, and then pulled her neck upwardly slightly. Suddenly, Rodrigue recalls, he twisted Rodrigue's neck to the right. She felt a sudden pain and then a feeling of spreading warmth in her neck.

Rodrigue got up from the adjusting table and went to pay for her visit. That's when she started having trouble holding her head up and her breathing became laboured. She sat slumped in an office chair as the feeling of warmth in her neck grew more intense. Her arms became floppy and her breathing grew steadily worse. According to Rodrigue, the chiropractor and his secretary were panicked. "I don't know why, but I wasn't," she recalls, "I was telling them what to do."

Dr. Nenonen, now practicing in Sault Ste. Marie, recalls that Rodrigue was his patient and that he did treat her that day. On the advice of the Canadian Chiropractic Association, he said he could not speak further about the incident.

Dr. Shepherd says she is completely confused about what treatment was given to Rodrigue that day. "What stumped me was to the best of my knowledge there was no adjustment of her neck, what you're calling a manipulation," she says.

"[Dr. Nenonen] said he did gentle traction, which he had done all along. I know it's not a case of him not reading her file. He knew it very well and he had done the same thing ... on two occasions before," she explained. "I have tremendous compassion for what it created in her life and what it created in the lives around her but I don't know what happened ... I trust completely Mike and I trust what she says so I don't know where to go from there."

Rodrigue was taken to a local hospital then flown by helicopter to Sudbury General. She stopped breathing on her own three days later. The hospital would be her home for eight months. She was on a ventilator and unable to speak for two years. Part of the settlement money she got went towards building the special apartment in her parents' house in Iroquois Falls, an hour north of Timmins, Ontario.

Today, she is still paralyzed but is no longer on a ventilator. She has implants in her sides that are connected to her phrenic nerve. Those implants send signals to her diaphragm, telling it to breathe. If something goes wrong with the implants, or she has a cold and gets a mucus blockage, she'll need suction or other immediate care. Rodrigue has around-the-clock care, including a registered nurse for six hours a day and then a caregiver for the remaining eighteen hours of the afternoon and evening. They cost her one hundred thousand dollars a year. To help offset the cost, she receives a subsidy to cover forty hours of nursing care a week.

"I decreased my level of care in September 2000 to save money and be more independent," she said in a 2002 interview. "I don't have very much of the insurance money left. I will have to look at other options in two or three years," she said.

Rodrigue worries that she'll be forced to leave her apartment and move to an institution. "Some place way down south," she said. "Away from my family. They don't have places like that for me up here because of the constant care I need. My biggest concern is, where am I going to end up?"

The Stroke Consortium and New Numbers

When things go horribly wrong, as they did for Diane Rodrigue, it is neurologists, not chiropractors, who pick up the pieces. It is neurologists who are seeing otherwise healthy young people apparently suffering from the effects of minor strokes, and it is neurologists who are questioning the chiropractor's numbers on neck manipulation and stroke.

One such neurologist is Dr. John Norris. He's a professor of neurology in the Stroke Research Unit at Sunnybrook and Women's College Health Science Centre in Toronto. He is also head of the Canadian Stroke Consortium. The consortium is a national network of stroke physicians in sixty centres spread across Canada who are collecting cases of neurological damage caused by dissections of the arteries in the neck and head. Dr. Norris's work with the Stroke Consortium has gained widespread media attention, and his results have fanned the smouldering debate between physicians and chiropractors in Canada into a raging firestorm.

Norris is a soft-spoken, balding man with quick dark eyes and a light English accent. He left his home in London, England to come to Canada in 1968, and he has worked in neurological research for more than thirty years. Today, Norris says it feels as though his whole life is about chiropractic. But it wasn't always that way.

In 1997, he and a colleague, Michael Chan, a visiting physician from Hong Kong, did a study on stroke in young people. Chan's findings surprised Norris. "He concluded that the commonest cause of stroke in young people was dissection," he explained. At the time, Norris was not aware that dissection was so widespread, and he questioned his young colleague's findings. Check it again, he told him. Chan checked it and told Norris that 13 percent of strokes in young people were caused by dissection, a startling figure.[23] Chan noted that chiropractic neck manipulation was one of several causes of the dissections. Norris became interested. Like most doctors, he knew very little about chiropractic, so he assigned a summer student to do a survey of chiropractic. "And it was following that that I realized that dissection was a bigger problem than I thought and chiropractic was a bigger problem than I thought," he said.

As head of the Stroke Consortium, Norris has asked neurologists across Canada to collect detailed information on cases of vertebral artery dissection, including laboratory reports, angiograms, and follow-up reports. The survey by the consortium is trying to establish what causes cervical artery dissection and to record the fate of patients who have suffered such an event. It's difficult work. Neurologists are extremely busy, and few have time to collect files, go over records, and fill out the forms that Norris needs to document the cases.

Despite the reporting problems, the cases have poured in to the consortium's offices at Sunnybrook. In 1999, Norris had seventy-four patients in his records who had suffered dissection of either their carotid arteries or their vertebral arteries. Most were young — the mean age was forty-four — and more than 80 percent had suffered the damage after sudden neck movement, everything from a vigorous game of volleyball to neck manipulation. Stroke resulting from neck manipulation occurred in 28 percent of the cases Norris has uncovered.[24] Strokes in people under the age of forty-five are relatively uncommon, and in that age group, dissection of the cervical arteries was the main cause of stroke. The single greatest contributor to torn arteries in that group? Cervical manipulation. At last count, Norris's 35 centres had reported 180 neck manipulation stroke cases. Based on his figures and statistics provided by the Heart and Stroke Foundation, Norris says about eighty people suffer a chiropractic-induced stroke each year.[25]

"But that is a gross underestimation, I think," said Norris. He thinks the number of cases they are getting from neurologists is low — just the tip of the iceberg. "Ludicrously low," he said. He says there's good evidence to believe that most neck manipulation strokes go unreported for a variety of reasons.

First, the people doing the manipulation — mostly chiropractors — are naturally reluctant to report adverse effects. Second, many don't even recognize the signs of a stroke. "When chiropractors see patients and the patient has minor symptoms of stroke, they don't do anything about it, they don't recognize it. I thought it was just that they were suppressing it — maybe some of them do — but a lot of them just don't know it's a stroke." Third, explains Norris, physicians who deal with stroke victims often do not understand the risks of neck manipulation and seldom question patients about visits to a chiropractor or a physiotherapist, though thanks to the Stroke Consortium that is now changing. Finally, it is likely that many minor strokes caused by dissection of the arteries in the neck are simply missed entirely, by patient, chiropractor, and doctor.

Neck pain is often misdiagnosed, and if there are residual minor deficits after the stroke, such as loss of peripheral vision, the patient may never associate the symptom with their chiropractic treatments. In other cases, the symptoms naturally resolve on their own, and the entire incident may go largely unnoticed and unreported.

Norris admits the limitations of his own study. He thinks most of the dissection-induced strokes that neurologists are treating simply do not get reported to the consortium. "There are over 100 centres that could be reporting and hundreds of individual neurologists we haven't heard from."

Part of the problem is that doctors are largely unaware of the problem of dissection caused by neck manipulation. Like Norris a few years ago, most physicians have no interest in, and no knowledge of, chiropractic. As well, most emergency room doctors are unaware that dissection is a potent cause of stroke. Based on all these factors, Norris feels that many, perhaps hundreds, of strokes are missed each year. "All these minor things are suppressed," he explained. "The patient goes home dizzy and gets better after a few days and doesn't realize what happened." And Norris is not alone in his fears.

Professor Edzard Ernst thinks the number of strokes induced by chiropractic manipulation is grossly underreported. Dr. Ernst is a professor in the department of complementary medicine in the School of Sports and Health Sciences at the University of Exeter and the author of a recent commentary in the *Canadian Medical Association Journal*. His group conducted a survey of all neurologists in Britain, asking them whether they had seen cases of serious neurological complication twenty-four hours after cervical spinal manipulation over the past year. Twenty-four respondents had observed thirty-five such cases, none of which had been reported. Ten cases were of vascular accidents.

Ernst admitted the data were not free of bias, that the findings are not conclusive, and that a prospective study would be better. In fact, Ernst examined six prospective studies that included more than two thousand patients. Not a single case of a serious adverse event after manipulation was reported. However, about 50 percent of the patients experienced mild and transient adverse effects (e.g., local discomfort, headache, tiredness, and radiating discomfort) after the procedure.[26] Ernst also points out that the study design was problematic in that serious complications were to be evaluated during follow-up, but, as he pointed out, "Almost by definition, patients who experienced a severe adverse effect would simply not return for such a follow-up visit. It is therefore hardly surprising that only mild complaints were registered in these studies."[27]

Ernst thinks that chiropractic estimates of neurological events following neck manipulation are not accurate and that chiropractors seem unable or unwilling to get to the truth. "One gets the impression that the risks of spinal manipulation are being played down, particularly by chiropractors. Perhaps the best indication that this is true are estimates of incidence rates based on assumptions, which are unproven at best and unrealistic at worse. One such assumption, for instance, is that 10 percent of actual complications will be reported. Our recent survey, however, demonstrated an underreporting rate of 100 percent. This extreme level of underreporting obviously renders estimates nonsensical."[28] So, Ernst is suggesting that only one in one hundred chiropractic complications is being reported.

A 2001 study by three Ontario researchers again challenged the chiropractors' notion that neck manipulation was inherently safe. Their study found neck manipulation to be ten to twenty times more dangerous than chiropractic estimates. The study concluded that one in every one hundred thousand patients under forty-five who are given a neck adjustment by a chiropractor will suffer a stroke.

The researchers relied on OHIP data and Ontario hospital admissions data. The study was carried out by the Toronto-based Institute for Clinical Evaluative Sciences and appeared in *Stroke* — *Journal of the American Heart*

Association. The study also determined that vertebral artery stroke sufferers under forty-five were five times more likely than a control group to have visited a chiropractor in the previous week. They were also five times more likely to have visited a chiropractor three times or more in the previous month.[29] The authors of the study were extremely cautious, noting that the association between neck manipulation and stroke was not conclusive evidence that one caused the other.

Is one in one hundred thousand the real number? It's impossible to tell without further studies. One thing is for sure — no researcher we spoke to believes the one-in-a-million number anymore. It appears to be a chiropractic fiction. Mounting evidence indicates that upper neck manipulation causes far more damage than chiropractors want to admit. In the winter of 2002, a young neurologist sent that message out loud and clear.

Dr. Brad Stewart and the Neurologists' Letter

While Norris was working hard in Toronto, Dr. Brad Stewart was in Saskatoon exploring the issue of stroke and chiropractic neck manipulation. Stewart remembers being called in to help the other doctors try to save Laurie Mathiason the day after her stroke. He was also involved in her autopsy. Stewart is absolutely clear about how Laurie died. "There was no question what happened. Her artery was dissected and she died as a direct result of that," he said.

Like Norris and other neurologists, Stewart knew little about chiropractic in general and even less about their particular brand of neck manipulation.

Stewart has been a neurologist since 1998. He was born in British Columbia, did his undergraduate degree at Queen's University in Kingston, and attended medical school at the University of Saskatchewan. Today he runs a practice, is an assistant professor of neurology at the University of Alberta, and works out of the University Hospital in Edmonton, Alberta. He is by his own admission very busy — too busy, he thought, to research chiropractic or fill out Stroke Consortium forms. He really needed to spend more time with his wife, a radiologist, and their young daughter. But Laurie Mathiason's death had affected him. He had become more aware and more vigilant. He began to ask questions, to keep a watchful eye. He didn't have to wait long for the problem to surface.

"When I first came to Edmonton, in my first month, I had a young woman who had been dissected by a chiropractor a year or two earlier and proceeded to have another little TIA (transcient ischemic attack) and then one of my very first patients had his neck manipulated and ended up with a big disc in his neck compressing a nerve. He ended up undergoing surgery," said Stewart. "That was my introduction to Edmonton. After that, every month or two we would have another stroke. I had a span where in two months we had four strokes and a myalopathy — compression of the spinal cord — all of that in a very short period of time."

Though his evidence is anecdotal, Stewart is quick to emphasize that these cases were not based on his suspicions. "This is not speculative, these are people who have had angiograms that clearly demonstrate dissections and MRIs and infarcs and the patients had history of neck problem and marked problem with neck pain."

At last count, Stewart was closing in on two dozen patients who had suffered chiropractic mishaps. "I have 20 patients — a little over half are stroke, and the rest are compressed spinal cords, compressed nerves in the neck, and compressed nerves in the back."

All this occurred in little more than a year, since Stewart began documenting the cases. In the last year he has called chiropractors each time he encountered a problem and has been rebuffed each time. "I wrote the Alberta College of Chiropractic. I included the angiograms and the reports. They would not respond because it was not the patients who were making the complaints."

All of this convinced Stewart that the problem was larger than documented and that chiropractors and their organizations were uninterested in really dealing with the issues. He decided to speak out. "This was something I had been thinking about doing for years and I just got pissed off seeing more and more young people disabled," he explained.

In the winter of 2002, spearheaded by Stewart, sixty-three Canadian neurologists signed a statement warning the Canadian public of the dangers of chiropractic neck manipulation and calling into question many chiropractic practices, particularly the treatment of babies and children. The press release, issued on the fourth anniversary of Laurie Mathiason's death, was a "statement of concern to the Canadian public regarding the debilitating and fatal damage manipulation of the neck may cause to the nervous system." The statement used Norris's data and outlined six concerns, including the need for the Canadian public to be informed of the dangers of neck manipulation and for individual patients to be made aware of those risks. The neurologists raised their concerns that autopsy procedures fail to diagnose cases of death due to neck manipulation. They also called on the government to recognize and act upon the issues raised by pediatricians about chiropractors treating children. The letter writers asked for an immediate ban on all spinal manipulation of infants and children and criticized chiropractors for the "unscientific claims" they make for the benefits of neck manipulation.

Denials and Threats

Not surprisingly, the statement outraged chiropractors, who came out swinging. What had been simmering in the background as a journal-driven feud between physicians and chiropractors suddenly erupted into a very pubic debate. Once again, the chiropractors challenged the latest stroke studies, calling them incomplete and flawed, maintaining that there are many causes of strokes and that the causal link between the strokes and chiropractic manipulation remained unproven. In the United States, leading members of the chiropractic profession said the new data lacked scientific value and was speculative and unsupported.

Norris calls the attacks "nonsense." He explained, "Most stokes are painless. This is different, quite different." Because arteries are extremely sensitive, stretching or tearing them causes pain, a lot of pain. The patients in Norris's study reported neck pain, then characteristic symptoms of brain damage (dizziness, vision problems, unsteadiness, nausea, and vertigo). Finally, all the patients in the study had angiograms that confirmed dissection of the artery. "So you get a chiropractic manoeuvre, you get pain in the neck, you get characteristic symptoms and the angiogram is positive for dissection," said Norris.

In questioning Norris's data, chiropractors were, ironically, demanding a level of evidence they seldom, if ever, demand of themselves. But in this case, as in others where chiropractors see an assault on the profession, science took a back seat to legal manoeuvring and public relations. In its response to the letter by neurologists, the Canadian Chiropractic Association threatened them with legal action. "This letter highlights the seriousness of our concerns and the need for you to respond in a timely manner. If you fail to respond, due to the serious nature of what has taken place, we intend to take every appropriate and necessary legal step to have this matter remedied," wrote CCA president Mireille Duranleau.

But the letters, threats, and spin-doctoring could not stop the risk debate, and the statement from the neurologists publicly raised questions that had been brewing in the scientific literature for years, even decades. How often do chiropractors adjust the necks of their patients? Why do chiropractors manipulate necks at all? And what evidence is there that it provides any benefit?

The Risk at Hand

Chiropractors love to crack necks. Every day, in Canada and in the United States, chiropractors perform millions and millions of neck manipulations.

Exact numbers are impossible to calculate because chiropractors do not track every manipulation they perform, but estimates provided by chiropractors give us a fairly good picture of how many neck manipulations take place every year.

About 10 percent of the American population consults chiropractors, and the average number of office visits annually is ten. That means that there are approximately 250 million patient visits per year to chiropractors in America.[30] Several surveys suggest that 66 to 69 percent of chiropractic visits include cervical manipulation, so that means that 165 to 172 million patient visits in the United States include a neck manipulation.[31] In fact, chiropractors may adjust the neck more than one time per visit, so that number could be much higher.

In Canada, figures are difficult to determine, but a recent study suggests that chiropractors perform about 13.4 million neck manipulations per year.[32] In an earlier 1993 report, chiropractor Paul Carey examined provincial health insurance data and estimated conservatively that chiropractors performed about 20 million adjustments a year. Of those, Carey assumed half were to the cervical spine, resulting in about 10 million neck manipulations per year in Canada.[33] Carey does not explain why he uses the 50 percent figure, but surveys indicate a wide range of figures surrounding neck manipulation. In an information pamphlet by Saskatchewan chiropractors on the safety of chiropractic it was noted that, "Up to 3/4 of patients receive a neck adjustment as part of their individual treatment." Researchers at Life Chiropractic College assume that 30 percent of manipulations are cervical,[34] but other surveys indicate the numbers are much higher.[35] If we assumed that 69 percent of the manipulations were to the neck, then the number of cervical manipulations in Canada could be almost 14 million per year. It is well accepted that the manipulation most closely associated with stroke is the upper cervical adjustment, the one that targets C1 and C2. If half or a third of all neck manipulations are upper neck, then the risk ratio changes dramatically. But all of this is a guessing game because no one keeps track of what kind of adjustments chiropractors are performing, or why. Chiropractors, by their own admission, adjust a lot of necks, which is quite perplexing when you consider that according to the figures provided by chiropractors themselves, most patients — almost 70 percent — who visit a chiropractor complain of *low-back* pain.[36] So, why do chiropractors adjust the necks of most of their patients, no matter what their complaint? Like most things in chiropractic, the answer is a muddle of philosophy, belief, and history, with little, if any, scientific support.

B.J. Palmer's Second-Best Idea

To really understand why chiropractors are so dogmatic about adjusting patients' necks, we need to return to Davenport, Iowa, during the Great Depression.

It was late summer 1931, and B.J. Palmer's finances had barely survived the collapse of the American stock market two years earlier. Enrolment in the Palmer School of Chiropractic was in a slow decline and had been since the end of the First World War. Palmer had lost supremacy in the profession after his disastrous introduction of the expensive and useless neurocalometer in 1924. *(See "The P.T. Barnum of Chiropractic")* It was time for a new idea. Palmer had already used print advertising and his own radio station, WOC, to blanket America with a simplified version of his father's chiropractic theories.[37] Now he was about to make things even easier. Since 1921, Palmer had been the host of chiropractic lyceums — events that featured a parade through Davenport (featuring giant vertebrae), revival-like tent meetings, and, the pièce de résistance, an evangelical speech by B.J. Palmer himself.[38] It was at the 1924 Lyceum that Palmer had introduced the neurocalometer. But in 1931 he told the gathered, though dwindled, faithful about the next great advance in chiropractic: the Hole-in-One theory.

Despite the odd name, Palmer was convinced he had reduced chiropractic to its essence. Through extensive study of neurocalometer data, Palmer had decided that he and his father had been wrong about chiropractic after all. It wasn't necessary to adjust every vertebra in the spine to remove spinal subluxations — you just needed to adjust the vertebrae in the upper neck, the atlas and axis (C1 and C2). All the other subluxations would disappear in sympathy. So, according to Palmer's new idea, chiropractors could now cure almost all human "dis-ease" (as he liked to call it) by adjusting patients' necks only. The Hole-in-One technique was the "adjustment with extra something," B.J. Palmer told the Lyceum crowd, many of whom left confused by the bombastic sermon.[39] They were perplexed because not only had Palmer literally turned chiropractic theory on its head, he had also used the address as an opportunity to redefine the vertebral subluxation and once again pump the neurocalometer.[40]

Prior to the 1931 Lyceum, any misaligned vertebrae could cause a subluxation. Now Palmer had rejected the teachings of his father, D.D. Palmer, and summarily ignored his own earlier writings. He now proclaimed that a subluxation had to:

• be most often in the neck
• interfere with the transmission of the "mental impulse"

- cause an increase in skin temperature
- put pressure on the spinal nerves or spinal cord.

Not surprisingly, Palmer felt the neurocalometer could best detect the newly defined subluxation. And, writing in the *Fountain Head News*, he clearly connects the two ideas:

> [The Hole-in-One theory] has greater health benefit than anything we have ever said or done except the introduction of the Neurocalometer ... Chiropractic has evolved through many stages on its way to the present, or scientific specific state.[41]

This was also the first time Palmer mentions that subluxations can appear in a part of the brain just above the spine: the brain stem. The brain stem, as the name implies, is the lowest part of the brain just before it extends into the spinal cord. Palmer came to believe that "cord pressure" on the brain stem could cause subluxations that responded well to upper cervical chiropractic adjustments. This idea was central to the Hole-in-One theory.

Why this shift in attention to the brain stem and "cord pressure"? By the early 1930s, Palmer was coming under increasing pressure from the medical community to demonstrate that misaligned vertebrae could really pinch spinal nerves. As we've seen, this is anatomically impossible in all but badly damaged or diseased spines. By 1934, it is clear that Palmer was searching for a new mechanism for subluxations in the pressure that misalignments of the first two vertebrae put on the brain stem and spinal cord. Again, not surprisingly, this type of pressure was harder to prove, or disprove, than spinal nerve subluxations. Palmer went so far as to have the Dresden Hygienic Museum in Germany create a translucent specimen of the first cervical vertebrae and a portion of the lower skull, the occiput. This is known as the "wet specimen" and is still on display at the Palmer School in Davenport, Iowa.[42] He also obtained photographs showing that the spinal cord almost fills the spinal canal even after death. This, he suggested, showed that his theorized "spinal pressure" was possible. In fact, the spinal cord is protected in the spinal canal by three membranes and a protective fluid in which it almost floats. Despite Palmer's efforts, he was unable to show that subluxations exist, that spinal pressure is real, or that adjusting the cervical vertebrae can correct subluxations in the neck or anywhere else. And, after eighty years of trying, chiropractic researchers have not made any real progress on these fronts — but the widespread practice of adjusting cervical vertebrae continues nonetheless. As for the supposed therapeutic benefits of neck manipulation, chiropractors have little evidence that their beliefs are true.

Neck Manipulation — What's the Benefit?

Though chiropractors have been doing neck manipulations since the birth of chiropractic, they have little evidence that they are effective for anything.

In 1999, The RAND Corporation conducted a review of the appropriateness of manipulation and mobilization of the cervical spine. They assembled a panel of nine experts: four chiropractors, four medical doctors, and one doctor-chiropractor. The panel did an extensive search and review of all the literature published and rated cervical manipulation for appropriateness and effectiveness for specified clinical conditions such as tension headaches and neck pain. The report's first conclusion was that there was a lack of research on the effectiveness of chiropractic and that there was not enough data to validate chiropractic's effectiveness for many conditions.[43] Second, the panel considered 1,436 indications for cervical manipulation and mobilization, and of that total only 122 (16 percent) were considered appropriate. The panel found 632 (43 percent) to be inappropriate and were uncertain about the remaining 586 (41 percent). In other words, the panel concluded that 84 percent of the indications for cervical manipulation were either inappropriate or dubious. In the 16 percent of cases where manipulating the neck is appropriate, the evidence of benefit is weak or non-existent. The RAND study concluded that for acute neck pain "there are no RCTs (randomized, controlled trials) or case series presenting data about the efficacy of cervical spine manipulation specifically for patients with acute neck pain."[44] For subacute and chronic neck pain, the study found that manipulation and or mobilization "may provide at least short-term pain relief and range of motion enhancement for persons with subacute or chronic neck pain."

For patients suffering from muscle tension headache, the researchers found that "the literature is sparse but suggests that cervical spine manipulation and/or mobilization may provide short-term relief for some patients with muscle tension (and other nonmigraine) headaches. The evidence for long-term benefit is much less conclusive."[45] Two Danish researchers who conducted a randomized controlled trial of chiropractic manipulation for tension headaches found that "it did not seem to have a positive effect."[46] For migraine headaches, RAND found there was not enough research to come to any conclusion about neck manipulation.[47]

In short, the evidence for manipulation and mobilization for these conditions is weak or non-existent. As well, it is important to point out that RAND was looking at spinal manipulative therapy, not specifically at chiropractic adjustment.

Add to that the reality that neck pain and headache pain are in most cases self-limiting, that is, they go away on their own in a matter of hours or days. So chiropractors, who deliver 90 percent of manipulations, are twisting necks with little evidence of benefit of any kind for conditions that get better on their own.[48] Based on the evidence from the RAND analysis and other studies, some experts question the wisdom of *any* cervical neck manipulation and call for a halt to the procedure until further study is done. Chiropractic critic Dr. Murray Katz has called for a ban on neck manipulation. Dr. Brad Stewart agrees. "It should be stopped and stopped now. And until they can demonstrate unequivocally that the benefits outweigh the risks, which they have been unable to do for a hundred years, it should cease."

Dr. Norris, whose work has renewed the debate on the matter, does not favour a ban. Unlike many of his colleagues, Norris wants to study the procedures to establish what particular manipulation is causing the dissections. "How can we understand it if we don't study it?" he asks. For Katz, the situation is clear. The longer chiropractors continue to adjust necks, the more people will be injured unnecessarily, he says. The National Council Against Health Fraud (NCAHF), in their review of chiropractic neck manipulation, states that when a therapy has no important medical benefit, then any risk of serious complication, such as stroke, paralysis, or death, no matter how small, is unacceptable.

The Case of Kim Barton

That's certainly how Kim Barton feels. Today, watching Barton talk to you in the living room of her Grimsby, Ontario home, you wouldn't suspect she was the victim of a stroke. She's an animated, intelligent forty-year-old woman with a quick wit and great comic delivery. But in her brain, she says, it's a different story. Barton used to be a parole officer and was on a variety of volunteer committees. She was taking part-time courses at McMaster University in Hamilton and mothering two young children. "I could juggle 50 balls at once," she explains. "Now I have trouble tossing three."

Barton's life changed in early October 1996. She had just given birth to her second daughter. One night she woke up with a pounding headache. Years earlier she had gone to a chiropractor for treatment after an inmate struck her. "I was a believer," she says. The chiropractor had helped her, so, with a throbbing headache, she went to visit him again in Stoney Creek. The treatment helped only marginally. She returned to the chiropractor for four more treatments.

On October 4, she was given a neck manipulation. The chiropractor twisted her neck sharply left then right. "I got to the waiting room and I felt so dizzy," she said. As she was paying for the treatment, she suddenly felt weak and disoriented. She struggled across the street to a variety store and bought an orange juice. "The guy behind the counter must have thought I'd been drinking at nine in the morning," she recalls. "I couldn't keep my balance and I was having trouble keeping my thoughts straight."

She drove home with a hand over one eye so she didn't see two of everything. "I crawled into the house and called for my husband who was upstairs with the kids," she says. By 4:00 P.M., Barton had a severe ringing in her ears and the vertigo was worse than ever. Her neurologist told her later that the vertigo and tinnitus were symptoms of a stroke caused by the dissection of her vertebral artery.

Despite her problems, five days later Barton went to another chiropractor. She lay face down on the new chiropractor's table and let her crack her neck in both directions. Her face and left arm went numb.

"Right away, I couldn't talk," Barton recalls. "I thought she had broken my neck. I was thinking, 'You don't know what you've done,' but I couldn't say a thing. But, I could feel the fear in that woman's hands. Everything sort of disconnected."

She was rushed to the West Lincoln Memorial hospital. She was told she'd had a brain stem stroke, her second in less than a week. She suffered extreme vertigo and her headache and partial paralysis persisted. An angiogram revealed that both vertebral arteries had been dissected. Her family and her best friend, who flew in from out west, gathered at her bed. "I'd never seen my mother ashen in my life," Barton said. "I thought, 'You think I'm going to die.'" Her girlfriend fed her breakfast, one bran flake at a time, because Barton couldn't swallow well. Barton says she fought to recover for the sake of her children. "I couldn't leave them," she recalls.

Nine days later she was discharged from hospital, and slowly, after months of work, she got most of her motor skills back. She and her husband sued the Grimsby chiropractor. One day, after a grueling eight-hour negotiation session, they agreed to a settlement that was much less than they had hoped to receive.

"As I was getting into the van afterwards," recalls Barton, "I said 'We've just made a deal with the devil.' I felt they had raped my character."

The Canadian Chiropractic Protective Association did not admit liability, and they did not apologize, explained Barton. As well, a condition of the settlement is that she not name the chiropractor in question.

Today, she says, her brain is still damaged as a result of the stroke. She says she has mood swings. "I can't control my anger," she states. During the interview tears well up and disappear frequently. "I still drool a bit on one side," Barton explains, touching the left side of her mouth. She tires easily, can't focus her attention, and is distracted by too many things happening at once.

"My husband says it's like he's been remarried," Barton explains. "The old Kim is gone....My children will never know the mother I was; they have a new one now."

Most of Barton's brain functions have come back. In December 2001, after two false starts, she returned to work. She looks fine, but she'll tell you that she still experiences intense fatigue, can only focus on one task at a time, struggles for words, and occasionally falls or drops objects. "Although the physical disabilities are masked, the injury to my brain is glaring to myself and my family," she says. Today, Barton continues to write about her experience and to speak out. She authored a first-person account of the incident for *Chatelaine* magazine and recently sent a letter to the chief coroner of Ontario. It read in part: "I think that it's about time these 'doctors' are held accountable for what they do in their 'practices,' ...Since my injury, I have never been so appalled by a bunch of 'professionals.' People are dying. This is not about money; this is not about politics; this is about a mother having to watch her daughter die on a chiropractor's table (Laurie Mathiason) ... and this is about me — and all the others out there who have been recklessly injured by these self-proclaimed 'doctors.'"[49]

Politics and Public Relations

In one respect, Kim Barton is wrong. For chiropractors, the issue of neck manipulation is all about politics. They see the journal articles, the public statements, and the media coverage on neck manipulation and stroke as a campaign against chiropractic, just another part of an ongoing attack on their profession. Some of their complaints are valid. A study by an Australian chiropractor found that in dozens of studies on injuries caused by cervical spinal manipulation, the authors — mostly medical doctors — incorrectly identified the practitioners as chiropractors when they were not.[50]

Nevertheless, chiropractors administer more than 90 percent of manipulations in North America; more importantly, only chiropractors routinely manipulate the neck, and it is only chiropractors who use the high-velocity, low-amplitude manipulation most often connected to arterial dissection. Despite these facts and the clear evidence that the safety of neck manipulation is in question, chiropractors have responded to the information not as science-based practitioners who need to re-evaluate the risks and benefit of a particular therapy, but rather as a group whose beliefs have been challenged by outsiders. The World Chiropractic Alliance in the United States called the stroke reports "media and medical attacks" and characterized them as "an attempt to discredit chiropractic" and a "deliberate and unethical scare tactic."[51]

Chiropractors have always emphasized how safe their treatments are for patients. Their brochures, books, commercials, and Web sites all portray chiropractic as the safe alternative to medicine's drugs and surgery. And, for the most part, the safety of most spinal manipulation is well documented, particularly for low-back pain.[52] So when the safety of neck manipulation was raised again in the 1990s, the chiropractic leadership stuck to their guns, maintaining that, as far as they knew, their procedures were safe and effective. Dr. Greg Dunn, the chief operating officer for the Canadian Chiropractic Protective Association, says that studies have also shown that in only one or two cases per million chiropractic adjustments is there a coincidence in time between the manipulation and a stroke. And Dunn, along with many other chiropractors, says he hasn't seen definitive evidence that the neck manipulation *causes* the arterial dissection. Dunn says he has two daughters and both receive neck adjustments with his blessing. "The research done to date is very inconclusive about how serious the risk is," he says.

As usual, what chiropractors were saying to the public and what they were saying to each other were two very different things. A confidential International Chiropractic Association (ICA) "Malpractice Alert" demonstrates clearly that the chiropractic community has been aware of the serious risks of neck manipulation for nearly twenty years and has ignored or suppressed that information.

The November 1981 alert, written by the ICA's general counsel, James Harrison, states:

> Evidence has now accumulated to the point that the chiropractic profession can no longer ignore the increasing incidents of strokes occurring concomitant with cervical manipulation. The reports of chiropractors, the settlements of patients, and the results of medical examinations and autopsies cumulatively compel serious consideration of the problem. Possible injury to the patient overshadows the cost element and demands that we take immediate and decisive action to curtail the number and severity of these incidents.

Dr. Charles DuVall is a third-generation American chiropractor and an expert witness on chiropractic in the United States. He was not aware of the 1981 alert until we brought it to his attention and was amazed by its content. "It is the quintessential smoking gun," he said, "that [shows] the political arms of the chiropractic profession knew of the hazards associated with cervical manipulation and the potential of injury and death to the population and suppressed it." In fact, after the Mathiason case and the negative media reports that surrounded it, the chiropractic leadership stressed the safety of their procedures to Canadians. In doing so, they sometimes stretched the truth. In one pamphlet, consumers were told:

> Your chiropractor will only include neck adjustments in your treatment if there is an objective clinical reason for treating your neck as part of our overall spinal care."[53]

In fact, the opposite is true. Chiropractors routinely do neck adjustments on patients who have complained about only low-back pain, and there is no credible evidence that adjusting the cervical vertebrae does anything for the lower back. As well, chiropractors have been aware for decades that neck manipulation, particularly upper neck manipulation, is a culprit in stroke cases. Chiropractor Allan Terrett warned that cervical manipulation with rotation was most likely to injure a patient,[54] and Canadian Memorial Chiropractic College instructor Brian Gleberzon recommended, in a student handbook, the use of "low amplitude techniques, and to always err on the side of caution…"[55] Terrett warned chiropractors that the evidence suggested that a specific type of neck adjustment was more commonly associated with arterial damage: "The vast majority of cases involve a particular type of SMT, the high velocity–low amplitude manipulation." Later in his book, he provides even more specific detail:

> The movement most likely to produce VA [vertebral artery] wall injury between C1-C-2 (with or without SMT) is rotation, which applies stretching, compression and torquing forces on the vessel wall resulting in either damage and/or vasospasm."[56]

While the chiropractic community debated among themselves the relative safety of their own widely used adjustments, patients were simply reassured that all was well. Anticipating the negative media attention it would get during the inquest in the death of Lana Dale Lewis, a forty-six-year-old Toronto woman who died of a stroke after receiving a chiropractic neck manipulation, the Ontario Chiropractic Association (OCA) planned to launch a marketing campaign aimed at women over thirty-five a few months after the inquest.

The ads were slated to appear in women's magazines, on television, and in newspapers in the late summer or fall of 2000. *(See "The Forgotten Death of Lana Dale Lewis")*

Critics like Dr. Katz, who in some cases were merely repeating what chiropractors such as Terrett were telling their colleagues, were accused of waging a campaign against chiropractic. And it wasn't just critics who came under fire.

The Ontario Chiropractic Association issued an information sheet titled "Are There Risks to Chiropractic Treatment," in which they accused the media of "greatly exaggerating" the risks of neck manipulation.

In the spring of 2002, as news from the Lewis inquest spread, the safety of the procedure again fell under media scrutiny. This time reporters didn't have to look far for a personal story to dramatize the issue. Avis Favro, the health reporter for CTV News, featured the stories of Diane Rodrigue and a more recent victim, Les Limage, in her special report on chiropractic neck manipulation.

Les Limage

At sixty-six years of age, Les Limage was a man who seemed to have it all. He ran a successful car dealership, where his wife of many years worked with him. He had a beautiful home in Waterloo, Ontario, six grown children, and thirteen grandchildren he could spoil. His health was good, except for the nagging pain he experienced from the hip replacement surgery he had had years before. In November 2001, he decided to visit a Waterloo chiropractor to see if he could get some relief from the pain in his hip. He had several sessions, which seemed to help. In late November, he went for what would be his final visit. Flo recalled that when Les came out to the car after his appointment, he told her the chiropractor had, without his permission, manipulated his neck. That evening, Limage got a headache that went on for a few days. On December 5, as he prepared to go back to the chiropractor's office, he began to show signs of a stroke. His wife drove him directly to the hospital, where it was confirmed that he was having a stroke. He suffered a second stroke while in hospital. Paralyzed from the neck down, Limage was placed on a respirator and put into intensive care. He had suffered a stroke brought on as a result of damage to his vertebral arteries. An MRI confirmed that Limage had suffered a dissection of his vertebral artery. In the following days, Limage fought for his life. Fed intravenously because he could not swallow, he eventually recovered some of his strength, and in March 2002, he was moved out of intensive care. Today, he spends most of his time bedridden in a small room at the Freeport Health Centre, with his wife Flo at his side. He can barely speak, pushing out short sentences in a barely audible whisper. He tires easily and rests most of the day. Flo describes Les today: "My husband suffered pneumonia, suffered kidney failure. He cannot speak. He has suffered paralysis and loss of sight. He cannot see clearly. He has lost his balance. He cannot walk."

The Limages have launched a lawsuit against the chiropractor who performed the neck manipulation, a suit being handled by the same lawyer,

Amani Oakley, who is representing the family of Lana Dale Lewis at the Coroner's Inquest.

His story, told powerfully in a segment of the show *W5*, was the kind of media exposure chiropractors dread. A few weeks later, in a Toronto press conference, a tearful Flo Limage pleaded with chiropractors to take steps to protect Canadians. "I just want to say for myself, my husband and my family that neck manipulation should be stopped. This should not be going on. The chiropractic association and the chiropractors are aware that the possibilities of stroke are there. They should be making the public aware."

Useless Screening Tests

During the show, and in interviews surrounding the Lewis case, the chiropractic leadership maintained that, while a very small number of people did suffer strokes following neck manipulation, the procedure was extremely safe. And chiropractors were doing everything they could to make it even safer, including tests to screen patients who might be at greater risk of a blood vessel accident. In the *W5* segment, an instructor at the Canadian Memorial Chiropractic College demonstrated on camera a screening test she uses to see if patients are sensitive to the rotation position used in neck manipulation. The test, and others like it, are useless, a fact chiropractic researchers have been telling the profession for years.

During the Mathiason inquest in Saskatoon in 1998, David Cassidy, a chiropractor and researcher, testified that there was no evidence that chiropractors could effectively screen patients before neck manipulation. Cassidy, who was involved in a study of the "extension-rotation test" commonly used by chiropractors to screen for neck manipulation, told the inquest that the test was useless. "We found the positive predictive value was zero. So, in other words, it has no predictive value."[57] The lawyer questioning Cassidy then asked an important question, "So, I guess then what you are taught in the Chiropractic College about the ability to use tests to screen as a protection for your prospective patients really means nothing, because you're telling us there's no effective screening?" Cassidy agreed, saying the literature has shown that the test simply does not work.

Terrett, in his book on complications after neck manipulation, says the "tests have little or no value." He calls the procedures "invalid" and says:

> It makes no sense to subject the patient to a "screening procedure" that is invalid and only gives the practitioner a false sense of security regarding the degree of risk for SMT [spinal manipulative therapy]. This can only lead to the conclusion that the tests should be

abandoned, for clinical and medico-legal purposes, and should not be used for non-clinical risk management reasons."[58]

In 1995, chiropractor Paul Carey, the president of the Canadian Chiropractic Protective Association, wrote, "there is no predictive value to ascertaining the risk of stroke by performing these tests on the patient prior to manipulation,"[59] but he continued to recommend them because they could benefit the chiropractor in the eventuality of a lawsuit.

Chiropractor Igor Steiman revealed the real purpose of the tests when he wrote: "To the best of my knowledge, these tests are only useful to lawyers, ever since they were imposed as a standard of practice upon those who manipulate cervical spines as a premature 'something is better than nothing' measure by panic-stricken insurers."[60]

In July 1999, David Chapman-Smith, the editor of *The Chiropractic Report*, told practitioners that "pre-manipulative tests of vertebral artery functions are invalid and unnecessary" and he strongly suggested that the best way for chiropractors to proceed was to always obtain informed patient consent — in writing.[61] So, why were chiropractic leaders telling Canadians, as late as spring 2002, that chiropractors were taking every precaution — including pre-testing — to safeguard patients? Were they trying to placate the public, to present a caring and concerned image, regardless of the facts?

Data Blindness and Denial

Perhaps most disturbing about safety and neck manipulation is the strong evidence presented by Terrett and others that chiropractors appear, in many cases, unwilling or unable to respond to clear signs that their patients are in trouble. In some cases, the chiropractors re-manipulated necks in the same session or performed manipulations days or weeks later on patients who displayed clear signs of arterial damage. Terrett presents fifteen chilling cases of chiropractors who continued to manipulate patients' necks even after they complained of severe pain, ordered the chiropractor to stop, or displayed symptoms of dizziness, headache, weakness, blurred vision, nausea, unsteadiness, or vertigo. That's what happened to Kim Barton, Diane Rodrique, and Laurie Mathiason.

In those cases and many others, the chiropractors seemed "data blind," unable to accept clear signs that their patient was in serious trouble. Many delayed proper emergency treatment, sent patients home, or waited hours before calling an ambulance.

Norris saw this time and again in his research. "When the patient starts getting dizzy and sick and is having a stroke, they give him a cold compress on his neck and tell him to lie back down for an hour. They [chiropractors] are not proper doctors you see. If they were, they would put that patient in an ambulance and send him off to hospital, but they don't do that. That's the problem," he said. Back in Edmonton, Dr. Stewart agrees. He maintains that the risk to patients is exacerbated because chiropractors are ill equipped to deal with the complications that can arise from their own treatment. "If you do not know how to look after an acute stroke, or an acute myalopathy, or an acute radiculopathy, get the hell out. You shouldn't be doing it. You have to know how to intubate a patient, you have to know how to start central lines, you have to know how to do advanced cardio life support. The chiropractors can't do anything like that," he said.

Many chiropractors seem to be operating in a paradigm that maintains they can do no harm and so, when confronted by evidence of harm, they cannot process it. "Chiropractors have been very poor at accepting that there is an inherent risk involved in providing care to patients," writes Greg Dunn, the CEO of the Canadian Chiropractic Protective Association. "Most chiropractors see their mode of treatment as being non-invasive and 'low-tech' care, therefore carrying little or no risk."[62] Perhaps, because chiropractors have been told so often that neck manipulation is safe and that vascular complications are a rarity, they are unable to accept evidence of damage even when they are staring straight at it. "Chiropractors will often tell me they just never expected it would happen to them," comments Dunn. What Dunn seems to be missing in his commentary seems obvious to most people — the stroke happens to the patient, not to the chiropractor.

Risk per Patient, Not per Chiropractor

When you look at chiropractic articles and commentaries on the risk associated with chiropractic neck manipulation, you notice an odd thing. In many of the articles, the authors talk about the risk *for* chiropractors, not the risk *to* patients.

Terrett notes in his book that the rate is "about one case per 1,000 practitioners per year" or "one case for each 25 practitioners who all practice for a 40-year period."[63] As well, critics say expressing the risk per manipulation is misleading because in real life, chiropractic patients seldom get one manipulation. And comparing the risk to risk for an angiogram or for neck surgery is absurd because people don't get neck surgery every week for a year.

Norris points out that looking at risk per manipulation is like looking at risk of lung cancer for each cigarette smoked. It doesn't make sense, because no one smokes one cigarette and no one, it seems, receives one neck manipulation. Most chiropractic patients have their necks repeatedly manipulated

— on average about ten times a year — so the more meaningful statistic is the risk of stroke per patient. That, according to Norris, is about one in one hundred thousand, ten times higher than the one in a million figure offered by the chiropractors. And it could be higher than that. No one is sure whether chiropractic neck manipulations have a cumulative negative effect, but they might, speculates Norris. "We don't know but we believe it may be cumulative. In some patients when they are operating on the artery to sew it back together again, they find scars of previous dissections. It is quite likely that when you manipulate someone you get little tears and little tears and finally the big tear. So it is probably a cumulative effect," said Norris.

But the real issue for both critics and patients is the question of benefit and risk, not of neck manipulation in general, but of the chiropractic neck adjustment. Chiropractors are fully aware that the manipulation that is most often associated with injury involves rotation of the neck, sometimes with extension, twisting, tilting, or stretching. It is usually a high-velocity, low-amplitude move, the typical chiropractic manipulation, which causes the well-known "crack" or "pop" associated with chiropractic adjustments. Stewart says his patients who have been injured all describe an extension with rotation. Experts, like Terrett, have expressed concern about this and suggested that chiropractors consider "avoiding those techniques that appear to carry the greatest risk." Nevertheless, chiropractors all over North America continue to twist and crack the necks of patients, many of whom have no complaint regarding the neck or head. Millions of these neck adjustments are delivered daily, despite the fact that there is no credible evidence that this particular manipulation — a brisk rotation and snapping of the neck — is of any therapeutic value at all. But the dangers are many.

"There is no question that the risks are extremely well documented — ranging from compression of the spinal cord, compression of the nerves as they exit your neck, tearing of muscles, breaking of bones, stroke and death. These are unequivocally established," said Stewart. "The benefits are dubious at best — some of the literature says maybe there's a little bit of benefit. But when you do a risk-benefit analysis there is no doubt. One cannot rationally proceed with upper cervical manipulation."

If chiropractors were seeking true informed consent, they would tell patients that there was no evidence that neck manipulation helped acute neck pain and only a few studies saying it *may* provide short-term relief of headache and chronic neck pain. Patients do report that neck manipulation provides some relief, but it is transitory, sometimes lasting only a few hours. Who would trade that weak promise of temporary relief against the risk of stroke, permanent brain damage, paralysis, or death? Perhaps the better question, though, is not about the patient but the practitioner. Faced with the evidence that a procedure offers little or no benefit to patients, but potentially catastrophic damage, why do chiropractors continue to adjust necks?

Money may be one reason. Chiropractors in North American make tens of millions of dollars a year manipulating necks. The vast majority also believe that it works. To give it up would mean a huge financial loss, and it would be a monumental philosophical setback, because many chiropractors adjust the neck for myriad problems, including ones that have nothing to do with the neck. As Dr. Stewart points out, "No one in the world thinks the body works that way except the chiropractic community. Because they have the label doctor in front of them everybody believes them. If you took away neck manipulation, you'd be taking away a big part of business from them." Chiropractors are worried that information that is negative about neck manipulation could have a large impact on their livelihoods. They may be right. According to a July 2000 Ontario Chiropractic Association newsletter, the association is concerned that the Lewis inquest will have a negative effect on the patient volume and income of Ontario chiropractors. Chiropractic officials testifying at the Lewis inquest told the jury that business had declined substantially since the beginning of the proceedings.

More Adjustments, More Strokes

On June 12, 2002, the family of Dr. Ronald Samuel Grainger held simultaneous press conferences in Toronto and Calgary to tell Canadians that their father had died of a stroke following neck manipulation.

In Toronto, Grainger's young son Mark, also an MD, sat at a desk flanked by the relatives of Lana Lewis and Les Limage. Mark told reporters his father had gone to a chiropractor for neck and back pain and after his last neck manipulation had experienced severe neck pain. Two days later he was re-manipulated by the chiropractor. The sixty-nine-year-old father of six then experienced headache, nausea, and was unsteady on his feet. He was taken to hospital, where doctors found blood at the base of his brain — a sub-arachnoid hemorrhage. Neurosurgeons operated, but Dr. Grainger died on November 16, 2001.

Though the precise cause of the stroke had not been verified by angiogram, Mark Grainger and his siblings felt there was substantial evidence that he had died as a direct result of upper cervical manipulation.

At first, the family decided to keep the death private, but a few months later Dr. Grainger was told about a twenty-one-year-old Alberta woman who had suffered a massive stroke after a chiropractic neck manipulation. He and his family then decided it was important to speak out. In a letter he read to reporters and a half-dozen representatives of the chiropractic community who stood at the back of the small room in Women's Hospital in Toronto, he called for an inquest into his father's death, a ban on chiropractors treating children, and a halt to funding for any chiropractic treatment of infants and children. He also called on the ministers of health in every province to order an immediate ban on all chiropractic upper neck manipulation. "We are not alone in our belief that there is substantial evidence that chiropractic upper neck manipulation constitutes a significant and not-uncommon risk to the Canadian public," he said, under the glare of TV camera lights.

Dr. Grainger called on government authorities to step in because chiropractors had refused to act. "The college of chiropractors appears to dismiss this risk and has ignored previous medical concerns," he said. He told the press conference that chiropractors should be forced to adopt standards of practice in line with current medical-scientific knowledge and then suggested that chiropractors follow the lead of the physiotherapy profession in Canada, which has banned the use of all extension-rotation upper neck manipulation.

Grainger then articulated what many doctors and scientists understood already, that chiropractors were not fully informing their patients of the scant evidence of benefit of cervical manipulation and its concomitant risk. He noted that the solid practical advice that came out of the Mathiason inquest had been all but ignored. Grainger told the reporters that not one of the provincial chiropractic regulatory bodies enforced the recommendation that information about the risks of upper neck manipulation be made available in the office of every chiropractor. "This death was a tragedy that need not happen again if the proper scientific and medical evidence of the risk of such procedures balanced against the perceived benefits, were communicated effectively to both the Canadian public as well as health ministers."

After the press conference, Stan Gorchynski, the chairman of the Ontario Chiropractic Association, who has acted as the main spokesperson for chiropractic during the Lewis inquest, stood in a throng of members of the national media. He calmly stuck to the party line. He told reporters the risk of stroke after neck manipulation was between one in six million and one in one million. He then repeated a blatant falsehood, one that chiropractors and their supporters have been reciting for years: "International peer review has placed chiropractic as the number one form of health care for low-back pain, neck pain, including upper cervical, and headaches. What more substantiation do we need from international peer review?"

Though chiropractors lack scientific evidence that neck manipulation is beneficial, their history, philosophy, and empirical evidence have convinced them of its efficacy. Even when the evidence indicates that belief is, at best, unsubstantiated and, at worst, utterly false, the chiropractic leadership presents the picture they want Canadians and the world to believe. Finally, though Gorchynski and others have said that the chiropractic profession is seeking the truth, the reality appears to be far different. All negative information, all external criticism — and most internal criticism — is viewed by chiropractors as an attack on their livelihood and their profession that must be repelled at all costs, even if it means harm to patients.

6

THE FORGOTTEN DEATH OF LANA DALE LEWIS

How an Inquest Reveals a Different Kind of Chiropractic Truth

On May 30, 2000, Dr. James Young, the chief coroner of Ontario, announced an inquest into the death of Lana Dale Lewis. Lewis was a forty-five-year-old Toronto woman who died in 1996, seventeen days after having her neck adjusted by a chiropractor. Her family suspected the neck adjustment caused the series of strokes that led to her death. In November 1999, they called for an inquest.

An inquest is a public inquiry into an unusual death. Its purpose is to determine the cause of death and to decide how to prevent similar deaths in the future. It's not a trial — there are no sides, no winners and losers. Everyone involved is called together for one purpose — to figure out what happened. The six-member jury's job is to decide what they believe killed the victim and to come up with a list of recommendations they hope will prevent other similar deaths. All parties at an inquest are supposed to be working to protect the public. The credo of the Coroner's Office is "We speak for the dead to protect the living."

The inquest process is built on the expectation that all those involved will cooperate in order to find the truth. That's why the Lewis family (Lana had twelve brothers and sisters) called for the inquest in the first place. And because her son, Adam Lewis, a teenager at the time of her death, needed to know what killed his mother.

We reported on the Lana Dale Lewis story from its beginning and have followed every development in its tangled route to and through the inquest, which officially started late in 2001 but began in earnest in the spring of 2002. In some ways, the outcome of the inquest process is not as important as what it has revealed about the behaviour of the chiropractic profession.

From the moment chiropractic officials were first informed of Lana Dale Lewis's death, they went on the defensive. Internal chiropractic documents reveal they quickly rallied the troops, considering the inquest to be a trial of the profession rather than an inquiry and viewing the death as a threat that needed to be managed in the media. They even planned a marketing campaign deliberately aimed at women just like Lana Dale Lewis. The campaign was to follow the conclusion of the inquest. To the chiropractors, the inquest into Lana Dale Lewis's death was a battle, and a very public one at that.

Greg Dunn, the chief operating officer of the Canadian Chiropractic Protective Association (CCPA), announced the battle plan in the June 2000 issue of *Canadian Chiropractor* magazine:

> CCPA as well as OCA [Ontario Chiropractic Association], CMCC [Canadian Memorial Chiropractic College] and CCA [Canadian Chiropractic Association] will be prepared to meet all the media challenges surrounding this issue ... CCPA will be defending the rights of the practitioner involved with top legal representation. Legal counsel at the inquest will also protect the interests of the profession. We intend to bring forward all of the top experts to testify on our behalf. This will be a costly and time-consuming exercise but we are prepared. ... As chiropractic organizations we have banned [sic] together and formed a "Chiropractic Defense Alliance". We are combining our resources both human and financial to meet this challenge. We are also receiving help from outside experts to guide us through these difficult times. We can't do this alone though. We must have you join us in this defence.[1]

Nowhere in Dunn's guest editorial does he mention the responsibility of the chiropractic profession to help the inquest determine the truth, to help the Lewis family learn how Lana Dale died, or to ensure the future safety of the Canadian public.

That chiropractic defensiveness began a few months after the death of Lana Dale Lewis, when members of Canada's chiropractic leadership were first informed of her death. On December 5, 1996, chiropractors Jean Moss, Paul Carey, and Jaroslaw Grod attended a meeting at the Coroners Building in Toronto. Moss was the president of the Canadian Memorial Chiropractic

College, Carey was the president of the Canadian Chiropractic Protective Association, and Grod was the deputy registrar of the College of Chiropractors of Ontario, the profession's regulatory body. Dr. Robert Huxter, the Regional Coroner for Metropolitan Toronto, reviewed the Lewis file and called the meeting. Dr. Murray Naiberg, the investigating coroner on the Lewis death, also attended. As investigating coroner, the final decision to call an inquest rested with him. Dr. John Deck, who would do a detailed neuropathological examination of Lewis's body, also came to the meeting. The coroners, who believed it was extremely likely that a chiropractic neck adjustment had caused Lewis's death, called the meeting in hopes of avoiding a costly and time-consuming inquest. As Dr. Naiberg said in an affidavit to the inquest, "It was not an unusual step to take if it was felt that the coroner's office could effectively achieve the same goal by negotiation as would have been achieved by way of a formal coroner's inquest."[2] The Lewis family says they were not informed of the meeting.

At the meeting, according to a letter written by Naiberg, all three doctors agreed that the most probable cause of Lewis's death was the chiropractic neck manipulation. According to Naiberg, the three chiropractors had some reservations at first about the opinion because of the length of time between the manipulation and the stroke. Deck remembers it the same way: "It is my clear recollection that the chiropractors claimed that the six-day delay between the last chiropractic manipulation and the onset of neurological symptoms of stroke cast doubt on the causal connection between the manipulation and the stroke." But, Deck noted, "such a delay is common and almost characteristic of the clinical course following traumatic injury of the vertebral artery in the neck ... there is no significant doubt in my mind that the manipulation was the cause of the fatal stroke."[3]

Deck made this preliminary finding based on the evidence he had at that point. Later, he would complete a neuropathological examination that would confirm his evaluation.

The way Naiberg recalls it, in the course of the discussion, the chiropractors eventually agreed with the three physicians. Naiberg said, "Based on our conclusions that the death of Lana Dale Lewis was likely related to chiropractic neck manipulation, they agreed to inform their members of the possible risk involved with high-level chiropractic manipulation and further they would post some form of notice to the public in chiropractors' offices for the benefit of patients. On that promise, I did not order an inquest. As it happened the chiropractic representatives did not comply with their agreement."

Naiberg is clear about the meeting and clear about the arrangement that was made with the chiropractors. "Had these officials denied the danger or refused any action on their part, or could we have known they would not honour this commitment, we most certainly would have considered proceeding to an inquest in this matter."[4]

The chiropractors in the room have a very different recollection of the meeting. They would later say that they did not accept that Lana Dale Lewis died as a result of chiropractic neck manipulation and they certainly did not assure the coroners that they would inform their membership of the case and the risks of upper neck manipulation.

If you accept the chiropractors' recollection of the meeting, you have to believe that Dr. Naiberg made the decision not to call an inquest despite the chiropractors' doing nothing, and that he did so in the face of the fact that the meeting was held in the first place to get the chiropractors' cooperation in lieu of an inquest.

The chiropractors made one more point. They said they never got a copy of the final coroner's report on Lana Dale Lewis and so didn't know conclusively what the cause of death was. "We made the assumption that there was no connection because we never got a response," Moss explained to us in a 1999 interview. "We had not been given any information that linked the two [the death and the chiropractic manipulation] together." The reason the chiropractors never got the report is that, by law, they're not entitled to one, since they're not family members.

Less than two years later, a twenty-year-old Saskatoon woman named Laurie Mathiason died after a chiropractic neck manipulation. During the 1998 inquest into her death, the chiropractic profession seemed to have forgotten all about Lana Dale Lewis. Chiropractic officials would say in Canadian media that the Mathiason death was the first case of its kind in Canada. In fact, they said it over and over again:

- A Canadian Chiropractic Association news release on October 6, 1998, quotes the association's president, David Peterson, as saying, "Although [the Mathiason death] was the first such event associated with chiropractic care in Canada."
- *The Chiropractic Report*, a publication edited by David Chapman-Smith, in March 1999, said, "In 1998 a patient died following chiropractic treatment in Canada. This event, a first in the history of the Canadian profession..."
- An Ontario Chiropractic Association letter sent out to family physicians in February 1999 calls the death of Laurie Jean Mathiason "the first such incident in the history of chiropractic practice in Canada."
- The newspaper *Dynamic Chiropractic*, in its November 2, 1998 issue states, "This was the first time in the 103-year history of

chiropractic in Canada that a patient had died after a chiropractic adjustment."
- A letter to patients on November 1, 1998, from a Saskatoon chiropractic office told readers, "This case represents the first time an incident such as this has ever happened in Canada."

Even two of the chiropractors who were in the 1996 meeting with the coroners about the Lana Dale Lewis death told journalists they knew of no similar incidents in Canada.

- In September 1998, Paul Carey appeared on the television station CFQC in Saskatoon and told reporter Robert MacDonald, "There's no other recorded death associated with chiropractic in Canada."
- On an episode of *This Morning* on CBC Radio that aired on December 7, 1998, Jean Moss, the president of the Canadian Memorial Chiropractic College, told host Michael Enright, "This was as far as we are aware, the first death in Canada."
- On an episode of *As It Happens* on CBC Radio that aired on September 13, 1998, Paul Carey says, "It's the first time there's been a death associated with chiropractic … in Canada."

So, ironically, rather than informing the Canadian public about the Lewis incident, the profession as a whole circled the wagons, denying any knowledge of a previous case. Rather than warn the public about the dangers of chiropractic neck manipulation, they took the opportunity to assure Canadians of its safety. Carey, as a senior official with the Canadian Chiropractic Protective Association, had not only written about chiropractic neck manipulation strokes as early as 1988[5] but would also have been aware of the cases of Diane Rodrigue and Kim Barton, two women who suffered strokes as a result of neck manipulation by chiropractors. *(See "Neck Manipulation and Stroke")* He didn't mention them.

Denials Lead to Family's Call for Inquest

The news of Laurie Mathiason's death and the chiropractic denials that followed infuriated the family of Lana Dale Lewis and prompted them to call for an inquest into Lewis's 1996 death.

They were aided by Dr. Murray Katz, a Montreal physician and a vocal critic of chiropractic. Dr. Katz helped them prepare their petition and their press conference. For decades, Dr. Katz, who specializes in treating children, has been an informed and persistent thorn in the side of organized chiropractic. He has taken chiropractic courses, attended seminars, and written about his experiences. Although originally concerned about pediatric chiropractic, Dr. Katz has more recently focused his energy on the dangers of chiropractic neck manipulation. He was a witness at the inquest into Laurie Mathiason's death, and he actively seeks out people who may have been harmed by a chiropractor.

He was vilified in the September 2001 issue of *The Chiropractic Report*,[6] which called him a "long-discredited medical critic," and he is viewed by chiropractors and their supporters as an aggressive opponent of the profession — a zealot waging a relentless battle. In reality, Dr. Katz is a tall, grey-haired, gregarious physician who frequently talks about his family, his practice in Montreal, and his love of golf. An early experience with a hydrocephalic child being treated by a chiropractor prompted the then-young Katz to investigate what to him was the unknown world of chiropractic. What he found changed his life. Intelligent, well-read, and with a near-photographic memory, Katz quickly became the most informed physician in Canada about the history, theory, and practice of chiropractic. And unlike most other doctors, Katz did not hesitate to speak out.

He has written about chiropractic, lectured widely to medical students and doctors, and prepared briefs for federal and provincial government officials. He has also traveled across Canada identifying and helping chiropractic victims and their families. He does all this for free, often devoting hundreds of hours to the cause that has become an important part of his life. That energy and focus has made Murray Katz chiropractic's worst nightmare. He is so reviled that the editors of the *Journal of the Canadian Chiropractic Association* allowed this insult to stand in an otherwise scholarly paper published in 2002: "...all the way from lowly life forms like amoebas, viruses and Murray Katz to the more complex organisms we call humans."[7]

Early in November 1999 at Toronto's Inn on the Park Hotel, in a brightly lit conference room, Dr. Katz sat in the audience while nineteen-year-old Adam Lewis stood nervously behind a microphone facing a group of reporters. He was there, along with his uncle Michael Ford, to announce that the Lewis family was launching a $12-million lawsuit against the chiropractor they say manipulated his mother's neck. The suit would also include Jean Moss, Paul Carey, and Jaroslaw Grod, along with the chiropractic establishments they each represent.

In their statement of claim, the Lewis family maintained that after their 1996 meeting with the three coroners, chiropractors Moss, Carey, and Grod ignored "their professional and civic responsibilities to widely disseminate the facts and findings surrounding the death of our beloved family member Lana Dale Lewis so as to ensure the safety of the Canadian public." The family also claimed "they reneged on the express commitment which they made during that meeting to do so." The Lewis family included the Canadian Memorial Chiropractic College itself in the lawsuit for teaching what the family's statement of claim calls "unsafe and inappropriate procedures that are dangerous and life threatening to the general public."

But their suit against the chiropractic organizations was soon rejected. In early April 2000, Ontario Superior Court Justice John Carvarzan ruled they could not take legal action against the CMCC, the College of Chiropractors of Ontario, or the Canadian Chiropractic Protective Association. The family was also prevented from suing the heads of those organizations.

In his ruling, Carvarzan stated there was "no reasonable cause of action" against the organizations. As well, the judge noted, "The plaintiff's conspiracy claim is wholly inadequate." He awarded costs to the defendants, ordering Adam to pay six thousand dollars in court costs. However, the family's entire suit was not thrown out. They were free to proceed with their action against Philip Emanuele, the chiropractor who they say performed the controversial neck manipulation on Lana Dale.

The Inquest Flip-Flop

Chief Coroner Dr. James Young assigned Dr. William Lucas to explore the possibility of an inquest into Lana Dale Lewis's death. In late January 2000, Dr. Lucas determined an inquest would not be necessary.

Lucas told us in a 2000 interview that during his deliberations he had met with the three chiropractors who had attended the 1996 meeting with the coroners. They told him, "so far as they were concerned, there was no definitive resolution in terms of the cause of death. They also have no recollection of any undertaking on their part that they would notify their profession of this particular case and the inherent risks of the procedure."

In the interview with us, Dr. Lucas could not explain the radically different views of the same December 5, 1996 meeting. He said there were no minutes taken of the meeting. "The chiropractors have one position and there is some documentation that adds some credence to their point of view," he said.

"Although I am not trying to undermine the position of my colleagues in the office of the chief coroner, I'm trying to look at this impartially and fairly. Other than [the doctors'] recollection three years after the event, there is nothing to support their position." Dr. Lucas did not speak with Drs. Huxter, Deck, or Naiberg about the 1996 meeting prior to determining that no inquest should be held. Both Dr. Deck and Dr. Naiberg wrote letters in 1999 in which they recall details of the meeting.

Dr. Lucas made it clear that his decision not to call an inquest did not call into question the earlier conclusions about what killed Lana Dale Lewis. Lucas believed that no one in the room contested the cause of death. Dr. Lucas said chiropractic leaders told him they were taking steps to inform their membership and the public about the risks of chiropractic neck manipulation. "If we feel that the substantial issues are being addressed already, we feel those are valid and legitimate reasons for not holding a full and open public inquiry," he explained.

Once again, the Coroner's Office took the chiropractor's statements at face value. And, once again, it would be confronted with that error in judgment. The day after Dr. Lucas announced there would be no inquest, the Lewis family appealed the decision. Five months later, they got what they wanted.

On May 30, 2000, Dr. James Young dramatically reversed himself. There would be an inquest into the death of Lana Dale Lewis after all. The inquest was to focus on "the association between high cervical manipulation and stroke," according to the Coroner's Office.

The main reason for the stunning flip-flop? Misleading information was published by chiropractors across Canada. In the months after Dr. Lucas's decision not to call an inquest, chiropractors had claimed in the media that Lana Dale Lewis did not die of a chiropractic neck manipulation, had misrepresented statements from the coroner's office, and had extolled the safety of chiropractic neck manipulations. In short, they did the opposite of what Dr. Lucas was convinced they would do.

In their appeal to Dr. Young, the Lewis family brought the following items to his attention:

- In February 2000, Dr. J. Ronald Carter, a member of the Calgary Chiropractic Society, stated in the *Calgary Herald*, "The case of Lana Dale Lewis is simply not true. The coroner's decision was that an inquest into this death would not be necessary."[8]
- On March 20, 2000, thirteen Burlington, Ontario-area chiropractors ran an advertisement in the *Burlington Post*. The ad stated, "In recent weeks, there have been media reports suggesting that chiropractic treatment may not be safe. There are some risks associated with chiropractic care as with all healthcare treatments, however the media reports have, we believe, exaggerated these risks ... the coroner has reviewed all relevant information and has decided not to call an inquest into [the Lana Dale Lewis] death."[9]
- On April 10, 2000, Roland Bryans, the president of the Canadian Chiropractic Association, wrote in a letter to the *Montreal Gazette*, "the tragic death of Laurie Mathiason was,

indeed, the first known case of its kind in Canada. Your article implies that the [chiropractic] profession had prior knowledge of another [chiropractic related] death. This is simply not true. Correspondence from the Office of the Coroner in the province of Ontario states that the profession had no such knowledge."[10]

During a May 2000 interview with us, Dr. Young made it clear that the media reports were a central reason for the inquest. "There was some debate in some areas in the press that weren't necessarily representative of the facts, as I knew them. And I thought that on the basis of all of it, the best way to handle this particular case was to have an inquest," he said.

Even chiropractic officials admitted, to their own membership, that the ads and press statements sparked the inquest. In the June issue of *Canadian Chiropractor* magazine, chiropractor Greg Dunn, the CCO of the Canadian Chiropractic Protective Association, wrote that:

> ...some well meaning chiropractors placed a large ad in a local newspaper to set the record straight about cervical adjustments. What they didn't bargain on was the same newspaper giving Mrs. Mathiason a whole page to respond and raise unfounded safety issues about chiropractic treatment. Not only that, it created an environment in which the Chief Coroner for Ontario reviewed the need for an inquest into the death of Lana Dale Lewis. The misinformation contained in this ad was a key factor in deciding to hold an inquest.[11]

In fact, had the chiropractic profession actually been in control of its membership and been informing its membership as it had assured Dr. Lucas it would, the inquest would never have been called. The chiropractors had no one to blame but themselves.

And despite Dr. Lucas's belief that no one was contesting the cause of death, it's clear chiropractors across Canada were doing exactly that — as a remarkable plan for an ad campaign was about to demonstrate.

Hide Your Brochures, Attract Older Women

As 2001 began, it was expected that the start of the Lana Dale Lewis inquest was imminent. In fact, it would be another year before it got underway. But in January 2001, a stunning item appeared in the Ontario Chiropractic Association newsletter. The item announced an upcoming marketing campaign for chiropractic.

The campaign, developed by Toronto-based Manifest Communications, was planned to target blue- and white-collar female workers over thirty-five who didn't currently use chiropractors but did use other remedies for back pain and muscle aches. It was intended to focus on professional women over thirty-five who had visited a chiropractor before but hadn't seen one lately.

In short, the campaign was aimed at women much like Lana Dale Lewis. It was being developed prior to the inquest into Lana Dale's death. But the OCA newsletter item makes it clear chiropractic officials planned to launch the campaign "in late April, allowing sufficient time to pass following the inquest."[12] The cynical campaign was being planned by the same group that had promised Dr. Lucas it was informing its membership of the dangers of neck manipulation.

The ads were slated to appear in women's magazines, on television, and in newspapers. The campaign was intended to create a strong chiropractic "brand" in Canada and to "present chiropractic to the public in a fresh, exciting and timeless manner," according to an OCA publication.

When we broke the story on canoe.ca about the planned campaign, OCA executives declined to be interviewed. However, we did get a fax from Marlene Paulin, the acting executive director of the OCA, stating that its new communications materials were "currently in development" and will be available at "a date yet to be determined."

But the ad campaign wasn't the only public relations action the inquest sparked. The OCA was also concerned that the inquest, which was now stumbling from delay to delay, would have a negative effect on the patient volume and income of Ontario chiropractors. According to the association, the September 1998 inquest into the chiropractic death of Laurie Jean Mathiason of Saskatchewan resulted in a 38 percent decrease in chiropractic income and patients in the year following the event. The OCA didn't want to see a repeat of those dismal numbers in Ontario after the Lana Dale Lewis inquest.

In an October 2000 OCA newsletter, the association told its members that during the inquest, members should tuck away promotion that makes outlandish claims in case reporters should come calling. The issue for the OCA wasn't whether its membership was offering services outside of its scope of practice. It just didn't want them to get caught at it. Even before it began, the inquest was seen as a public relations battle that had to be won based on appearances.

The "Plain Brown Envelope"

It took two years for the inquest Dr. James Young announced in May 2000 to get underway. But in the months leading up to the official inquest start, the Lewis family, its legal counsel, Dr. Murray Katz, and a phalanx of chiropractic lawyers faced off in a series of confrontational pre-inquest hearings. Dr. Katz was acting as a medical advisor and, eventually, legal agent for the family. The Lewis family found itself taxed by the expenses the often-delayed inquest was demanding.

The chiropractic profession, on the other hand, was represented by a half dozen advocates. They included high-profile trial lawyer Tim Danson, who represented the CMCC and the Canadian Chiropractic Association, and Chris Paliare, who spoke for the College of Chiropractors of Ontario. The pre-inquest hearings were presided over by coroner Dr. Barry McLellan, assisted by coroner's counsel Tom Schneider.

The presence of Dr. Katz at the pre-inquest hearings was a constant source of friction for the chiropractic officials and their counsel. That rancour only increased in February 2001, when Katz took on the role of legal agent for the Lewis family after they parted company with their legal counsel. The family was struggling, trying to find someone to represent them at the inquest. Katz agreed to act for the family at no cost. Agents can represent parties in legal proceedings and inquests despite having no legal training.

But in April 2001, Katz's role came to an abrupt end. Tim Danson presented the court with the contents of what he called a "plain brown envelope." Danson would not say how the "plain brown envelope" came into his possession. He told the court it contained dozens of private e-mails, faxes, and letters from Dr. Katz to a variety of friends and colleagues. One of those friends was Dr. Murray Naiberg, who had been the lead investigator for the coroner's office on the Lana Dale Lewis case back in 1996.

It was that private letter to Dr. Naiberg from Dr. Katz that caused presiding coroner Dr. McLellan to make the unprecedented ruling that Katz should be removed as the legal agent for the Lewis family. It was the first time in Canada that a legal agent had been removed from an inquest.

Katz sent the letter to Naiberg on January 30, 2000. That was just a few days after Dr. Lucas had decided not to hold an inquest into Lana Dale Lewis's death. In the letter, Katz urges Naiberg, who was near retirement, to press for that inquest and raises concerns about Naiberg's role in what was becoming an increasingly embarrassing and divisive process. "I want to help you and give you the best advice on how to extricate yourself from this mess," Katz wrote to Naiberg. "The reputation of the coroner's office is at stake. Do not end your career waiting for the next death to happen. The family WILL drag you into court," he added.

In reference to the autopsy and pathology report Naiberg did on Lewis, Katz wrote, "You acted as their physician in the making of a diagnosis as to the cause of death. You did not properly collaborate with them ... The family is now considering an official complaint with the Ontario College of

Physicians. You will have to extricate yourself from that. It is not a way to end a career."

In reference to the 1996 meeting between the coroners and the chiropractors, Katz wrote, "The family has sued all the chiropractors who attended the meeting on Dec 5, 1996. They could easily have sued you, in particular, as you were the main person involved. They saw you involved in a cover-up then and they see you involved in another one now."

In his ruling, McLellan called Katz's letter "threatening." He said, "Dr. Katz demonstrated poor judgement in sending the letter" to a public official.

Danson called Katz a "zealot" for his ongoing campaign against chiropractic and the proposed affiliation of York University and the CMCC. "Dr. Katz has demonstrated he cannot act professionally," Danson told the court.

Katz, who was shaken by the dismissal, said he sent the letter to Naiberg as "a friend to a friend," thirteen months before he became the agent for the family. "I was pouring my heart out to him," Katz said. As he left the court-room after his dismissal, he turned to a chiropractic lawyer and said quietly, "The phoenix will rise again."

After the hearing, Danson said the Lewis family had been manipulated by Dr. Katz and did not get proper legal advice. "I believe that anybody viewing that letter objectively would conclude that [the] letter is blackmail, it is threatening. It is egregious, it is scandalous, and in my 21 years of practice I have never seen this. I think the ruling speaks for itself ... the court has expressed its outrage and indignation."

But Dr. Naiberg himself couldn't agree less with Danson's opinion of Katz's letter. In an affidavit he submitted to the inquest, he recalls a friendly dinner in his Toronto home with Katz, during which the topic of the inquest came up. A couple of days later, he received the letter from Katz. Naiberg's affidavit says:

> I took absolutely no offence to [Katz's] comments although I cer-
> tainly appreciated their force and purpose. I had already deliberated
> all of his points in my own mind and concluded that I should make
> a further attempt to convince the Coroner's Office to [call an
> inquest]. Dr. Katz's letter of January 30, 2000, as referred to in the
> motion by Danson Recht & Freeman [Danson's law firm] seems
> to be used by them to suggest that I was in some fashion being
> intimidated or forced to bring about a new inquest. This cannot be
> further from the truth. Dr. Katz's comments are simply a dose of
> reality of which I was quite aware at the time.
>
> At the time of my dinner with Dr. Katz and his letter of January

30, 2000 I was close to mandatory retirement and it was of personal and professional concern to me that positive action should be taken given the failure of Chiropractor representatives to live up to the commitments made to me and the Coroner's Office in 1996. It was also of grave concern to me that the Coroner's Office do what is right. ... I have nothing but the highest regard for the Lewis family's interest and Dr. Katz's perseverance in the face of unwarranted insult to get to the bottom of a serious medical risk.

It is my opinion that Dr. Katz is a man of high integrity and considerable medical knowledge in this area and that the criticisms alleged against Dr. Katz have nothing whatsoever to do with the circumstances surrounding the death of Lana Dale Lewis and are solely designed to obstruct the course of justice and to prevent getting to the truth of the matter.[13]

In another affidavit, Michael Ford, Lana Dale Lewis's brother-in-law and the Lewis family spokesman, also stands strongly behind Dr. Katz:

We have the utmost confidence in Dr. Katz's integrity and knowledge of the matters that will be at issue. ... I verily believe that a summary decision to remove Dr. Katz at this preliminary stage is both unwarranted and prejudicial and will irreparably harm my family's ability to make a meaningful contribution to this proceeding.[14]

But the most blistering rebuttal to the removal of Katz came again from Dr. Naiberg in a letter to the College of Physicians and Surgeons after the chiropractic associations launched a complaint about Dr. Katz for unprofessional behaviour.

... the characterization of Dr. Katz's letter to me as coming "perilously close to blackmail" is egregious misrepresentation. They do not know the context or intent in which the comments were made, nor was an effort made to determine this by contacting me ... it has become obvious that the Canadian Chiropractic Association will countenance no scientific questioning of their methods. Any such is de facto considered heretical and scandalous.

As they are apparently concerned about any scientific debate, their tactic is to denigrate, insult, vilify, intimidate and threaten any and all who would bring evidence or raise concerns about their rationale or practice. Failing rational defence of their position, they resort to character assassination, the classical argumentum ad hominum [personal attack]. It is obvious they fear any breath of reason will blow away their house of cards.[15]

The removal of Dr. Katz as their agent left the Lewis family with no legal counsel and left the inquest in limbo. It was delayed again, this time until the fall of 2001, so the family could try to find a new lawyer. When it started again, another delay, caused by a faulty report and a block of missing evidence, would postpone the stuttering embarrassment of an inquest yet again.

The Case of the Missing Tissue

On October 10, 2001, the first official day of the Lana Dale Lewis inquest, in the lobby and on the wide sidewalk in front of the Grosvenor Street coroner's building in downtown Toronto, the banter was crackling with tension. Something strange had gone wrong. Something big was coming down. Police were involved. No one could say much. Everybody knew it. As soon as the inquest was called to order, coroner's counsel Tom Schneider dropped the bombshell.

Tissue samples from Lewis's neck had gone missing from the coroner's office. Schneider launched an immediate investigation, but it would be weeks until the samples were recovered.

The wayward samples were key slices of Lewis's vertebral artery, which the family believed was damaged when her neck was adjusted by a chiropractor. The chiropractic legal team, however, planned to argue that Lewis died of natural causes as a result of her weight, drinking, smoking, and medication. Evidence for either argument might be locked inside tissue that had now mysteriously vanished.

What, exactly, the paper-thin slices of Lewis's arteries told pathologists had already become a major source of conflict in the inquest. The missing tissue was just the latest gaffe in a series of bad fumbles and conflicts surrounding medical evidence.

The tissue problems for the coroner's office actually began in 1997. That's when coroner Dr. John Deck and his medical student protégé, Michael Pollanen, did a neuropathology report on Lana Dale Lewis. It was Pollanen who, despite his inexperience, actually cut and analyzed the samples from which the report's conclusions were drawn. Pollanen had also removed some important samples but had neglected to examine them. However, in the report completed by Pollanen but signed by both men, Deck and Pollanen said they had found no evidence of "microscopic or gross dissection" in the left vertebral artery of Ms Lewis's neck. A dissection is a tearing and bulging of an artery's inner wall. They did conclude, however, that it was extremely likely that Lewis's death was caused by chiropractic neck manipulation — a conclusion Deck continues to support.

That pathology report, although based on an incomplete examination of the neck tissue, was key to pre-inquest legal preparations. It had been used by chiropractic lawyers as they searched for, and briefed, expert witnesses for the inquest. The chiropractic experts submitted reports on the understanding that no dissection had occurred. The chiropractors considered that an absence of dissection could exonerate chiropractic in Lewis's death. Chiropractic neck manipulations that result in stroke often damage the lining of the artery at the point of neck rotation, frequently at the top two cervical vertebrae known as C1 and C2.

Fortunately, much of the tissue that had been taken from Lewis's neck was carefully preserved and waiting for other pathologists to let it tell them its story. And tell them it did.

During the summer, the Lewis family found a new lawyer willing to take the inquest on for free. She was Amani Oakley, a former medical technician who was familiar with pathology, evidence, and inquests. During the late summer of 2001, she devoured the Lewis file, bringing her medical and legal expertise to bear on what was now pounds of detailed documents that had been piling up for years. She wanted to know exactly what the tissue in Lewis's neck had to say about what killed her. She knew just whom to ask.

She approached Dr. John Richardson, against whom she had previously squared off when she was a union rep, for help with the case. Dr. Richardson is the director of neuropathology at the Montreal Neurological Institute. At Oakley's request, he examined the work of Deck and Pollanen, then later the samples themselves. He submitted a written report, and two of his conclusions were dynamite:

> Third conclusion is that there was a dissection of the intimal layer of [Lewis's] left vertebral artery.
>
> Fourth conclusion is that these events were initiated and took place at the cervical one to cervical two vertebrae, the place where the neck manipulation was administered.[16]

In short, Dr. Richardson, a leading neuropathologist, was saying that Deck and Pollanen were wrong, that there was a dissection and it took place at the location where, it's alleged, the chiropractor had rotated the neck. The coroner's report on which all the chiropractic experts had based their testimony had just been shredded by a feisty lawyer and a sage physician.

When Oakley submitted Richardson's report to the pre-inquest hearing on September 21, she began a process that would bring the stumbling inquest to a screeching halt. And the report sent Dr. Pollanen, now working in the United States, back to the tissue samples to take another look to see if he could see the same evidence of dissection Dr. Richardson had seen. He could.

Pollanen's new report, completed in early October, just before the inquest was about to officially begin, said that he had re-examined tissue from Lewis's neck and had found evidence of a "classic dissection" in her left vertebral artery just inside the skull. On October 10, Tom Schneider told the court that the new report from Pollanen had caused a "seismic shift in evidence" in the case. "This is a 180-degree-turn in evidence," Schneider said in court. He explained that all parties had a right to expect that the original coroner's pathology report be correct and that they could act on that information. Now, that information appeared to be wrong. Schneider called for another delay, this one months long, after the family had already waited years.

But Schneider told the court something else. He explained that Pollanen was unable to do as extensive an investigation as he would have liked because it appears that there were some tissue samples missing.

According to Oakley, the Lewis family lawyer, only two parties had signed out slides and tissue blocks from the coroner's office — experts for the family and experts for the College of Chiropractors of Ontario (CCO). The CCO regulates chiropractors in Ontario and acts to protect the public.

In an interview, Oakley recalled that on October 10, a few minutes before the Lewis inquest officially began, she was called to a meeting with Schneider and Constable John Rowett, a Toronto police detective assigned to the Lewis inquest. That's when she learned tissue was missing. She assured Schneider that her experts had returned all tissue they had taken out for examination.

That left the College of Chiropractors and their expert, Halifax-based neuropathologist Dr. Robert Macaulay. Macaulay, who had been an expert witness at the Mathiason inquest, had been approached by the CCO lawyers to provide some medical expertise for them.

Karen Jones was a lawyer who was working on behalf of the CCO along with its main counsel, Chris Paliare. In January 2001, Jones picked up slides and tissue samples from the coroner's office. She was to deliver them to Dr. Macaulay. That's clear from a portion of legal correspondence read into the court record by Amani Oakley: "Karen Jones has now picked up the requested histological samples for review by Dr. Macaulay," says a January 17, 2001 letter from the coroner's office.

The tissue samples sent by Jones to Macaulay included the tissue block where Pollanen later noted slices were missing. Lawyers for the College of Chiropractors told the court that Macaulay was sent slides to assist him in acting only as a medical interpreter for them — to help the lawyers for the chiropractors understand the highly technical language of the pathology reports.

But at a pre-inquest hearing on August 22, Oakley challenged the idea that Macaulay was retained only as a translator. She asked Paliare what report Macaulay had made about the tissue samples he had been sent. Paliare told the court that Macaulay had produced "no written report" and that he was simply asking the neuropathologist to interpret the medical language of the reports. "We've asked him to assist us with terminology.... Dr. Macaulay acts as a translator for us," Paliare told the court and Oakley.

In an interview with us, Oakley said that it "makes no sense whatsoever" that Macaulay would not only examine the slides of Lewis's neck, but also cut new tissue samples if he was only acting as a medical translator. "[Dr. Macaulay] shaving extra tissue when the submissions made by Chris Paliare were that he was only retained to advise on terminology [is] rather illogical," said Oakley. "You don't even need the slides at all ... but he absolutely would not need to slice new tissue to do it," she explained.

We contacted Macaulay, who said he was restricted from commenting because of issues of confidentiality. What Dr. Macaulay, did, or didn't do, with the slides and what he may have seen if he examined the slides are important for two reasons. First, if Macaulay did, in fact, examine the slides in January, he may well have seen the same dissection as Richardson and Pollanen had seen. That would have meant that in January, the chiropractic lawyers would have been aware of the dissection. We do not know if Macaulay looked at the slides, though we tried to find out. That's the second reason the issue of the missing slides is so important. When we asked the CCO about the missing tissue and Macaulay's role, they had their lawyer, Chris Paliare, act as their media spokesman. He refused to comment on the tissue samples or on what, if anything, Dr. Macaulay told him about them.

So, let's unravel this. In January 2001, the CCO, a body set up in part to serve the public interest in regard to chiropractic, has tissue from the coroner's office (though actually property of the Lewis family) sent to a distinguished neuropathologist in Halifax. They refuse to say what the neuropathologist did with the tissue samples and why they went missing for so many months, even though they're in an inquest that is supposed to get to the truth about how Lana Dale Lewis died.

Oakley believes the CCO has an obligation to the public to ask Macaulay what he found. "The college's role is that of public protection. So, it's completely wrong if they did find something to not follow through with Macaulay," she argues. "Their job isn't to find good things, their job is to find whatever is necessary to safeguard the public."

One of the CCO's stated strategic goals is "ensuring that all College activities are open, accessible, equitable and fair to all parties." When we tried to speak to the CCO about their obligation to protect the public, we were referred to Paliare, who refused to comment.

The news of Pollanen's second report and the debacle of the missing tissue delayed the inquest again, this time until the spring of 2002. When it started in April, chiropractic lawyers continued to treat the inquest as an aggressive criminal trial. They were just being loyal members of what Greg Dunn had called the "Chiropractic Defense Alliance." The CCO, however, didn't have that excuse. It had forgotten whom it was supposed to be protecting.

7

COURTING YORK – THE UNSUITABLE SUITOR
How the CMCC Tried to Win Academic Acceptance and Wound Up Empty-Handed

For more than thirty years, the administrators of the Canadian Memorial Chiropractic College have been tantalized by an unfulfilled dream. They want, desperately, to forge a relationship with a Canadian university and to have that university grant chiropractic doctorates. The CMCC, Canada's only English chiropractic school, has wooed nearly a dozen Canadian universities in pursuit of that goal, and has been turned down flat every time. The college's most recent bid for affiliation, to York University in Toronto, is a textbook example of the ease with which chiropractic officials don the insincere shell of science to help them get what they want. In documents and presentations to York's administration and faculty, CMCC officials painted a picture of chiropractic and chiropractic education that bore faint resemblance to reality. They exaggerated hospital affiliations, claimed a scientific basis the profession lacks, and underplayed or ignored scientific studies that have pointed out that chiropractic treatments are of little or no benefit for various disorders. As they had done before in front of government bodies, other universities, and the media, they presented a construct of chiropractic they were perfectly aware was as thin as a papier mâché mask.

This is the story of how Canadian chiropractors almost seduced York University into a disastrous marriage of convenience.

York Senators Caught with Hands and Pants Down

It was two days before Hallowe'en in 1999. An audience of fifty, including a handful of York University senators and a smattering of faculty members, sat in the Vanier College Dining Hall listening to the speakers at a conference on the planned marriage between York and the CMCC. The presenters were dry, but informative. Then came a very strange moment for everyone in the room. Dr. Stephen Barrett, a high-profile American critic of chiropractic, asked all the York senators to stand up. About a dozen men and women stood.

The senate's Academic Policy and Planning Committee had been considering the proposed affiliation since 1994. The proposal to offer a doctorate of chiropractic at York University, in co-operation with the CMCC, was approved by the senators by a vote of fifty-seven to thirteen in May 1998. They had waded through numerous proposals, reports, and submissions from their faculties, the senate's policy and planning committee, and the CMCC itself. With the senators still standing, Barrett asked them to raise their hand to respond to this question, "How many of you have a really good understanding of what chiropractic is all about?"

No hands went up.

"How many of you know what the term subluxation means to chiropractors?" asked Barrett.

No hands went up.

He then admonished the senators, saying, "How could the senate vote on whether or not a chiropractic school should come in if the senators don't know what is chiropractic and what is a subluxation? ... Why don't you know? What's wrong with the evaluation process that has been going on since 1995 that not a single person in this room from the school can say, 'Yes, I know what chiropractic is and what is a subluxation'?"

That uncomfortable moment crystallized a problem that flowed through the reports and submissions that had piled up around the CMCC/York affiliation bid. Barrett went on to explain the flimsy basis of subluxation theory and provide proof that CMCC's teachings still supported it, a fact that CMCC had denied during its courtship of York.

An examination of the bid documents shows that York administrators did not do sufficient research to get a comprehensive and clear picture of chiropractic education and practice in Canada, despite being warned the previous March by members of the university's science faculty that the university's investigation was lax and was not challenging CMCC statements. In fact, on March 17, 1999, members of the science faculty chastised York administration officials for simply handing serious questions about "misrepresentations" back to CMCC officials for response.

The science faculty was right to raise the alarm. In its desperation to affiliate, CMCC officials overstated, and, in some cases, misrepresented the CMCC's associations with Canadian universities and hospitals. They also misused studies into the efficacy of chiropractic manipulation. As well, they underplayed the influence that unscientific thinking has on the practice of chiropractic in Canada and misrepresented the scope of practice of chiropractors. Finally, they fudged the reasons for the failure of CMCC to affiliate with other Canadian universities in the past.

Bearing Little Relationship to the Truth

CMCC officials told York University in official submissions:

> Research has been and is conducted in-house and offsite through collaboration with faculty from many institutions, including the University of Toronto, University of Waterloo, McMaster University, University of Western Ontario, University of Calgary, University of Saskatchewan, the Institute for Work and Health, Wellesley Central Hospital, St. Michael's Hospital and Sunnybrook Health Sciences Centre.[1]

CMCC officials also stated:

> CMCC currently maintains collaborative activity with the University of Waterloo, University of Toronto, University of Calgary, McMaster University and the University of Saskatoon, a number of chiropractic colleges, and the Institute for Work and Health.[2]

But many of those institutions painted a more subdued picture of the relationships or stated clearly that no formal relationships existed. A November 1998 letter from Dr. Donald Livingston, the vice-president of Professional Affairs for Sunnybrook Health Science Centre, specifically addresses the relationship between Sunnybrook and CMCC. It states:

> ... it has been claimed that '...scientific investigations have been and are being conducted in collaboration with a variety of institutions of higher education, including the University of Toronto' ... At the Sunnybrook site such research has been limited to information consultation on one occasion, providing consultation to the college in research design on a contract basis in a single instance, and in a further instance providing an opportunity for members of

the college to send out questionnaires in a supervised manner to a subset of patients in the hospital. ...

It has been claimed that, '[chiropractic] interns and graduate students work as part of teams at ... Sunnybrook Hospital.' Such a claim is without foundation. At no time have chiropractic under-graduate or postgraduate students been part of any clinical service provided at Sunnybrook.[3]

The letter concludes, "In summary, there is no relationship of substance between Sunnybrook and the Canadian Memorial Chiropractic College."

While CMCC claimed that its students worked in teams at Sunnybrook and other hospitals, its own internal communications reveal that, at Sunnybrook, the relationship was an informal one with Dr. Richard Hu, a hospital staff member who was supportive of chiropractic in the health care system and who let students come on rounds. "During these sessions our residents acted purely as observers," Dr. Hu writes to Jean Moss, the president of the CMCC. "At no time was there any independent assessment or treatment provided by the chiropractic residents and ... the primary and only care during that time would be provided by me."[4]

In September 1998, Dr. Harry Shulman, the director of the Department of Medical Imaging at Sunnybrook Health Science Centre wrote, forcefully, about the claims of a CMCC association with Sunnybrook.

A number of communications have been forwarded to me which state there is an association or educational relationship of some kind between the Canadian Memorial Chiropractic College and the Department of Medical Imaging at Sunnybrook and Women's College Health Sciences Centre. No such relationship exists.[5]

The letter goes on to say that a radiologist hired by Sunnybrook had trained as a chiropractor and had taught at CMCC. "It was this association that led to chiropractic students attending some of the rounds," Dr. Shulman writes. He adds, "Most of our staff and residents have always felt uncomfortable about this loose arrangement because of the differences in our basic approach to the cause and treatment of disease. This discomfort has been greatly exacerbated by the public claim that part of the radiology training of the chiropractic students occurs at Sunnybrook." Shulman concludes the letter by making it clear that CMCC students are no longer welcome to attend rounds at Sunnybrook.

A January 1999 letter from Dr. James Waddell in the division of orthopedic surgery at the University of Toronto states:

I have reiterated on every possible occasion that there is no official link between the division of orthopedic surgery, University of Toronto and any college of chiropractic; furthermore, there is no official relationship between St. Michael's Hospital and any members of the chiropractic profession.[6]

In a November 10 letter, Waddell states that he has written to Dr. Robin Richards, chief of orthopedics and program director for neuromusculoskeletal medicine at St. Michael's Hospital, requesting any information regarding chiropractic involvement with the hospital. He concluded:

To my knowledge, there are no chiropractic students in the hospital at the present time nor have there been for many, many years. There are no chiropractors practising at St. Michael's Hospital.[7]

St. Michael's Hospital does have a chiropractic clinic operated by CMCC. "We provide the facility and that's it. No money changes hands with us and they don't charge us for the services," explained Nicole Ireland, a spokesperson for St. Michael's Hospital.

A September 15, 1998 letter from Dr. Ken Yong-Hing, the head of orthopedic surgery at the Royal University Hospital, University of Saskatchewan, states that some chiropractic students had access to the hospital as a personal favour to Dr. David Cassidy, a former chiropractor who heads up the Institute of Health and Outcomes Research at the Royal University Hospital. However, those chiropractors "did not participate in decision-making or in the treatment of patients on the hospital premises where the clinics were held." He also states:

No chiropractic college, including the Canadian Memorial Chiropractic College, to my knowledge, had a formal relationship with the College of Medicine, or the University of Saskatchewan. The Canadian Memorial Chiropractic College did not have any formal relationship with any academic unit, division, department or college of the University of Saskatchewan. No individual or college at the University of Saskatchewan, to my knowledge has participated in granting certificates or degrees, setting standards, setting courses evaluating students or evaluating programs for Canadian Memorial Chiropractic College (CMCC) students.[8]

A March 14, 1999 e-mail from Dr. Caroline Quartly, an assistant clinical professor at McMaster University Medical Centre (MUMC), stated, "I am not aware of any proposal by the MEDICAL community to bring chiropractic into the hospital service model." Quartly explained that the business school had suggested chiropractors be brought into the McMaster centre, but that many physicians polled were "categorically and vehemently opposed to embracing any idea of bringing chiropractic service into the hospital system." She added that chiropractic residents were allowed to do some pain management training at a cognitive/behavioural-basic chronic pain program, and that one chiropractor was brought in on a third-party payer basis by administration, but "when the health-care community realized that the administration had apparently acted unilaterally in the original initiative to bring chiropractic into hospital service (seemingly without consultation or consideration of existing services) there was a bit of an uproar." She concludes by saying, "So, other than the third-party payer pain program model where one chiropractor has been employed by David Montgomery, administrator, chiropractors are not at present in the hospital system."

Dr. Stuart McGill, a professor at the University of Waterloo, said he's conducting research on chiropractic manipulations. "We don't train chiropractors. They come here and do what they do and we make scientific measurements of their work on patients in the community," McGill explained. The two-year-old program is designed to evaluate the effect of chiropractic. "The mandate of our research clinic is to conduct studies using scientific instruments on the patients to try to understand what it is that chiropractors do," he said. "The reason the chiropractic clinic is here is purely to conduct a research investigation."

Dr. Walter Herzog, a professor of biomechanics at the University of Calgary, has been working on research into the biomechanics of the spine and spinal manipulations since 1985. The Canadian Chiropractic Association, the Chiropractic Foundation for Research, the College of Chiropractors of Alberta, and the Medical Research Council of Canada fund the research. Herzog said the University of Calgary runs a program with the CMCC for one to two chiropractic residents to spend six months in his lab each year. "The CMCC sends their best students to us for research training. The CMCC pays for the salary of these chiropractic residents and we pay the operational costs of the research," Herzog explained.

So, while the CMCC was portraying itself as working hand in hand with medical researchers across the country, those same researchers were making it clear that they wanted to have little or nothing to do with the chiropractors or that their relationships were extremely limited. In fact, some said clearly that the CMCC misrepresented the tenuous relationships.

Not surprisingly, the CMCC did the same with studies about chiropractic itself.

Taking Studies for a Spin

In presentations and reports to York University, CMCC officials cited numerous papers and studies that seem to support chiropractic care. But if you actually look at those studies, they tell a very different story. They demonstrate that CMCC misled York officials about the reports, conveniently failed to mention studies that didn't support chiropractic treatments, and misrepresented research data.

In general, CMCC presented reports of studies to York that supported spinal manipulative therapy (SMT) for low-back pain as though they were supportive of chiropractic. Although chiropractors spend much of their time on back pain and do perform spinal manipulative therapy, these studies are not, in fact, endorsements of chiropractic. Many other practitioners, including doctors, physiotherapists, and osteopaths, deliver SMT.

Perhaps the best study of the effectiveness of SMT is the RAND report on "The Appropriateness of Spinal Manipulation for Lower-Back Pain."[9] After analyzing twenty-two controlled trials, the RAND panel concluded that manipulation was useful for acute low-back pain in patients showing no sign of lower-limb nerve root involvement. They recommended trying two different types of manipulation for two weeks each, and discontinuing therapy if there was no improvement.

The CMCC, and chiropractors in general, cite RAND as supportive of chiropractic, but the report's writers have been clear that the study is no such thing. In fact, the report's lead authors have criticized chiropractors for inappropriately using the study to support their treatments and ideas. In 1993, Dr. Paul Shekelle wrote an article for the *American Chiropractic Association Journal of Chiropractic* chastising chiropractors for misrepresenting the RAND findings and explicitly told them, "RAND's studies were about spinal manipulation, not chiropractic, and dealt with appropriateness, which is a measure of net benefit and harms. Comparative efficacy of chiropractic and other treatments was not explicitly dealt with."

Despite these clarifications, CMCC used the RAND study in its submissions to York to bolster its case. CMCC officials also didn't mention another important RAND study, "The Appropriateness of Manipulation and Mobilization of the Cervical Spine." The 1996 study is a parallel to the low-back study much touted by chiropractors and uses similar evaluative techniques. But its conclusion is not as favourable to the use of manipulation and mobilization for the upper spine. The panel found only 11 percent of 736 indications for cervical manipulation were judged appropriate. The most important finding was the lack of evidence for the benefit of these procedures.

Another study used by CMCC to bolster chiropractic's status in the world is the 1979 "Chiropractic in New Zealand" commission report, which contends, "chiropractors are included as partners in the general health care team." What they leave out is that the New Zealand Commission rejected the title "doctor" for chiropractors, rejected the notion "that chiropractic treatment will necessarily cure or alleviate any organic or visceral disorder," and finally recommended that patients not see a chiropractor without a medical referral.

The chiropractic college also notes the 1993 Ontario Ministry of Health report (known as the Manga Report, after its author, economist Pran Manga), which stated that chiropractic manipulation is safer, more effective, and more cost effective than medical management of low-back pain. Again, this is not an endorsement of chiropractic in general, but only as a treatment for low-back pain, and the conclusions of the report are not supported by other researchers who have examined the same studies Manga did.

Perhaps most damning of all is the fact that CMCC officials were fully aware that their own researcher, Howard Vernon, had written that the subluxation itself, which is the basis for chiropractic, has not been proven to exist. They were also aware, from the debates raging in the pages of the *Journal of the Canadian Chiropractic Association* and other journals, that many chiropractors reject the entire idea of scientific validity. They're more comfortable with the pre-scientific ideas of D.D. and B.J. Palmer. Like B.J. Palmer himself, many chiropractors already believe chiropractic works; they don't need any scientist to tell them that.

In fact, the CMCC's own attitude towards studies, as demonstrated in its presentations to York, was anti-scientific. They were content to reject any studies that didn't support their hypothesis and to distort, to their benefit, any that hinted at efficacy. In the process, they led York to believe chiropractic was both effective and science-based. But the very evidence they claimed to hold in such high regard did not support either idea.

Pseudo-science in Plain View

In its presentations to York, CMCC officials took great pains to paint a picture of the college and chiropractic as embracing the scientific method and evidence-based practices. In a response to questions from York officials, Jean Moss, the CMCC's president, writes, "researchers at the CMCC know of no other philosophy of science than that which informs research conducted by university scholars."[10] She says that CMCC has embraced the "modern biomedical model." But had York officials visited the CMCC bookstore in 1999, they would have seen evidence to the contrary.

There, homeopathic remedies were stocked next to herbal nostrums. Many homeopathic products are so dilute that it is unlikely that they contain even a single molecule of active ingredient. Across the aisle, reflexology charts vied for attention with stickers used by pediatric chiropractors, a text on pediatric chiropractic, and a book about the dangers of immunization. Neither reflexology nor homeopathy has been proven effective in dealing with health problems.

The bookstore also contained a thick text on acupuncture. In submissions to York, CMCC officials said that, "acupressure is taught as a soft tissue technique involving pressure over trigger/tender points in myofascial structures responsible for local or referred pain."

But while those submissions were being made, the college offered a 220-hour advanced training program in clinical acupuncture. The textbook for the course, *The Foundations of Chinese Medicine*, presented students with acupuncture as an alternative medical model completely unlike the "modern biomedical model" the CMCC was supposed to have embraced. That alternative model includes the ancient Chinese notion of moxabustion — the burning of herbs on the ends of acupuncture needles to facilitate the energy flow along meridian lines. This is done to balance Yin and Yang and the five elements: fire, earth, wood, metal, and water. The book also discusses a life force called Qi. The text says this about the organs of the body:

> The Spleen is the mother of the Lungs: Spleen-Qi provides Food-Qi to the Lungs where it interacts with air to form the Gathering-Qi. The Lungs are the mother of the Kidneys: Lung-Qi descends to meet Kidney-Qi. The Lungs also send fluids down to the Kidneys.

Despite the CMCC's explanation to York, the brochure for the course went much further than just trigger points and localized pain relief. The brochure told would-be students that the course covered, among other things, acupuncture and moxabustion treatment of painful conditions, the pathology of Qi, Chinese dietary therapy, and the integration of acupuncture into an existing chiropractic clinic.

In the submission, CMCC states that acupressure "may also be used along with acupuncture meridians and this use is supported by a significant body of knowledge which substantiates the underlying benefits and mechanisms of acupuncture." In fact, numerous scientific studies have failed to find any support for the notion of "meridians." Acupuncture, as described in the text used at CMCC, has not been substantiated by modern science in any way. But acupuncture is just one of the pseudo-scientific treatments Canadian chiropractors, most of whom graduated from CMCC, offer.

A 1993 survey of Canadian chiropractors by the National Board of Chiropractic Examiners found that:

- 27.4 percent used homeopathic remedies;
- 31 percent used applied kinesiology (a bogus form of allergy testing that has nothing to do with kinesiology);
- 66.3 percent used acupressure/meridian therapy.

The "modern biomedical model" has discounted both homeopathy and applied kinesiology. Despite that, and despite what it told York, CMCC did nothing to distance itself from those practices. A chelation therapy information session by CMCC graduate Katrina Kulhay, of the Kulhay Wellness Centre in Toronto, was advertised on a bulletin board near the CMCC library while CMCC was hoping to affiliate. Chelation therapy, used by alternative practitioners to reduce arteriosclerosis, has no scientific validity.

A 1999 issue of *Primary Contact*, the magazine put out by CMCC, contained a back-page ad for homeopathic remedies. The advertisement noted that they are easy to sell because "the claim is right on the bottle." The homeopathic remedies are advertised as "available at the CMCC Supply Centre and Bookstore."

But the most obvious proof of CMCC's inability to shed chiropractic's unscientific past comes from a 1997 position statement signed by the members of the Association of Chiropractic Colleges. The "Paradigm" section reads:

Chiropractic is concerned with the preservation and restoration of health, and focuses particular attention on the subluxation. A subluxation is a complex of functional and/or structural and/or pathological articular changes that compromise neural integrity and may influence organ system function and general health. A subluxation is evaluated, diagnosed, and managed through the use of chiropractic procedures based on the best available rational and empirical evidence.

In other words, the association members believe that there are subluxations and that they may cause general disease. No non-chiropractic researcher believes that, and there's no science that supports it. The statement says nothing about treating the spine to treat low-back pain.

The association is made up of chiropractic colleges in North America, including the CMCC. Jean Moss signed the statement on behalf of the CMCC.

A Cad Comes Calling

It turns out that it was just that sort of evidence that has made it so hard for CMCC to affiliate with a university. For decades, CMCC officials have seen affiliation as essential to the development and recognition of the profession and the college itself. Affiliation would also give them access to government research money. But every time they popped the question to a Canadian university, the answer was always a polite, but firm, "No."

In 1999, CMCC officials told York University that past failures have been because of "lack of government funding." They offered no other explanation. But while funding certainly played a role, the CMCC's sorry dance card is also due to extremely serious concerns the medical community and universities have had about the philosophy, training, and practices of chiropractic. These concerns went unmentioned by the CMCC, although officials would have been painfully aware of them.

According to a history of CMCC's persistent university courtship by chiropractor Dr. Douglas Brown,[11] CMCC started pursuing university affiliation in Ontario in earnest in 1965. Ironically, one of its first targets that year was a small university in north Toronto called York. But York, a university that was busy "improving its educational facilities and standards," rebuffed its initial overture.

That same year, CMCC also paid a call to the University of Guelph, hoping for some sort of engagement. Guelph officials thought the chiropractic suitor was too lowbrow. "We find that with only one exception, all your teachers received their primary training in a course in chiropractic," a Guelph official wrote. "We feel that this reveals a serious weakness in your educational program."[12] Guelph officials did not mention funding as any impediment.

In 1971, the college knocked on the door of Queen's University. A letter from CMCC Dean Herbert Vear after a Queen's meeting states, "… the long held identity of chiropractic as a 'cult,' 'dogma,' 'non-scientific,' etc. is the same stigma that requires we advance cautiously and soundly."[13] Nothing came of the Queen's courtship, which ended in 1974 when CMCC was informed that policy problems and a small clinic base precluded Queen's taking on new health-care initiatives.

In 1972, the tireless would-be groom paid a visit to the University of Toronto. This time the dean expressed concern about "the lack of any commitment from a health sciences centre to accept chiropractic education into their fold." Over a decade later, in 1984, the university again slammed the door, saying it was facing difficult financial circumstances. That same year, the University of Ottawa told its beau plainly that it did not wish to pursue an affiliation.

At that time, CMCC was also finding the Ministry of Education was complicating its courting. Dr. Bette Stephenson, the Ontario Education Minister from 1978 to 1985, laid down firm guidelines for how the college could become part of a university. She demanded that a detailed proposal be put together for an affiliation with a university that "had a major role in health care education." The proposal had to be approved by the university's senate and administration. It would then have to be given the nod by a variety of provincial government bodies, including the ministry of health, with the minister of colleges and universities making the final decision.

The conditions that Stephenson placed on the affiliation prompted a CMCC board member to write, "The profession feels discriminated against by the never-ending conditions required for university affiliation." This is not a complaint about funding, but a concern about the procedural roadblocks it felt Stephenson was placing on its bridal path. Nevertheless, the CMCC trudged on and got turned down by the University of Western Ontario in 1984, which raised Stephenson's conditions as a reason for not uniting. In 1980, Wilfrid Laurier University also turned down the CMCC offer.

That same year, the Ontario Medical Association passed a motion that stated, "the OMA is opposed to the merger of chiropractic training with a university and the subsequent granting of degrees, and that the OMA take an active role in attempting to prevent this union of the college of chiropractic with a university."[14] Resistance from Ontario universities with medical schools, which would have been the princess brides for the CMCC, would now be coming, in part, from the OMA, because of issues of science and medicine, not finance.

In 1984, the Health Sciences Legislative Committee, which was made up of Ontario universities with health sciences centres, decided that, "owing to limitations in funding and other scarce resources, the development of an arrangement with CMCC was not a priority at this time. In addition, some [universities] indicated that differences in philosophy between them effectively precluded any association. None of the universities with a health sciences centre was prepared at this time to enter into an arrangement with CMCC." Once again, money wasn't the only issue; there was also the problem that the bride and groom couldn't see eye to eye.

By the end of the 1980s, CMCC got the message loud and clear. The Ontario government and medical associations were going to be stern parents, dishing out what the CMCC felt were arbitrary and restrictive rules about who could and could not affiliate with universities.

In December 1988, in frustration over what the CMCC felt were capricious and discriminatory restrictions, the college "entered into discussions with the University of Victoria in British Columbia." At first, the West Coast university was open to the idea, but the mood out west soured quickly after a group of professors visited CMCC in Toronto. In September 1989, a committee from the university visited the CMCC campus to review the admission standards and curriculum of the college. They also planned to check out the equipment and meet with some of the staff. According to Professor Charles Picciotto, the chair of physics and astronomy at the University of Victoria and a member of the visiting team, the four-person committee did its homework prior to the visit and understood the history and philosophy of chiropractic.

When they arrived they were, according to Picciotto, disappointed by the "quality of the entering students." They were also unimpressed by the amount of research CMCC had produced and felt the research labs were poorly equipped. But they were even more dismayed because early chiropractic philosophy was still being taught. Picciotto writes:

> We were hoping that the original tenets of chiropractic which are necessarily anti-scientific (and proud of it!) had given way to a serious scientific study of what benefits might result from the physiotherapy aspects of the chiropractic treatment. The reality is that this simply is not the case. Although there was an effort by some of the administrators to tell us what we wanted to hear, the fact is that the majority of the staff that we interviewed was committed to pursuing chiropractic as an alternate primary-care methodology, with a "medical" professional path which parallels conventional medicine, i.e. an anti-scientific system which private citizens use as first-contact care providers for anything from the flu to cancer, from cradle to grave. Mixed in with the general anti-rational approach to health care, there were particular procedures that were advocated which might make one think that we are living in the Middle Ages.[15]

After the visit, the University of Victoria voted to reject affiliation with CMCC. It cited concerns that "research in chiropractic at this time is not consistent with contemporary standards of university research" and questioned "the subject of subluxation and its influence on the practice of chiropractic," among other problems.

After the failure of the University of Victoria bid, CMCC tried a new affiliation model, in which the college would remain financially independent but would be affiliated so graduates would receive a university degree. Armed with this new financial model and renewed optimism, CMCC again appealed to York.

In all, counting York, CMCC has made at least thirteen bids for a dozen scholarly hands. The experience left CMCC officials feeling bitter, frustrated, and marginalized. In the end, CMCC found itself back where had it started over thirty years earlier, on bended knee in front of York University.

CMCC Still Waiting

Despite York's dismal lack of diligence, on March 28, 2001, a slim majority of the faculty of York's Atkinson College voted against any affiliation with the CMCC. That decision was in good part due to the work of four York scientists: Michael De Robertis, James Alcock, Diethard Bohme, and Stanley Jeffers. They consistently called CMCC's bluff on misleading statements and chiropractic's unscientific underpinnings. Dr. Murray Katz helped the scientists. The Montreal physician and longtime chiropractic critic met with senior York officials and explained why affiliation with CMCC would be a disaster for York. In the end, despite support for the union from some of the most senior York administrators, clearer heads ruled the day.

The CMCC has made strides to improve the quality of its education. They require at least three years of undergraduate university study, with a B to B-plus average. About 90 percent of CMCC students come to the college with an undergraduate degree, and only about 15 percent of applicants are accepted. Students then receive four years of instruction and must pass provincial and national board exams before they enter practice. However, the college seems unable to publicly renounce pseudo-science and has failed to distance itself from techniques that are not supported by evidence. In fact, surveys of CMCC students' attitudes show that they want more pseudo-science, not less. But for decades, universities have told CMCC that their unscientific teachings and pseudo-scientific methods are unacceptable in a university.

Doubtless the CMCC will make another bid for affiliation elsewhere, possibly Ryerson University. When they make their next attempt, it's likely they will use the same tactics, putting a false face on chiropractic in order to win the hand that remains just beyond their grasp.

8

ARE CHIROPRACTORS BACK DOCTORS?
Why Low-Back Pain is a Happy Accident for Chiropractors

Most people think of chiropractors as back specialists. They're viewed by many as the health practitioner best suited to deal with back pain and other musculoskeletal problems. That's no accident. Chiropractic organizations in Canada and the United States have for years promoted the profession's success at treating back and neck problems. Brochures, information sheets, and radio and television advertisements have tried to position chiropractors as the obvious and best choice for treating one of the most common complaints in society — back pain, particularly low-back pain. But are they?

Chiropractic, as we've seen, is actually focused on the spine as a source of disease, not the back as a source of pain. D.D. Palmer believed manipulating the spine was the key to treating all human ailments and the secret to maintaining good health. According to chiropractic legend, his first adjustment cured a man's deafness. Palmer claimed that he could cure diabetes, heart disease, stomach problems, and more with spinal adjustments. Back pain was, perhaps, the least of his concerns. So how did legislators, lawmakers, and the public come to view chiropractors as back doctors?

Telling the Truth: A Lesson Learned

The answer is complicated and covers decades of manoeuvring by chiropractors before countless boards of inquiry, committees, and the public. But the key to understanding what chiropractic has become may lie in what happened one day in Ontario, almost a century ago.

First, a little background. Before the First World War, there were only about forty chiropractors in Ontario, and even at this early stage in chiropractic's evolution, they were divided among no fewer than three associations.[1] Chiropractors were, for the most part, considered to be cultists and charlatans, still operating on the fringes of health care, but events overseas were about to change that image.

Thousands of soldiers were injured and maimed in the bloody battlefields of Europe. Hospitals were crowded with men whose injuries and protracted recoveries had left them with wasted muscles and stiffened joints. But optimistic reports of the beneficial effects of a new branch of treatment called "physical therapy" were making their way back to Canada. The therapy had many names — mechanotherapy, thermotherapy, kinesitherapy, bonesetting, and manipulation — but the results were startlingly consistent. Functionally disabled soldiers were regaining use of their limbs and, in some cases, even returning to active duty. Recovery rates were high and costs were surprisingly low. None of the manipulations was done by chiropractors.

At the same time, the premier of Ontario appointed the Honourable Mr. Justice Hodgins to preside over a royal commission on medical education in Ontario. Hodgins had read the reports coming from Europe and was highly impressed with these new therapies, suggesting that they could play a significant role in health care in Ontario and across the country.

Chiropractors and osteopaths were delighted with the news. Chiropractors saw this wave of favourable attitudes towards manipulation and physical therapy as something they might ride toward recognition and official regulation. But they made an enormous strategic mistake, one that they would never make again. They told the commission the truth about chiropractic.

The two leading proponents of chiropractic, Dr. Ernst DuVal, representing the Canadian Chiropractic College in Hamilton, and B.J. Palmer himself, appeared before the commission. They were enthusiastic about the success of manipulation on injured soldiers, although DuVal was quick to point out that chiropractic was not physiotherapy, but rather a "unique science" with "nothing in common with any other method, class, school or cult, neither in its science, philosophy, art, doctrine or principle...."[2] He went on to explain to Judge Hodgins that chiropractic did not claim to treat, cure, or heal any ailment or disease and that it had no use for diagnosis at all.

When B.J. made his submission to the commission, he too explained fully and clearly the true nature of chiropractic. He even went so far as to tell the judge that chiropractors did not believe in bacteria and that "bacteriology was the greatest of all gigantic farces ever invented for ignorance and incompetency" and that the analysis of blood and urine was useless.

The outcome was predictable. Judge Hodgins was appalled by chiropractic's rejection of diagnosis, chemistry, and bacteriology and its total reliance on the principle of adjustment in all cases. In his decision, he stated that he must withhold status from a profession that "denies the need of diagnosis, refers 95 percent of disease to one and the same cause, and turns its back resolutely upon all modern scientific methods as being founded on nothing and unworthy even to be discussed."[3]

He recommended that the chiropractic colleges of Ontario be closed, and no provision was made for any regulation or licensing of chiropractors in the future. It was a huge setback for the fledgling profession in Canada. But the judge found value in the care that soldiers were getting overseas and he made a recommendation that physical treatment methods be developed as part of medicine. Doctors for the most part ignored Judge Hodgins's advice and in doing so inadvertently left the door open for chiropractors. As chiropractic historian Donald Sutherland writes:

> It is quite possible that if the medical profession had acted in accordance with the recommendation of the Hodgins Commission and had demonstrated a greater interest in developing and utilizing manipulative therapy following the impressive record established in the care of injured soldiers, chiropractic history would have been quite different.[4]

In many ways, the chiropractic profession today remains as DuVal and Palmer described it to Judge Hodgins in 1915. A significant proportion of chiropractors believe in subluxation as the cause of disease, many reject immunization, many believe in the power of Innate to heal the body, and almost all adjust the spine for conditions unrelated to the musculoskeletal system in the belief that a well-adjusted spine is the key to good health. Though the profession did not change that day, how chiropractors would present the profession to panels, committees, and the public changed forever. Never again would chiropractic leaders tell the whole, unvarnished truth about chiropractic to lawmakers or regulators. And they recognized an opportunity when they saw one. They jumped on the success that rehabilitation therapists had established during the war for various physical therapies, including manipulation. From this point forward they would present themselves publicly as manipulative therapists skilled in the treatment of back and limb pain for injuries sustained in war or in the workplace. They would claim for themselves the benefits ascribed to joint manipulation and have continued to do that up to the present day. For public consumption, the spine men would become back experts if that's what it took to get ahead. That tactic, still in operation today, was, and is, a smashing success.

Back Pain — The Billion-Dollar Problem

Low-back pain is an enormous problem in Canada and the United States. About 80 percent of adults will have an episode of low-back pain in their lives. Two to five percent of those people will have it at any given time. The good news is that most low-back pain is self-limited, meaning that it resolves on its own within a few weeks. Though it can recur and is usually painful, it is seldom serious. Only a tiny minority of low-back pain sufferers require surgery. For most people, low-back pain is a temporary annoyance, and only a small group of those afflicted — between 5 and 10 percent — become chronic sufferers.

The majority of people who "put out" their back carrying a child or lifting a box simply manage the problem themselves. Rest, ice packs, and over-the-counter pain remedies such as Ibuprofen are often effective treatments for simple low-back pain. Experts agree that in most cases, consulting a health professional is unnecessary, but almost 40 percent of people who have acute low-back pain seek help from a health care practitioner, most often their medical doctor. Back pain complaints are the fifth most common reason people consult a physician in the United States and the number one reason they go to see a chiropractor. Statistics in Canada are similar. In 1996, about three million Canadians visited a chiropractor. Studies indicate that the majority of people — between 40 percent and almost 70 percent — see chiropractors for back pain or injury.[5] Canadians spent about $500 million on approximately 30 million patient visits to the country's more than five thousand chiropractors in 1995. Those numbers may have increased slightly, but studies show that between 8 and 15 percent of the population use chiropractic care annually.[6]

What this means is that back business is big business. In Canada, musculoskeletal problems ranked second only to cardiovascular disease in terms of cost to Canadians. In 1993, the direct and indirect costs of musculoskeletal problems came to $17.8 billion.[7] And it is a business that chiropractors have claimed almost by chance. Unlike dentistry, which was created to deal with teeth, or optometry, which focuses on the eye and vision, chiropractic was never envisioned by D.D. Palmer, nor developed by his son B.J., as a profession focused on the back. Chiropractic is unusual in that it is defined not by what it is (in fact, chiropractors cannot agree what it is) but rather by what it does. "Chiropractic is a unique profession in that it is a profession driven by the main therapeutic procedure practiced by its members," writes Meridel Gatterman, a professor at the Canadian Memorial Chiropractic College.[8] That procedure is the "adjustment," in chiropractic parlance, or "spinal manipulative therapy," in general. When it became apparent through clinical practice and studies carried out by other health professionals that manipulation of the spine might be of benefit in the treatment of acute low-back pain, chiropractors were quick to exploit the support of science and moved to position themselves as the most skilled purveyors of manipulation. For the most part, chiropractors have had little time for science or scientific evidence.[9] They have openly derided the importance of scientific experimentation and evidence for more than a century, and continue to do so today, but they are happy to use it when it serves their purposes. So, though they cling tenaciously to the position that chiropractic remains a form of health care separate and distinct from medicine, they have been equally aggressive in marketing themselves as experts in back care.

The Canadian Chiropractic Association states:

> Industry, insurance and governments can save millions of dollars annually, with a shift in policy to prefer chiropractic services for patients with low back pain, since it has been scientifically proven time and again that for low back pain, chiropractic provides clinical results, cost-effectiveness and patient satisfaction.[10]

The Ontario Chiropractic Association, the single largest provincial chiropractic body, published a pamphlet on low-back pain telling Canadians that chiropractors are "the doctors that have been proven to get the best results in the relief of back pain."[11] The pamphlet goes on to assure the reader that chiropractic adjustments will "correct spinal problems and offer long term relief." As well, in outlining symptoms, the OCA lists symptoms such as leg pain with numbness, tingling, or weakness, and pain in the hip, buttock, or thigh, and then says, "IF you've answered 'yes' to any of these symptoms, it's time you got help from a doctor. A doctor of chiropractic." Some of those symptoms could be signs of nerve involvement and are indications, in fact, that you should not be manipulated.

Much of the profession's marketing efforts are directed at convincing the public that chiropractors should be the first contact for back pain, not the family doctor. But are chiropractors' claims that their treatment has been scientifically validated true? Has chiropractic been shown to be both safe and effective in the treatment of back pain?

The Studies: Yes, No, and Maybe

In the 1990s, several major studies on back pain were published, and chiropractors quickly used them to support the idea that chiropractic is an effective treatment for back pain. Chiropractic organizations in Canada and the United States declared that these studies — The Meade Study, the RAND study, and a Canadian government report called the Manga Report — had legitimized chiropractic treatment. They boasted that chiropractic was now scientifically proven to be effective. Long an enemy of chiropractic, scientific data was now warmly embraced by the profession, and these studies' findings were widely promoted — an evidence windfall for chiropractors. Whereas earlier, chiropractors had relied on anecdotes and clinical experience to persuade the public that chiropractic care was effective, their marketing efforts now boasted that they had scientific proof that chiropractic worked. But did they?

In the last decade, at least thirty-six controlled trials of spinal manipulation for low-back pain have been conducted. *(See "Neck Manipulation and Stroke")* Some, like the one conducted by T.W. Meade in England, showed long-term benefit of chiropractic for low-back pain,[12] others have shown modest benefit, and still others have shown no significant benefit beyond placebo.

Two major meta-analyses (studies which gather and evaluate all other similar studies) came to different conclusions about whether spinal manipulation was beneficial. Koes looked at all the available evidence in 1991[13] and 1996[14] and found that the studies ranged widely in quality and design. The reviewers concluded that, while there were indications that spinal manipulation might be beneficial for some subgroups of patients with low-back pain, the efficacy of spinal manipulation for patients with acute or chronic low-back pain had not been demonstrated with sound randomized clinical trials.[15] Another set of scientists looked at the same studies and, by analyzing the combined results, came to the conclusion that spinal manipulation is more efficacious than the comparison treatments.[16]

Since those two examinations of the data, several additional studies have been conducted looking at spinal manipulation and other treatments for low-back pain. Unfortunately, the results were mixed, and while the studies added fuel to the debate, they did little to clarify the situation. There was no convincing evidence that spinal manipulation helped with chronic back pain or sciatica. As for acute low-back pain, some studies showed manipulation was effective for short-term pain relief, but others showed no significant benefit. Shekelle, in his review of all the data, concludes that the view he expressed almost a decade earlier still stands:

The addition of these new trials would not seem to alter the conclusions of the prior review and meta-analysis. Based on the available evidence, convincing conclusions cannot be made regarding net benefits of spinal manipulation for patients with chronic low back pain or sciatica.[17]

All of these studies looked at spinal manipulation, not chiropractic. Although chiropractors deliver the vast majority of spinal manipulation — estimates run as high as 90 percent — in Canada and the United States, spinal manipulative therapy is not chiropractic. Most of the studies reviewed by Koes and Shekelle involved manipulation performed by doctors and physiotherapists, not chiropractors. These two reviews did not support chiropractic treatment or the chiropractic profession.

When it is in their interest, chiropractors like to equate spinal manipulation with chiropractic, but they are not one and the same thing. Other practitioners — osteopaths, physiotherapists, and physical therapists — are trained to deliver manipulation and mobilization, and they do so with none of the anti-scientific and pseudo-scientific beliefs that characterize the chiropractic profession.[18] The propensity for chiropractors to use any study supporting spinal manipulation as evidence for chiropractic is clear, and it is nowhere better demonstrated than in the profession's consistent and ongoing misrepresentation of the RAND studies.

Spinning the RAND Studies

The RAND Corporation is a non-profit health science research centre in Santa Monica, California. In the early 1990s, two chiropractic research organizations — the California Chiropractic Foundation and the Foundation for Chiropractic Education and Research — commissioned RAND to study spinal manipulation and back pain.

The highly respected research firm assembled a team of expert physicians and chiropractors, led by Paul G. Shekelle M.D., M.P.H. The multi-part study was named "The Appropriateness of Spinal Manipulation for Low-Back Pain." The panel examined all the published studies on manipulation and low-back pain and analyzed them for effectiveness and complications. They reviewed more than fifty studies; including twenty-five randomized controlled trials of spinal manipulative therapy performed by a variety of health professionals. Only four of the studies involved chiropractic care. In a review of those findings, Shekelle found that for acute and sub-acute uncomplicated low-back pain, "manipulation increased the probability of recovery after two to three weeks of treatment...The benefit disappeared within a few weeks, which is consistent with the natural history of the disease." For chronic low-back pain, or back pain with sciatica (involvement of the sciatic nerve, which runs down the buttocks and legs) the "data was insufficient to evaluate efficacy."[19]

In a commentary that accompanied the study published in the *Annals of Internal Medicine*, San Antonio physician Valerie Lawrence put the findings in perspective, saying that manipulation provides "some early benefit for acute and sub-acute nonspecific low-back pain, but no known long-term benefit: efficacy is unclear for chronic pain or pain with sciatica." She also noted, "This therapy is one of several effective modalities for acute low-back pain including analgesics, 2 days bed rest, physical therapy, and back school [instruction on exercises and techniques for reducing back pain]," adding that the study had not shown any one therapy "clearly superior" to any other.

The nine-member panel (physicians and chiropractors) then studied when manipulation was appropriate in the treatment of low-back pain. They found that out of 1,550 instances, manipulation was appropriate for 112 situations, or about 7 percent of the time. The panel found that manipulation was inappropriate in about 924 circumstances (60 percent of the time) and equivocal for the remaining 514 situations (33 percent of the time).

When was manipulation appropriate? The panel noted that manipulation may be beneficial in cases where the patient has:

- low-back pain for less than three weeks,
- no sciatic nerve irritation (shooting pain in the buttocks, back of thigh and calf),
- no or minor neurological findings,
- and no evidence of a negative reaction to an earlier manipulation.

As well, the panel concluded that care should run for two weeks for each of two different types of manipulation. If there is no improvement, manipulation should stop. The study found no benefit in extended or long-term manipulation. The authors also outlined a long list of situations in which spinal manipulation was not appropriate, including when the patient has:

- no response (or negative response) to manipulation,
- inflammatory arthritis,
- osteomyelitis,
- herniated disc,
- central spinal stenosis,
- spondylolisthesis,
- malignant tumour,

- evidence of infection (such as fever),
- any kind of fracture,
- severe osteoporosis,
- pain for longer than six months,
- or any major neurological findings.

In other words, manipulation may be effective only in the treatment of acute, simple, uncomplicated low-back pain. Shekelle was careful in his conclusion, stating that: "…spinal manipulation is of short-term benefit in some patients, particularly those with uncomplicated acute low-back pain, but that data are insufficient concerning the efficacy of spinal manipulation for chronic low-back pain."[20]

Despite what the authors clearly wrote, chiropractors all over North America viewed the RAND studies as vindications of chiropractic and as scientific evidence supporting chiropractic for back pain. They wasted little time telling the media and the public that RAND has "endorsed" chiropractic. Even today, chiropractors misuse the RAND findings in their claims about the effectiveness of chiropractic and back pain. In fact, RAND says nothing about the effectiveness of chiropractic, but only about spinal manipulation, which in their review was administered for the most part by physiotherapists, doctors, osteopaths, and other manipulative therapists. RAND in no way supported general chiropractic principles or the subluxation theory, long-term manipulation, preventative "maintenance" adjustments, or the wide variety of unproven chiropractic techniques and tools. Chiropractors, at least those who read the study, knew this, but that didn't stop them from using RAND to promote their profession and to drive business. The report's lead authors have criticized chiropractors for inappropriately using the study to support their treatments and ideas.

In a 1993 open letter to the chiropractic profession, Dr. Paul Shekelle said:

> Through RAND's process of monitoring the popular media, we have become aware of numerous instances where our results have been seriously misrepresented by chiropractors writing for their local paper or writing letters to the editor. RAND vigorously defends the integrity of its work, and we have had to write letters to these same newspapers pointedly correcting the misrepresentations. In order to avoid future similar embarrassments to the chiropractic profession, we would like to describe for your readers some common misinterpretations of our work.
>
> **The RAND Study showed that chiropractic is the most effective treatment for low-back pain.**

RAND's results were about spinal manipulation, not chiropractic, and dealt with appropriateness, which is a measure of net benefits and harms. Comparative efficacy of chiropractic and other treatments was not explicitly dealt with.

The RAND study showed that chiropractic is the most cost-effective form of treatment for low-back pain.

Again, RAND's results are specific to spinal manipulation, and cost was specifically excluded from our analyses.

The RAND study showed that patients with low-back pain should first seek care from a doctor of chiropractic.

No mention is made from whom patients should seek care in our work.

The RAND study showed that chiropractic is the best form of care for many common musculoskeletal conditions.

We dealt only with low-back pain, and our results cannot be extrapolated to any other condition.

Any statement that links RAND research with care delivered to injured workers or workers' compensation.

We did not consider injured workers as a separate entity.

RAND showed that there is more good scientific evidence supporting chiropractic than there is for medical procedures.

Again, our work was specific to spinal manipulation, not the practice of chiropractic.

It is true that there is more evidence to support the use of spinal manipulation as a treatment for some patients with low-back pain than there is for many medical procedures currently being used. It is not true that there is more evidence to support the use of spinal manipulation (or chiropractic) than there is to support the practice of medicine.

What can be concluded from RAND's research is:

There is enough scientific evidence to justify the use of spinal manipulation for some patients with acute low-back pain. It is the judgment of a multi-disciplinary group of back pain experts, based on the scientific literature and their clinical experience, that spinal manipulation is ... appropriate ... for some patients with low-back pain.[21]

Shekelle's conclusions in the RAND studies are in no way an endorsement of chiropractic, yet today, ten years after their publication, they continue to be misrepresented by the profession.

Chiropractic Reviewed and Found Wanting

Only a few studies have specifically examined the benefit of chiropractic treatment on low-back pain. In 1996, Assendelft systematically reviewed the literature and, after an exhaustive search, found eight randomized clinical trials involving chiropractic. Four examined patients with chronic pain, and the remaining four looked at chronic and acute low-back pain. All the studies had design flaws, and the results were mixed. In the end, the study's authors concluded that their review failed to find convincing evidence for the effectiveness of chiropractic for acute or chronic low-back pain, and that higher quality studies would be needed before firm conclusions for or against the effectiveness of chiropractic could be reached.[22]

More recent studies have confirmed those findings. A 1998 study compared patients with low-back pain who were treated by being given either chiropractic manipulation, McKenzie method physical therapy, or simply a book on back exercises to read.[23] The two treatment groups reported marginally better short-term pain relief at the four-week mark, but there were no significant differences among the three groups through the fifty-two-week study in their ability to function or in disability.

It would appear, based on the evidence, that people with acute low-back pain get better at pretty much the same rate no matter whom they see for treatment. Timothy Carey, a researcher at the University of North Carolina, looked at what happened to 1,633 low-back pain patients who saw a primary care practitioner, a chiropractor, or an orthopedic surgeon over six months. He found that the recovery time and the time in which patients returned to work was similar for all practitioners.[24]

Carey concluded that, in general, research does not support manual or physical therapy as the primary intervention for acute low-back pain, though he found it was not harmful and sometimes led to greater patient satisfaction.

Carey's study is also consistent with the recommendations issued by the Agency for Health Care Policy and Research (AHCPR) in 1994, which advocated simple treatments (such as nonprescription painkillers and mild exercise followed by conditioning exercises, beginning two weeks after pain first occurs) for most cases of acute low-back pain. The guidelines noted that nine out of ten patients with acute low-back pain will recover on their own within a month.[25]

So, according to the best scientific evidence available, almost all people suffering from low-back pain get better on their own, with no help from health care professionals. If they seek help, the evidence indicates that the results are similar no matter what kind of treatment they receive, including just reading a book about back care! And finally, despite all the claims of the chiropractic community, there is not any convincing evidence that chiropractic specifically is effective for either acute or chronic low-back pain.

Yeah, But It's Cost Effective

The chiropractic community makes claims in their advertisements, brochures, and Web sites that chiropractic care for low-back pain is not only effective, but cost-effective. For example, promotional material put out by Alberta chiropractors under the title "Chiropractors: Here to help you Get Back into Action!" claims, "Numerous research studies have confirmed that chiropractic care is one of the most effective, safe and cost-efficient methods of health care available."[26] In fact, no studies have concluded that chiropractic care specifically is effective for low-back pain. And more cost-efficient? Though chiropractic promotional material often states that chiropractic is more cost-effective, the evidence around cost is mixed. Chiropractors often use a 1993 report funded by the Ontario Ministry of Health to bolster their claim of cost-effectiveness. The report, known simply as the Manga Report, after its lead author, economist Pran Manga, is actually called "The Effectiveness and Cost-Effectiveness of Chiropractic Management of Low-Back Pain." The report makes a number of sweeping conclusions, including:

- spinal manipulation applied by chiropractors is shown to be more effective than alternate treatments for low-back pain
- there was some evidence in the literature to suggest that spinal manipulations are less safe and less effective when performed by non-chiropractic professionals
- there is an "overwhelming body of evidence" indicating that chiropractic management of low-back pain is more cost-effective than medical management
- and hundreds of millions of dollars would be saved annually if the management of low-back pain were transferred from doctors to chiropractors.[27]

The problem with Manga's report is that he arrives at conclusions that are unsupported by the studies he examined. First, major reviews of the literature like the one done by epidemiologist B.W. Koes in 1996 looked at all the randomized controlled trials and concluded, "The efficacy of spinal manipulation for patients with acute or chronic low-back pain has not been demonstrated with sound randomized clinical trials. There certainly are indications that manipulation might be effective in some subgroups of patients with low-back pain. These impressions justify additional research efforts on this topic."[28] Like the RAND researchers and others, Manga examined studies on spinal manipulation performed for the most part by doctors and physiotherapists, not chiropractors. Yet Manga claims that spinal manipulation may be "less safe and less effective when performed by non-chiropractic professionals."[29] Other researchers looking at the same material did not find evidence that chiropractors deliver safer manipulation than physicians or physiotherapists.

And finally, other researchers who have examined the same data did not find, as Manga did, "overwhelming" evidence that chiropractic is cost effective. A review of the data by Shekelle found that "The relative cost-effectiveness of chiropractic care and medical care has not been convincingly established,"[30] and another overview of the profession by Cherkin and Mootz similarly noted that "it is not yet clear if chiropractic care is more cost-effective than the various forms of conventional medical care (e.g., medications, physical therapy, exercise programs) or alternative care (e.g., massage or acupuncture) used to treat back pain."[31]

Advertisements for chiropractic care note that patients are very satisfied with the care that chiropractors provide and research supports the idea that patients are often pleased with chiropractic care for their low-back pain. In several studies comparing treatments, recovery and recurrence rates were similar for all providers, but the patients treated by chiropractors reported greater satisfaction with their care.[32] [33] But researchers such as Carey raise an interesting issue. If the benefit of manipulative therapy for acute low-back pain is "minimal" or "modest," as he points out, is it worth the extra cost to private and public health insurance plans? He asks, "Is improved satisfaction worth an additional several hundred dollars per patient? Are resources better spent on patients with spinal disease who might receive more benefit?"[34]

Why were patients who visited chiropractors more satisfied? One of the answers may be that chiropractors are more confident than doctors and other health care practitioners about their ability to help back pain.[35] But is their confidence supported by the facts? Chiropractors are more confident than medical doctors about what they can do for low-back pain, but that confidence does not translate into faster recovery. Chiropractors' high patient satisfaction may stem from their communication skills, the amount of time they spend with patients and the effect of a "hands-on" treatment, particularly for patients with chronic pain.

So, chiropractic care for low-back pain is not more cost-effective than other treatments, despite the repeated claims by chiropractors and their organizations. And it is considerably more expensive than simpler treatments that have the same results.

As physician Valerie Lawrence wrote in a journal commentary after considering the latest evidence, "Because no therapy is clearly superior, economic evaluation is important. To fully assess cost-effectiveness, we need more information on benefits and potential risks. Without proven benefit in preventing recurrences or chronic disabling pain, bed rest may remain the most cost-effective, conservative therapy."[36]

The bottom line is that the vast majority of people who have acute low-back pain get better all by themselves. The 1994 Agency for Health Care Policy and Research (AHCPR) guidelines noted that nine out of ten patients suffering from acute low-back pain will recover on their own within a month. The report said if patients use over-the-counter pain medication and do some basic back conditioning exercises, they'll do just fine, and they'll save the system in the United States as much as $5 billion annually.[37]

Appropriate Care?

A generous assessment of the scientific evidence would be that spinal manipulation may be of benefit to some patients with uncomplicated acute low-back pain. And even that conclusion is based on studies in which patients were carefully examined and screened for any contraindications to manipulation. What kind of treatment they received and how many treatments they received were was also carefully monitored and controlled. Unfortunately, none of these safeguards is in place in the real world.

Chiropractor and author Samuel Homola recommends seeing your family doctor first to establish that your back pain is mechanical and uncomplicated. If you and your physician can identify a "rational chiropractor who uses spinal manipulation appropriately," then you may want to try the treatment. "But," warns Homola in his book *Inside Chiropractic: A Patient's Guide*,[38] "you must be prepared to deal with the nonsense that is so often associated with chiropractic treatment." And there is a lot of nonsense in chiropractic today. Just finding a chiropractor who does not make false claims and who practices scientifically may be difficult. A recent study showed that the largest chiropractic organizations in Canada and the United States, representing the majority of working chiropractors, continue to make unsubstantiated and sometimes outlandish claims for chiropractic.[39]

As well, only about 19 percent of chiropractors in Canada limit their practice to manipulation for musculoskeletal problems.[40] And even if they limit their practice, there's no guarantee that they are using the kind of hands-on spinal manipulation evaluated in the studies. In Canada, most chiropractors use a grab-bag of therapies, including many so-called "name techniques," that have little or no evidence of effectiveness. For example, almost 38 percent of chiropractors surveyed in Canada use a hand-held tool called an Activator to deliver so-called chiropractic adjustments to the spine.[41] There are no scientific studies that support the effectiveness of Activator, or any other "Name techniques" for low-back pain. *(See "Gizmos, Parlour Tricks, and Nonsense")*

Critics of chiropractic have also accused chiropractors of overtreating. Most studies indicate that if spinal manipulation helps, it will be of benefit within a month. There is currently no evidence that ongoing manipulation, known to chiropractors as "maintenance care," is of any benefit for back pain. Despite this lack of evidence, many chiropractors recommend maintenance care, which they believe will reduce recurrences, particularly for musculoskeletal problems.[42] Surveys of chiropractors in Australia and the United States reveal that more than 90 percent of them believe maintenance care is effective. Eight out of ten chiropractors believe that one of the functions of maintenance care is to identify and remove subluxations of the spine by chiropractic adjustment.[43] The problem is that repeated tests of chiropractors have revealed that none of the tests they use to find and correct subluxations is reliable or valid. As one study put it, "Because such tests have not been established, the presence of the manipulable lesion remains hypothetical."[44] In plain language, most chiropractors believe in unproven maintenance adjustments of an unproven entity — the subluxation — that they cannot reliably detect!

In addition, studies indicate that despite published guidelines, chiropractors continue to overuse x-rays on patients who report low-back pain. A British survey found chiropractors x-rayed 71 percent of patients with low-back pain, and an American survey indicated 96 percent of all new patients were x-rayed. "The usage of X-rays by chiropractors seems exorbitantly high, particularly considering that experts on low-back pain uniformly agree that plain radiographs are usually not useful in this condition," wrote a researcher who examined the issue.[45] Not only are radiographs rarely helpful in the treatment of low-back pain, but exposure to x-ray is indisputably a cause of increased risk of cancer. Despite these facts, studies indicate that some patients receive multiple x-rays when being treated by chiropractors.[46]

Finally, though the risk of serious harm from low-back spinal manipulation is extremely low, the treatment is not without side effects. A recent study examining the complications of spinal manipulation presented some surprising findings. The 1997 study looked at 102 Norwegian chiropractors who treated 1,058 new patients. "After an average of about 4.5 visits, 55 percent of the patients reported at least one reaction to the manipulation. The most commonly reported reactions were: local discomfort (53 percent), headache (12 percent), tiredness (11 percent), and radiating discomfort (10 percent). Only 15 percent of reactions were considered "severe" and no serious complications were reported."[47] Twelve of the patients considered their discomfort unbearable.

Backing Out of Back Treatment

While chiropractic organizations in Canada and the United States trumpet the expertise of their members in treating low-back pain and the "proven" effectiveness of chiropractic treatment, chiropractors themselves aren't really sure they want to be known as back experts at all.

In fact, chiropractors are not back experts. They are not back specialists in the way that orthopods or orthopedic surgeons or neurologists can be. Chiropractors cannot deal with a wide range of potential problems of the back and spine, including trauma, compression fractures, herniated discs, spinal stenosis (narrowing of the spinal canal), spinal arthritis, kyphosis, scoliosis, spinal tumours, or any kind of neurological damage or disease.

They are, by their own definition, a separate, alternative health profession "directed toward maintaining, improving, restoring or enhancing the health of the patient, through the use of chiropractic adjustments and related therapies, primarily to the musculoskeletal system, in order to affect the neural regulation of the body."[48] If that doesn't sound much like the treatment of uncomplicated, mechanical low-back pain using hands-on manipulation, it's because it isn't. Most chiropractors do not want to be considered "back doctors," and some are outspoken about it. A pamphlet put out by a Calgary chiropractor lists one of the "Top 10 Myths About Chiropractic": "Chiropractors treat back pain only. Some doctors do, but that is like changing your motor oil only when your engine is smoking. The best Doctor of Chiropractic corrects the subluxations of the spine."[49] In a letter to the editor of *The Medical Post*, one chiropractor objected to the inclusion of chiropractors in a list of practitioners dealing with low-back pain. "It [chiropractic] was not intended as a treatment for back pain...," he wrote. He then went on to explain that the role of the chiropractor is to remove "interference" in the nervous system so the body can regulate itself. "This has absolutely nothing to do with treating low back pain... Rest assured, low back pain is NOT our forte, nor is it our direction as a profession."[50] Though not quite as direct, official materials from the Ontario Chiropractic Association and the Canadian Chiropractic Association carry the same message. Chiropractors adjust the spine to ensure proper alignment so the nervous system can work properly and allow the body to heal itself. As an OCA pamphlet explains, "These adjustments help return your spine to optimum health by restoring and maintaining nerve and joint function.[51] In terms of chiropractic philosophy, the fact that spinal manipulative therapy may help with back pain is not much more than a happy coincidence.

In fact, some chiropractors feel that focusing on the treatment of back pain could not be a worse mistake. If chiropractors leave behind the philosophy of chiropractic — the belief in subluxation and Innate Intelligence in the body — and concentrate on exploring the possible benefits of spinal manipulative therapy they could be, as one chiropractic student warned, "destined to become third-rate medical doctors specializing in back pain and headaches."[52] Right now, they're not even that.

9

SO, HOW DID THEY BECOME DOCTORS ANYWAY?
Chiropractors Lobby Their Way to Legitimacy

Since chiropractors began practicing in Canada at the beginning of the twentieth century, they have had one overriding goal: to become recognized health professionals. Today, in every province in Canada, they have achieved the status of a regulated health profession with the right to use the title "doctor." In five provinces, their services are at least partially covered by provincial health insurance programs.

From the very start in 1900, when only a few chiropractors had offices in the province of Ontario, they began to lobby for legislative control, to fight for legal recognition of the profession. This is important because here, as in the United States, where the profession began, chiropractors have worked hard for legitimacy. Their efforts to legitimize themselves scientifically and to test their theories, validate their clinical procedures, and conduct research have been minimal (and, in some cases, non-existent). However, their work to curry public favour and to influence lawmakers has been relentless. Sociologist Leslie Biggs documents how chiropractors in Ontario intensely lobbied politicians and the public in their fight against restrictive legislation.[1] Ralph Lee, author of *At Your Own Risk*, writes, "From its infancy chiropractic looked to politics and licensing, not as a way of working with science but as a protection against science."[2]

The story of chiropractic's efforts to obtain legal recognition in Canada is characterized by a series of repetitive encounters with legislative bodies, committees, boards of inquiry, and commissions. After their appearance before a 1915 Royal Commission headed up by Mr. Justice Frank E. Hodgins, which was an "unmitigated disaster," the chiropractors became incrementally better and better at presenting their case. *(See "Are Chiropractors Back Doctors?")* The profession was set back, but over the next two decades, chiropractic in Canada grew and continued to push for standing. Two things helped them along: a recognition that the relatively new art of "physical therapy" helped injured people rehabilitate and organized medicine's general lack of interest in learning about it.

Chiropractors and chiropractic historians like to describe the development of chiropractic in Canada and the United States in terms of a battle with organized medicine. While it is true that doctors worked hard to block chiropractors' attempts to further their standing and scope of practice, it is incorrect to see their clashes as merely part of a professional "turf war." Many medical doctors opposed chiropractic then, as they do now, on grounds that the fundamental premise of chiropractic is unsupported by scientific fact.

Chiropractic histories paint medicine's charges that chiropractic was riddled with quackery as part of medicine's persecution of their profession. But the charge in the early twentieth century that chiropractic was largely quackery was factual. As chiropractic historian Joseph Keating Jr. states, the profession has a long tradition of making unjustified claims.[3] More than one hundred years later, despite their official standing in every Canadian province and American state, the leading chiropractic associations continue to make false and unsupported claims about the benefits of chiropractic. These claims in patient brochures — not much different from the exaggerated promises of benefit and cure of a century ago — "meet several of the formal criteria for quackery."[4]

Many Defeats and a Few Key Victories

On April 11, 1925, chiropractors in Ontario (where the large majority of Canada's practitioners resided), were registered along with naturopaths and osteopaths under the Drugless Practitioner's Act. The act restricted them from using the title "doctor" and gave them a limited scope of practice. After several practitioners were jailed for calling themselves doctors, chiropractors abided by the rules. In 1935, the Drugless Practitioners Act was amended to include physiotherapists, and at the same time osteopaths and chiropractors were given more rights, including diagnosis within their range of expertise.

Chiropractic grew rapidly in the next decades, particularly after the opening of the Canadian Memorial Chiropractic College in Toronto in 1945. Veterans, among others, took the chiropractic course, and their numbers grew so quickly that by the late 1940s there were about five hundred chiropractors in Canada. They were regulated in five of the ten provinces, with Manitoba, Alberta, Saskatchewan, British Columbia, and Ontario all having passed regulations that governed the profession.

Things remained more or less static until 1952, when Ontario granted each profession under the Drugless Practitioners Act its own board. The Board of Directors of Chiropractic came into being, but at the same time the government clamped down on unethical advertising and did not return control over advertising to the chiropractors for a decade.

In the late 1950s, the chiropractors in Ontario worked hard on a plan for chiropractic legislation, which recommended raising them to the same level as doctors and dentists. It was presented to the minister of health in 1957 and promptly dropped out of sight.

In the 1960s, two major inquiries looked at chiropractic, one in Quebec and one in Ontario. The federal government's Royal Commission on Health Services, chaired by Justice Emmett Hall and known as the Hall Commission, considered submissions by chiropractors and by the medical profession. The commission received papers from various medical bodies and academic institutions that rightly criticized chiropractic for its glaring shortcomings. The Faculty of Medicine at McGill University stated that the "theory which underlies chiropractic is false, and no consistently successful practice can be expected to result from a false theory."[5] A report prepared earlier by the College of Physicians and Surgeons of Ontario, written by Warwick Noble, stated that chiropractic was "built upon a foundation of sand" and that it would likely, along with osteopathy, "disintegrate and collapse."[6]

Hall also received evidence, in the form of printed material, that chiropractors were making claims for which there was no clinical justification. In response, "advertising regulations were strengthened and literature available through chiropractors' offices was reviewed, whether it originated in Canada or the United States. All printed material not meeting standards set by the Board of Directors of Chiropractic was banned."[7]

This undertaking to "clean up" advertising in the profession was no doubt impressive to lawmakers, but, as we have seen, had almost no effect on the penchant for chiropractors to make false and unsubstantiated claims.

Hall decided the scientific controversy surrounding chiropractic was bigger than his commission and deferred to a similar inquiry in Quebec, known as the Royal Commission on Chiropraxy and Osteopathy, being chaired by Mr. Justice Gerard Lacroix. In the meantime, despite not having ruled on the scientific validity of chiropractic, Hall recommended that chiropractic services be included on an interim basis in the province's health insurance plan as long as they were prescribed by a medical doctor. He would wait until the

Lacroix Commission, which he felt was conducting an independent scientific study, to make his final decision.

Unfortunately, Lacroix, who was a lawyer, was not conducting a scientific inquiry, but rather a survey of legislative issues. Once again, chiropractic was not evaluated scientifically, but rather from a legal and social point of view.

The Lacroix Commission found that a spinal diagnosis was not good enough to protect people, but that chiropractors were not skilled or educated enough to make a differential diagnosis. That's a diagnosis in which the doctor identifies the disease afflicting that patient from among the full spectrum of human ailments. He called for chiropractors to retain their manipulation technique and recommended beefing up their education. To protect the public, he recommended the profession be regulated and controlled. Eight years later, in 1973, the Chiropractic Act in Quebec was adopted, allowing chiropractors not to make a differential diagnosis but to conduct tests to determine if a patient requires chiropractic care.

In Ontario, though the Hall Commission had deferred to the findings of Lacroix, the government did not find the Quebec inquiry's findings very helpful. So, once again, another inquiry was launched, this one called the Committee on the Healing Arts. After hearing numerous submissions and conducting its own research, it ruled that it could not accept the soundness of chiropractic theory and expressed doubt about the ability of chiropractors to do a differential diagnosis. The committee proposed that before chiropractic treatment could begin, a patient get a differential diagnosis from a medical doctor. The chiropractors objected and the recommendation was never put into effect. The committee felt that there was benefit in manipulative therapy and cautioned doctors not to interfere with the rights of patients who wanted chiropractic care.

In 1970, a new health minister adopted the minority position of the Committee on the Healing Arts and granted coverage for chiropractic in the province's health insurance plan without a prior medical examination. This essentially gave chiropractors the ability to be front-line health care practitioners, able to see patients without a referral. This, and a later task force, both arrived at the conclusion that chiropractors were able to "distinguish disorders that fall within their scope of practice from those which should be referred to other health disciplines."[8]

It is clear in reviewing the Hall and Lacroix commission findings that both inquiries assumed that chiropractic would limit itself to problems of the musculoskeletal system. Their judgments make it clear that they saw chiropractic as a profession specializing in manipulation and focusing on the bones and muscles of the body. There is no indication anywhere in the long history of commissions and inquiries that lawmakers saw chiropractic as an alternative form of health care, in which removal of subluxations could cure disease and benefit overall health. Although this, as we have seen, is the very foundation of chiropractic, it is missing from any legislation surrounding the practice.

Oddly, it was Warwick Noble, the lawyer who wrote the report for the College of Physicians and Surgeons of Ontario in 1958, who understood the inherent dichotomy of chiropractic theory and practice that in some ways defied any kind of meaningful regulation. He warned that chiropractors were "limited as to method but unlimited as to the disease or diseases they might treat."[9]

Through the 1980s and 1990s, chiropractic grew in Canada, spreading from Ontario into every province and territory. In 1991, Ontario, the province where chiropractic began in Canada, granted it full self-regulation under the Regulated Health Professions Act. The other Canadian provinces have similar legislation in place, Newfoundland being the last to introduce regulations. Chiropractors continue to lobby for broader testing rights, the use of laboratory facilities, and hospital privileges. As in the past, they approach these challenges legally and legislatively.

Throughout its struggle for acceptance, the profession has focused its attention on the appearance rather than the reality of the profession. When, in the 1940s, the provinces began discussion of a national health insurance plan, the chiropractors responded quickly and decisively. Chiropractic leaders believed that chiropractic would disappear if it were not included in a government-sponsored plan, so they embarked on a campaign to improve their image and convince legislators and the public that they offered a valid service.[10] Similarly, the CMCC, which was first dominated by subluxation-based or "straight" chiropractors, realized in the 1950s that it had to clean up its image. Sociologist Leslie Biggs writes:

> CMCC adopted a secular and scientific definition of chiropractic that they believed would allow them to appear more credible before the various government inquiries into health care.[11]

Throughout their struggle for legitimacy and their battles with medicine, chiropractors have focused on political lobbying and pubic relations to advance the profession. Their victories in the legislative arena have papered over the deep and serious holes in their philosophy and clinical practice.

10

GIZMOS, PARLOUR TRICKS, AND NONSENSE
Many Chiropractors are Suckers for Gadgets and Outlandish Treatments

Techniques, Techniques, and More Techniques

Imagine for a minute that when you went to the dentist, you had to ask what kind of dentistry she practiced. Imagine that you needed to ask what specific technique of dentistry she used. Now, imagine that the list of dentistry techniques would fill a page in this book, and that none of them would have any scientific evidence showing that they actually worked. Nothing, not a single scientific study that showed that the particular technique or group of techniques that your dentist swore by was effective.

That's the state of chiropractic today in Canada, the United States, and abroad. Chiropractic is not only split over the subluxation (with the majority for it), it is a jumbled hodge-podge of techniques, most of which claim to locate and remove subluxations more effectively. They are called "Name Brand" or more simply "Name" techniques because most of them are named after the individual developer who cooked them up. Samuel Homola, a retired science-based chiropractor and author, nicely described the almost comical variety of conflicting theories and claims on the modern chiropractic landscape:

> Some techniques are focused on the head, some on the neck, some on the lower spine, some on several spinal areas, and some on the entire spine. Yet all are claimed to "work" and some chiropractic

educators suggest that all adjustive techniques that "remove nerve interference" have value. The claim that diametrically opposite techniques are equally effective in improving health is absurd and suggests that few have any real value.[1]

This aspect of chiropractic is seldom, if ever, mentioned in position papers or reports to government agencies, public or private insurers, academic institutions, or the general public. And in advertising copy or articles intended for public consumption, the chiropractic leadership either ignores or carefully slides over the fact that the profession is made up of hundreds of separate, incompatible, and often mutually exclusive techniques, all huddled under the umbrella of chiropractic. When Canadian Chiropractic Association president David Leprich wrote his article "Everything you wanted to know about chiropractic..." for *The Medical Post* in February 2000, he did not even mention the proliferation of Name techniques nor their ubiquitous presence in the profession.[2]

Chiropractic techniques, and the gadgets often associated with them, have a long history in the profession. Within a few years of its conception by D.D. Palmer, chiropractors began to introduce new versions, derivations, and spin-offs of the fundamental practice. Schools of chiropractic that were competitive with the Palmer school sprung up across America, each teaching and advocating their own version of his spine-centred therapy. This annoyed and sometimes frustrated D.D., but he too was guilty of profoundly changing his own views on chiropractic several times in the years after 1895. D.D's son, B.J. Palmer, invented a Name technique of his own (Hole-in-One, which is still practiced today) and one of the first widely used diagnostic gadgets, the neurocalometer, the offspring of which are used in chiropractic offices all over Canada and the United States. *(See "The P.T. Barnum of Chiropractic")*

But even the Palmers would have been amazed, and perhaps dismayed, at the hundreds of techniques used in the modern profession, all presented to patients as "chiropractic."

Homola estimates that as many as two hundred Name techniques have been developed, with about half that many still used in modern chiropractic. That number does not include the personal refinements or interpretations that many chiropractors apply to the techniques. Chiropractic historian Joseph Keating Jr. assembled a list of chiropractic techniques. It is worth reproducing, if only for its sheer breathtaking scope. The 1993 list, which Keating admits is incomplete, has doubtlessly grown since then:

Activator Methods

Anatomical Adjustive Technique

Applied Kinesiology

Applied Spinal Biomechanical
Engineering

Aquarian Age Healing

Atlas Orthogonality

BioEnergetic Synchronization
Technique (BEST)

Buxton's Painless Chiropractic

Carver Body Drop

Chiropractic Biophysics

Chiropractic Manipulative Reflex
Technique (CMRT/SOT)

Concept Theory

Cox Flexion Distraction

Cranial Therapy

Derefield Leg Analysis

Derma-thermograph

Dermathermoscribe

Directional Non-Force Technique
(DNFT/Van Rumpt)

Diversified Adjusting

Educational Kinesiology

Gonstead Adjusting

Gravel Integrated Chiropractic
Model

Grostic Technique

Harrison Dynamic Visualization
Procedure

Herring Cervical Technique

Hole-In-One (HIO/Palmer)

Inverse Myotatic Technique

Keck System

Life Upper Cervical Adjusting
Instrument (Williams)

Logan Basic Technique

Mears Technique

Meric System (Palmer)

Micro-Manipulation

Motion-Palpation (Passive)

Naprapathy (Oakley Smith)

Nervoscope

Neural Organization Technique
(NOT)

Neuro-Vascular Dynamics (NVD)

Neurocalometer, neurocalograph
(Evins, B.J. Palmer)

Neuropathy (A.P. Davis)

Nimmo Technique

Palmer Diversified

Palmer Upper Cervical Specific

Palmer System (Jim Palmer)

Pettibon Technique

Pierce-Stillwagon Technique

Postural Method of Adjusting
(Carver)

Receptor Techniques (DeJarnette)

Reflexology

RESULTS System (Pierce)

Sacro-Occipital Technique
(SOT, DeJarnette)

Soft Tissue Orthopedics
(STO/SOT)

Spears Painless Technique

Spinology (Gold)

Stressology (Ward)

Structural Approach
(Carver, Levine)

Sweat Adjusting Instrument

Thompson Technique
(drop-piece table)

Toftness Technique

Toggle-Recoil (Palmer)

Total Body Modification (TBM,
Frank)

Vector Point Cranial Therapy

Zone Therapy[3]

Who Uses Them?

Is this alphabet soup of techniques used only by fringe practitioners? No — in fact, various surveys of chiropractors have found that a large majority employ Name techniques in their practices. A 1993 survey of chiropractors in Canada found that although 87.3 percent used Diversified technique (a variety of adjustive techniques and the core of CMCC's teaching) many used Name techniques. The chiropractors surveyed utilized a wide variety of techniques:

- 44.2 percent SacroOccipital Technique
- 43.6 percent Activator
- 37.3 percent Meric
- 35 percent Gonstead
- 32.4 percent NIMMO/tonus receptor
- 31 percent Applied Kinesiology
- 30 percent Thompson
- 25.9 percent Logan Basic
- 22.4 percent Cox/Flexion-Distraction
- 22.3 percent Palmer HIO
- 22.2 percent Cranial
- 15.5 percent other

Chiropractors admit that there isn't much evidence for the main technique used by the majority of chiropractors in Canada, Diversified, but there's even less for everything else. Most techniques are part diagnostic and part treatment, and there's not much evidence to back up either part in all of these Name approaches. As Brian Gleberzon, a professor at CMCC, says, "...good quality research comprising this evidence is sparse for every technique, Diversified included."[4] When he did a literature search, he didn't find much to support the long list of techniques:

> Advocates of particular "Name Techniques" often assert that there is an abundance of evidence to substantiate their claims of a technique's clinical efficacy. Sadly, upon further exploration, this abundance of articles is often nowhere to be found...[5]

That wouldn't be so bad if the techniques were innocuous variations on spinal manipulation, but they are anything but. In fact, most Name techniques are based upon the notions of subluxation and Innate Intelligence, both of which are unproven theories underpinning chiropractic. The proponents of these techniques usually invent some inspired derivation on the idea of vitalism (the idea that organisms contain an unseen, immeasurable life force or energy).

This leaves chiropractic awash in what Keating calls "technique anarchy,"[6] in which anything goes. Chiropractor Lon Morgan says the profession has an almost infinite number of incoherent and conflicting methods to find subluxations and then an equal number of exotic ways to get rid of them. There is no scientific evidence to support any of them, says Morgan. He says the modern world is drowning in unproven alternative health fads and laments:

> To this could be added Concept and Network chiropractic, plus the rest of the chiropractic alphabet soup of NET, BEST, SOT, AK, etc. All claim to treat via Innate and all have utterly failed independent, objective examination.[7]

It is beyond the scope of this book to analyze all the Name techniques used by chiropractors, but a description of the origins and theories of a handful will provide some insight into the utterly bizarre world of chiropractic techniques.

Cranialsacral Therapy

Proponents of Cranialsacral Therapy believe that rhythmic impulses run through the fluid that surrounds the spinal cord and brain. They suggest that restrictions in the bones of the cranium or skull affect the rhythm and cause ill health, including colic, learning disabilities, and epilepsy. Therapists believe that they can detect imbalance in the rhythm of the cerebrospinal fluid and that they can manipulate the skull bones to correct it. The British Columbia Office of Health Technology Assessment commissioned a large-scale review and critical appraisal of cranialsacral therapy in 1999. The fifty-six-page study concluded that there was no evidence that therapists could detect rhythms, nor that practitioners could manipulate the bones of the skull. They found that some brain-injured patients had suffered adverse effects from the treatment and that there was no evidence of health benefit for anyone.[8]

Neural Organization Technique (NOT)

A spinoff of cranialsacral therapy, NOT was the brainchild of New York chiropractor Carl A. Ferreri. He decided that misaligned skull bones created blockages in the "neural pathways" and caused serious problems such as learning disabilities, schizophrenia, cerebral palsy, and even Down's syndrome. In 1988, NOT practitioners conducted a five-month "research" program in a Del Norte County, California school on children aged four to sixteen. The children endured painful "adjustments" to their heads, their eyes, and the roofs of their mouths. The treatments had no beneficial effects. The parents of some of the children filed a lawsuit over the treatment against Ferreri, and a jury ordered the chiropractor to pay half a million dollars in damages. Two other chiropractors involved settled out of court for a total of $207,000.[9]

Applied Kinesiology

Applied Kinesiology (AK) was founded by a Michigan chiropractor named George Goodheart. In his clinical practice, Goodheart began to believe that weak or dysfunctional organs had a corresponding weak muscle. Using a technique invented by chiropractor Terrence Bennett, Goodheart stimulated "reflex points" to make the weak muscles stronger. Then Goodheart treated a young woman with chronic headaches and noticed that her cranial bones seemed out of place. He knew of the work of another chiropractor, William G. Sutherland, who postulated that the "bones of the skull move like the gills of a fish as one breathes." Goodheart adjusted her head and cured her headache.

Goodheart went on to hypothesize that there were fourteen different kinds of cranial misalignments that were associated with particular problems in the body. But he didn't stop there. In the early 1960s, he integrated the work of several other chiropractors to come up with his main idea — that every organ dysfunction is linked to a specific muscle weakness. So, AK practitioners check for muscle weakness — usually by pushing down on an outstretched arm — to test for things like food allergies and nutritional deficiencies. Some practitioners even perform "surrogate" AK, by pressing down on the arm of a parent who is holding hands with a child.

Neurovascular Dynamics (NVD)

This form of treatment was created by chiropractor Terrence Bennett in the 1930s in California. Bennett was treating patients using the Aquarian Age Healing concepts of two chiropractors from Hollywood named Helen Sanders and John Hurley. Adapting their theory and adding his own ideas, Bennett came up with an extraordinary concept. He hypothesized that "remnants of the embryological pulse existed in humans and could be palpated at a fine rhythm of approximately 70 beats per minute." He felt that when pulse centres were activated by touching them, a stimulation of blood supply to specific areas of the body could be achieved and organ function enhanced or restored. His technique, also called Autonomic Nerve Control, was popular from the late 1940s to the 1970s.[10]

Logan Basic Technique

Created by chiropractor Hugh Logan, who ran his own school in St. Louis, the Logan Basic College of Chiropractic, this technique was founded on Logan's view that subluxations in the spine are a result of body distortions caused by unequal leg lengths, sacral subluxation, and problems in the fifth lumbar vertebra. Logan held that the lower spine, particularly the sacrum, had to be adjusted before any other subluxations could be corrected.

Grostic Procedure

Invented by chiropractor John F. Grostic, this technique focuses on the top of the spine, looking for subluxations between the atlas and the skull. The patient receives pre-treatment x-rays to detect the subluxations and x-rays immediately after the adjustment to confirm that the subluxation has been reduced. This whole area of treating subluxations of the atlas, considered the most important subluxation, is known as atlas orthogonality, and an entire association — the National Upper Cervical Association (NUCCA) — has developed around it. The cervical adjustments can be applied by hand or delivered by a tabletop adjusting device.

Activator Methods

Invented by chiropractor Arlan Fuhr, Activator Methods Chiropractic Technique (AMCT) uses a small, hand-held, spring-loaded device to deliver adjustments. Fuhr teaches that "pelvic deficiency" or "functional short leg" is a common problem and indicates subluxations in the spine. The technique also teaches that adjustment of subluxations in certain vertebrae can produce kidney problems, migraines, ulcers, and other conditions. Tapping the proper spot with the Activator removes nerve interference and allows the body to return to health.

Directional Non-Force Technique (Van Rumpt)

In the 1960s, a chiropractor named Richard Van Rumpt was using a "double thumb-lock" adjusting procedure and checking leg length before and after adjusting. This technique, still practiced today, supposedly corrects subluxations by applying thumb pressure to the spine and using a small wooden dowel to press between the vertebrae. Chiropractors using this technique recommend maintenance and preventative adjustments. In his seminars to chiropractors, Van Rumpt also introduced something he called "Dropping the Bomb," a procedure that "involved the chiropractor standing at and observing the patient's feet and mentally asking Innate Intelligence to communicate the locations and listings of subluxation via changes in the relative lengths of the patient's legs."[11]

Thompson Technique

Also known as Thompson Terminal Point Technique, this particular form of chiropractic was developed by J. Clay Thompson, a chiropractor who was the head of research at the Palmer College for years. Thompson based his work on the leg length testing technique of another chiropractor, Romer Derifield. Derifield believed leg lengths of some patients changed when they turned their heads left or right, indicating cervical subluxations. Similarly, testing bent-leg and straight-leg length helped Derifield determine back subluxations. Thompson used this test, but added in the drop-table, a special chiropractor's table that drops a short distance when an adjustment is made. Thompson postulated that subluxations "contracted" the leg, creating what he termed "leg length inequality" (LLI), but provided no evidence for this rationale. As well, many studies on the reliability of Thompson-like leg check procedures have failed. There are no studies that demonstrate clinical effectiveness of the Thompson Technique.[12]

The Meric System

This system of chiropractic relates subluxations at various levels of the spine with specific organs and diseases. Developed in part by B.J. Palmer, this system was based on the idea that clearing subluxations at specific joints in the spine would clear disease in the corresponding organ. All this was illustrated on large wall charts that the Palmer College supplied, which were popular in chiropractic offices in the 1960s and 1970s.[13]

Bio-Energetic Synchronization Technique (B.E.S.T.)

This system, taught by the Morter Clinic in Rogers, Arkansas, holds that there are internal communicating energy fields in the body traveling along innate pathways. If there is electromagnetic imbalance — manifested by uneven leg length — then the practitioner can correct these blockages by carefully applying his own electromagnetic energy through his hands at certain contact points on the patient's body. Two fingers on the hand are "magnetic North seeking" and two are "magnetic South seeking" and the thumb is neutral. The practitioner applies his hands and then waits until he perceives a synchronization of pulses in the cranial area at which point the patient's complaint should disappear.

The chiropractor may also establish a relationship with the patient's energy field by standing at the feet of a supine patient and mentally envisioning a series of questions along with a yes or no answer. "Clinical observations have revealed that if the practitioner inaudibly requests a yes response, the patient will respond by expressing a change in leg length."[14]

It should go without saying that all of this is pseudo-scientific nonsense. When chiropractor Brian Gleberzon searched for evidence for these Name techniques, he found 111 articles, most of which were descriptions and anecdotal observations, with almost nothing supporting or refuting their clinical effectiveness.[15] Chiropractic has entire schools of treatment built upon the unproven, often frankly absurd, notions of their inventor.

Are these blatantly pseudo-scientific diagnostic and treatment techniques challenged by the profession and exposed for the nonsense that they are? No, instead they are embraced by the profession now and are likely to play an even greater role in the future.[16] Students in chiropractic colleges, including the Canadian Memorial Chiropractic College, are exposed to these techniques, and many join "Technique Clubs" at school. After studying these techniques and researching their backgrounds, Gleberzon, a professor at CMCC, felt they met "the level of clinical competence required of a 'reasonable' chiropractor" and recommended that some be included in the college's curriculum.[17]

As well as these techniques, some chiropractors dabble in modalities beyond chiropractic, including homeopathy, acupuncture, holistic nutrition, mega-vitamin and supplement therapy, reflexology, iridology, hair analysis, energy medicine, live blood analysis, and a host of other unproven therapies. In 1988, chiropractor Paul Carey bemoaned the profession's seeming preoccupation with dubious health care practices: "For our numbers, we have far too many fools or people who get involved in fringe therapy — megavitamins, laser therapy, things that are clearly unproven."[18] Surveys demonstrate that many chiropractors use some of these modalities while treating their patients, in a kind of unscientific hodge-podge.[19]

Chiropractor Samuel Homola describes the situation:

Despite their senselessness, nearly all of the approaches described here have been promoted by articles or advertisements in chiropractic publications, and a few have been promoted through chiropractic schools and organizations. They are very much a part of the chiropractic marketplace and have been subjected to little or no criticism by their colleagues or by professional organizations.[20]

How can a profession that calls itself science-based be awash in so much pseudo-scientific, often bizarre beliefs and therapies? Chiropractic historian Joseph Keating Jr. suggests that many chiropractors, perhaps a majority, rely on "ways of knowing" that are not scientific. They believe chiropractic works because the Palmers said so, because it "just makes sense," because they see it in their practice everyday and hear anecdotes, read testimonials, and see non-experimental data such as clinical case studies. All this, Keating says, has been:

> ... bolstered by the proliferation of pseudoscience journals of chiropractic wherein poor quality research and exuberant overinterpretation of results masquerade as science and provide false confidence about the value of various chiropractic techniques.[21]

This lack of critical-thinking skills combined with a non-scientific and often anti-scientific attitude results in chiropractors adopting other unproven modalities in their practices.

Keating sees skepticism and a scientific attitude among a small group of chiropractors and schools, but he is far from optimistic. For one thing, to challenge the notion that "chiropractic works" is considered heresy in most of the profession, so instead of teaching skepticism and critical thinking to students, most chiropractic colleges instill strong belief in chiropractic, strengthening an already prevalent anti-intellectual tradition in the profession.[22] A questionnaire sent to chiropractic colleges in the United States showed the majority continue to teach students to locate and correct vertebral subluxations and to instruct that these subluxations can be related to disease and overall health.[23]

The quality and quantity of education in chiropractic colleges has improved dramatically since the days of D.D. and B.J. Palmer, and today the CMCC requires at least three years of undergraduate study to get in. Students then receive four years of instruction and must pass provincial and national board exams before they enter practice.

Nonetheless, entrance requirements are still low in the United States in comparison to other doctoral-level health care professions, says Keating Jr., and competition for admission is not much of a factor. He writes:

Many of the schools are magnets for New Agers, theosophists, magical and mystical thinkers, and those attracted by the low admission standards and the lure of a lucrative private practice. Almost anyone who can accumulate sixty credit hours of undergraduate liberal arts college work will be admitted to one of these schools and can become a chiropractor. Moreover, since the larger chiropractic colleges tend to have the strongest commitment to dogma, fuzzy thinkers are likely to fill the chiropractic ranks for decades to come.[24]

Gadget Freaks and Gizmos

But it's not just wacky techniques and alternative remedies that attract chiropractors. In fact, if the chiropractic profession in general were allowed to order only one magazine subscription, it would probably pick *Popular Mechanics* over *Scientific American*, hands down. That's because since the early 1900s, chiropractors have been avid gadgeteers and indifferent researchers. The chiropractic fascination with gizmos with strange-sounding names, lots of dials, and bizarre operating theories begins with B.J. Palmer, the profession's self-styled master promoter and diehard gadget freak.

It was B.J. who, in 1910, introduced the profession to the x-ray machine (then renamed it the spinograph). X-rays had only been discovered by Wilhelm Roentgen some fifteen years earlier and were still considered a near-magical phenomenon. Early x-ray machines looked like props from a horror film — as did the unnerving but fascinating images they produced. B.J. Palmer understood the power of showing patients the ghostly shadows of their own spines.

Not all chiropractors were as taken with the newly invented x-ray machinery as Palmer. In fact, B.J.'s fascination may have been one of the reasons several dozen Palmer School pupils, led by star instructor Joy Loban, walked out and formed the rival Universal Chiropractic College the same year x-rays were being touted by Palmer. Certainly many chiropractors were taken aback that B.J., who had advocated straight chiropractic "done by hand," was suddenly trumpeting a machine that could diagnose subluxations with no hands involved.

But despite the early reluctance, x-ray machines soon became common fixtures in chiropractic offices. Chiropractors came to see them as enormously valuable because they believed they could use them to actually show subluxations to skeptical patients. Within the first year of Palmer's school getting its Sheidel-Western x-ray machine, school technicians produced two thousand x-rays of the spine.[25] That was just the beginning. Soon chiropractors nation-wide would be generating thousands of x-rays, many of them full-spine radiographs, including the unshielded pelvic area. The problem was that the chiropractors were deluding themselves that they could see subluxations on x-ray film.

In 1966, officials with the National Association of Letter Carriers in the United States set up a test. They asked chiropractors from the two largest professional bodies, the American Chiropractic Association and the International Chiropractors Association, to examine twenty sets of x-rays. Each film was purported to show a subluxation, but the chiropractors present could not identify a single one. Full-spine x-rays, the kind favoured by "straight" (subluxation-based) chiropractors, are almost useless for diagnostic purposes. X-rays used to find so-called subluxations expose patients to the cancer-causing radiation for no purpose except that of a marketing tool.[26]

In 1973, the U.S. Congress agreed to Medicare payment only for subluxations "demonstrated by x-ray to exist." The move forced chiropractors to huddle and redefine the subluxation to include just about any spinal problem, most of which wouldn't respond to chiropractic adjustment — but looked great in an x-ray.

And the x-raying continued. Subluxation-based chiropractors ordered radiographs, even of children, for conditions that had nothing to do with the spine. Dr. Marvin Levant, an Alberta radiologist, saw proof of this every day in his practice. In 1997 he and his partners were getting x-ray referrals from chiropractors for all sorts of non-musculoskeletal conditions, including skin rashes. Dr. Levant noted that one chiropractic practice made 210 inappropriate x-ray referrals in two months.

In September 1998, that information led the Alberta Society of Radiologists to vote unanimously to refuse to take x-rays for chiropractors of patients in the pediatric age group. This was not a skirmish in a "turf war" between medicine and chiropractic. Radiologists made money making x-rays for chiropractors, and their stand was sure to cost the profession a lot of money. But Dr. Levant, who spearheaded the move, explained, "We had calculated that it would cost us, but the argument is simple ... you can't put a price on your own professionalism and you can't put a price on a clear conscience."

The pediatric section of the Alberta Medical Association agreed in 1998:

> Chiropractic use of x-rays of infants and children to diagnose so-called vertebral subluxations is unscientific and of no value whatsoever. Without any benefit to the child, these x-rays can contribute to the risk of cancers and genetic damage. Parents should never allow their children's spines to be x-rayed by a chiropractor.[27]

One of this book's authors, Wayne, recently visited a Toronto-based chiropractor. Wayne complained of allergies but said he had no back pain or back problems. The chiropractor not only said he could treat allergies, but expressed interest in x-raying Wayne's back to get a better idea of how his spine was misaligned. The chiropractor had an x-ray machine in his office.

The Granddaddy of all Gimcracks

But the x-ray machine was just the first gadget B.J. Palmer fell in love with. As we've seen, in 1924 he thrust the granddaddy of all chiropractic gimcracks, the neurocalometer, into the chiropractic limelight by insisting that followers of "pure" chiropractic lease the unproven device for about the price of a house. The neurocalometer was supposed to automatically detect elusive subluxations by means of a thermocouple input attached to a needle and dial. In fact, the pricey instrument could do no such thing. But that didn't stop thousands of chiropractors from snapping them up like eager computer enthusiasts buying the latest, fastest, feature-loaded machine. Even before its official introduction at the chiropractic Lyceum of 1924, the device had spawned a few relatively inexpensive clones. It also sparked a series of upgrades and improved models such as the Neurocalograph, a device that could automatically produce charts of neurocalometric readings. These scientific-looking printouts were interpreted using arcane methodologies based, at best, on chiropractors' wishful thinking. The problem was, depending on the type of chiropractor using the device, the interpretation of the readings could differ.

For example, a chiropractor who believed in B.J. Palmer's Hole-In-One (HIO) theory might detect subluxations along the length of the spine, but would only adjust the upper neck to remove them. Meanwhile, a chiropractor who used Gonstead adjustment methods might use the same readings to manipulate other parts of the spine.

To make matters worse, the neurocalometer's competition multiplied in the decades following its introduction. There were the Nervoscope, the Neuropyrometer, the Temposcope, the Dermoscope, the Thermodeltameter, and the Vasotonometer, to name just a few. There was even a tiny neurocalometer for detecting subluxations in babies. The gadgets all made the same promise: they would allow chiropractors to quickly and "scientifically" detect subluxations.

But there was no indication that the different subluxation-detecting devices could spot the same subluxations in the same place. Actually, they all failed miserably, for two reasons. First, they depended on detecting subluxations by picking up temperature variations on either side of the spine, an idea first suggested by D.D. Palmer in 1903 and based on the erroneous idea that excited nerves produce the heat that warms the blood. Second, they were trying to find something — the subluxation — that chiropractors could not then (and cannot now) prove exists. Descendents of these devices are still in use today. In fact, one of the chiropractors to whom we took eleven-year-old Judy Matthews used one on her back. But that's just one of many unproven gizmos used by chiropractors.

The Toftness Radiation Detector

In 1971, Irwing Toftness patented the Toftness Radiation Detector. The device looks like a plastic gavel. It's really just a length of PVC piping into which six plastic lenses have been inserted. The handle is made of a brass rod surrounded by a plastic sleeve. The top of the device is capped with a mylar disc. Toftness claimed that compressed spinal nerves gave off energy at a frequency of 69.5 gigahertz. The lenses in the device were supposed to focus that energy on the top disc. While moving the detector up and down a patient's spine, a chiropractor was to rub the disc with a finger. When it squeaked it revealed a subluxation. Chiropractors all over North America made use of the device. In 1984, the U.S. Federal Drug administration outlawed the Toftness detector in the United States, declaring it totally useless. Yet a 1993 survey found that 2.2 percent of Canadian chiropractors were still employing Toftness techniques.

The Subluxation Station

Many more chiropractors are still using other, more elaborate subluxation detectors. A chiropractor Judy Matthews visited tested her with a device called the Subluxation Station. That's a brand name for a surface electromyography (EMG) unit that chiropractors say can detect subluxations. The device scans the spine and produces a colour printout. That output portrays muscle activity along in the spine as coloured bars of varying lengths. Another chiropractor Judy visited used a different brand of EMG machine. Both chiropractors found different subluxations. That doesn't surprise critics, who say the devices and their printouts don't show anything useful about backbones.

Chiropractor Samuel Homola explains, "Some chiropractors claim that the test provides an objective measurement of overall spinal health by detecting electrical activity in the muscles along the spine enabling them to screen patients initially and to follow the progress of their treatment. This usage is invalid." Homola has more than forty years of experience as a science-based chiropractor in the United States.

Other chiropractic critics are more blunt. "Surface EMG is absolute garbage," says Charles DuVall, a practicing Ohio chiropractor and an outspoken critic of the profession. DuVall learned about EMG during his work on an investigation for the Ohio Bureau of Workers Compensation. DuVall took the twelve-hour EMG course mandated by the Ohio chiropractic licensing board. "The first three things that the man teaching the course said set the tone. A) This will increase your revenue by 30 per cent at minimum. B) The patients are impressed with the lights and the graphs. And C) you can show a patient they need treatment even if they feel good," he explained.

DuVall says the surface scanning EMG is not accepted as a valid diagnostic instrument by the American College of Radiology or the American College of Electro-Diagnosis. "None of these tests have any validity," he said. "It's all PR. It's lights and whistles. It looks good and it is a way they can talk the patient into treatment."

Until we did our investigation of pediatric chiropractic on canoe.ca in 2000, officials with Health Canada's Medical Devices Section were unaware the Subluxation Station was being used in Canada. After our feature ran, the device's manufacturer applied for licensing. It was granted. Health Canada officials explained that the device does no harm. The government body leaves the determination of diagnostic effectiveness to the chiropractors themselves, since they're a self-regulating profession.

The Activator Method

Many chiropractors test for subluxations by comparing the length of their patients' legs. They then treat the subluxations they say they've discovered with a device that looks like a small handheld pogo stick. They're using what's called the Activator Method. The Activator itself is a rubber-tipped, spring-loaded device that delivers a controlled "thump" to the vertebrae.

The Activator Method is based on the idea of "functional short leg." Conveniently, this doesn't appear to be an actual anatomical different in leg length, just an apparent one. During an episode of *Scientific American Frontiers* that aired on PBS in June 2002, former chiropractor John Badanes demonstrated the leg-length test. He explained that small changes in position side-to-side could throw off any such test. And, as Dr. Robert Baratz, president of the National Council Against Health Fraud, explained on the show, it's perfectly normal for one leg to be longer than the other. He added, "The length of the leg is not determined by the spine, it's determined by the bones of the leg. And by manipulating the spine or the back, you're not going to change that, because those bones aren't going to change their length by any form of manipulation, unless you break them."

But despite the anatomical realities, chiropractors who use the Activator Method employ the handheld Activator device to "thump" subluxations until a patient's legs appear to be the same length.

About 36 percent of Canadian chiropractors use the Activator Method, and 17 percent of them use it on children, according to the device's manufacturer, Activator Methods International. In Judy Matthews's visits to five Toronto-area chiropractors, two wanted to use Activator on the eleven-year-old test patient. While allowed in all other provinces, the Chiropractic Association of Saskatchewan prohibits its use. *(See "A Profession Out of Control")*

But despite the use of Activator in most provinces, medical experts say the device serves no medical purpose. It is purported to treat subluxations, unproven misalignments of the spine. "It piles one dubious claim on another," says Homola.

Again, until we brought the device to the attention of the Medical Devices Section of Health Canada in 2000, they were unaware that it was being used in Canada. After our stories appeared on canoe.ca, Activator Methods International applied for and received a Canadian license. The device is still in use today.

Off the Meter Devices

At the Kulhay Wellness Centre in the heart of Toronto, you can find another chiropractor enamoured with another type of bogus gadget — the Interro machine. The device, which looks like an ancient stereo receiver with probes attached, is purported to diagnose allergies. According to Katrina Kulhay, the chiropractor and self-styled nutritionist who heads up the centre, the Interro machine works on the principal of vibrational medicine. While working on a feature story for *Elm Street* magazine, we sent a female editor, Heather, into the Kulhay Centre to see what that actually meant. Heather was asked to hold a brass rod attached to the Interro machine in one hand. The technician then touched the index finger of her other hand with a small probe, also wired into the Interro. The Interro machine itself was connected to a desktop computer. Heather was told there was an acupuncture point on the tip of her finger, which was connected to her large intestine.

"It's a biofeedback machine," Kulhay told us when we interviewed her about the device after Heather's visit. "Every food has a molecular structure. And every food has a vibrational frequency. If you take a piece of food, put it under an electron microscope and magnify it 1,000 or 2,000 [times], you can actually see the difference vibrationally as well as molecularly. You can find the frequency wavelength, put it into a computer and it can be fed back to the individual, to their electronic frequency wavelength," she said. "It's called vibrational medicine."

But Dr. Stephen Barrett, a longtime critic of chiropractic, is clear about what the Interro is, and vibrational medicine has nothing to do with it. He says the Interro is just a fancied-up instrument that can measure electrical resistance. It can't detect the "vibrational frequency" of anything, he says. Dr. Arthur Leznoff, an allergist and immunologist at St. Michael's Hospital in Toronto agrees. "It can't do what it's said to be able to do," he explains. "There's no mechanism by which it's possible."

But the Interro is just one kind of "bio-electric" device used by chiropractors. This class of device has a long and ignoble history. Previous versions include the Ellis Microdynameter, the Rx-Micro-tabulometer, the Psychgalvanometer, the Galvanopsychometer, and the Psychroneurometer — all nonsense devices used by chiropractors.

A more recent incarnation, however, is the German-made Vegatest machine. Early in 2002, CBC Television's *Disclosures* told the story of a Laval-based chiropractor who used the Vegatest to diagnose and treat cirrhosis and other ailments. The show revealed that he bilked one family of $30,000 for two years' worth of treatments that included paper cards the patient was to wear under his clothes. Each card cost $2,500. The chiropractor told the patient, who had advanced liver disease, that he did not need a vital liver transplant. The chiropractor had been fined two thousand by the Quebec Order of Chiropractors for making exaggerated claims but was still practicing. The patient had the transplant. After *Disclosures* approached Health Canada about the device, it moved to ban four models of the Vegatest in Canada. Officials told the show they had no idea how many Vegatest-like machines are currently in use in Canada. "These devices should be confiscated," Barrett says.

Meanwhile, in Courtenay, British Columbia, another chiropractor, James Bare, is marketing the RifeBare Resonant Light System. It's a radio tuner and amplifier attached to an argon-filled glass tube. The device is based on the Rife Machine, developed in 1934 by Royal Rife, a German optical scientist who came to believe that pathogens could be destroyed by various frequencies of electromagnetic energy. After developing a powerful microscope, Rife went on to create a machine he thought could rid the world of disease by essentially exploding germs with highly tuned energy (he believed cancer was caused by bacteria). There is no evidence this is the case. The disciples of Rife believe that a systematic medical conspiracy has kept Rife's work from reaching the general public.

Rife's beliefs fall into the category of radionics, a pseudo-science that holds that zeroing in on specific frequencies can treat disease. Albert Abrams, called the "dean of gadget quacks" by the American Medical Association, first suggested the idea.

Bare's device is an updated version of Rife's original design. On his Web site, Bare calls his device experimental, but that doesn't put much of a limit on his claims for it. He writes:

> *Cancer* was the first disease we evaluated with the RifeBare System built for Batyah Elizabeth who had cancer which had metastasized to six places in her body. When the device was used, some tumors shrank, her energy levels improved and pain levels diminished. When the cancer frequencies were stopped for three months, the cancer tumors returned along with intense pain.
>
> Since then others deemed terminal with cancer have used the RifeBare and reported similar successful results. Of those who died, the cause of death was often from other complications such as pneumonia, heart failure or pancreatic breakdown. All these volunteers were stage 4 Cancer victims who used the technology as a last resort. Many lived far longer than anyone expected and some are still alive today.
>
> The RifeBare **will not cure cancer** and neither will surgery, radiation, chemo or drugs. Cancer is the "effect" of something else; it is not its own cause. RifeBare Technology is not a magic wand although it certainly improves the quality of a person's life. In the case of cancer, it provides a "window of opportunity" for the person to make the necessary changes to diet and lifestyle which bring about good health.[28]

Cancer sufferers can buy an assembled RifeBare Resonant Light System for about five thousand dollars. Bare also sells a two thousand dollar model. He claims to have ten thousand of the devices worldwide.

The RifeBare Web site also suggests other uses for the technology:

> The control of insects, purification of water, decontamination of food processing facilities, germ free operating rooms, control of contagious diseases, agriculture and veterinarian uses — are just some of the future benefits of RifeBare technology.[29]

But Bare isn't the only chiropractor who's developed treatment devices. When Wayne visited a Toronto chiropractor, he noticed a small handheld device in a cabinet near the chiropractor's reception desk. The device was called the Triggerizer. The chiropractor said it did the same thing as acupressure but didn't require a technician to use their thumbs. "I'm an inventor," he said.

The Toronto chiropractor is right; he is an inventor, as are many chiropractors. But what they invent are the reasons why the bogus devices they use work and how they can detect subluxations and treat disorders. Many use the devices to convince their patients that the subluxations exist or have responded to treatment. Meanwhile, any well-read chiropractor knows that the subluxation itself is unproven, as are the devices and techniques they use. But though they're using a useless apparatus to treat a chimera, the gadgets let them look like scientists while they do it. When it comes to chiropractic, whether it's gizmos or scientific-sounding techniques, appearance is everything.

11

A PROFESSION OUT OF CONTROL
Why the Real Regulation of Chiropractic is Impossible

You don't have to be an investigative journalist to find out that chiropractic in Canada is a profession out of control. All you have to do is what *Toronto Star* reporter Robin Harvey did: go out and visit a handful of chiropractors' offices in the city or town where you live. Chances are that, like her, you will find a troubling mix of quack claims, exaggerated benefits, misleading brochures and information sheets, useless diagnostic tests, dubious electronic machines, and a host of wacky alternative therapies that are either unproven or have been disproved.

When Harvey went to fifteen randomly selected chiropractic offices across Toronto in October 1999, she found:

- all the offices said they treated children
- pamphlets claiming chiropractic could treat ear infections, allergies, and asthma
- eight offices with pamphlets claiming babies should be treated with chiropractic from birth
- a pamphlet indicating that chiropractic could help constipation, recurring ear infections, bed-wetting, colds, headaches, poor concentration, sinus problems, stomach aches, and scoliosis in infants and children
- four chiropractors offering live blood cell analysis to test for immune deficiencies, microbial overgrowth, and metabolism problems

- three offering hair analysis to diagnose nutrition imbalances and diseases such as MS, cancer, and Cystic Fibrosis
- four offering ear candling to suck out impurities, toxins, and poisons in the ear
- five offices with brochures or charts claiming subluxations caused most or all disease, including serious problems such as hypertension and heart arrhythmia
- offices offering Radionics, an energy-based healing system; meridian therapy and neural emotional therapy (NET); Interro machine testing for nutritional imbalance and organ and tissue weakness; cranial sacral therapy for learning disabilities, chronic fatigue, and emotional difficulties; and Omega Acubase System testing for "energy imbalances."[1]

In the same year, a journalist at the online news organization Canoe did a telephone survey of fifty randomly selected chiropractic offices in Toronto to ask about treating an infant for ear infections. A majority of chiropractors surveyed said they treated children and could help with ear infections. *(See "The Not-So-Well-Adjusted Child")*

When confronted with the results of simple field tests like these, chiropractic officials blame the media for sensational and negative reporting and counter that the profession should not be judged by a handful of fringe practitioners. Some chiropractic officials in Canada promulgate the notion, expressed in a 1999 *Globe and Mail* feature, that chiropractic gets a bad rap because of the "outlandish claims of a few bad eggs." As the *Globe* piece put it:

> Chiropractic officials admit that a small proportion of chiropractic services are "experimental", but what line of work doesn't have skeletons in the closet? "In every profession, there are people who do things not considered mainstream," says Greg Dunn, executive director of the Canadian Chiropractic Protective Association in Toronto, which covers chiropractors for malpractice.[2]

In the same piece, Ed Barisa, executive director of the Canadian Chiropractic Association, supports that view. "Yes, it's worrying," he says of the chiropractic fringe. "The association's position is that chiropractic needs to be evidence-based."[3]

Chiropractic association leaders and educators have repeatedly suggested and supported the idea that only a small minority — "the fringe" — of chiropractors in Canada make false claims about the benefits of chiropractic and operate outside the legislated scope of practice.

Rotten to the Top

The largest chiropractic agencies and associations in Canada and the United States make quack claims for the validity and effectiveness of chiropractic theories and methods.[4] That conclusion comes from three prominent chiropractic educators in a recently published study titled "Unsubstantiated Claims in Patient Brochures From the Largest State, Provincial and National Chiropractic Associations and Research Agencies." The study, published in 2001, dropped like a bomb on chiropractic, exploding for good the myth that a responsible leadership was working hard to clean up the profession.

The researchers, including Jaroslaw Grod, a professor at CMCC in Toronto, requested patient brochures from eleven groups, including the national professional associations in the United States and Canada, the three largest state associations and the three largest provincial associations, and the two largest research agencies. They are: the American Chiropractic Association, the International Chiropractors' Association, the Canadian Chiropractic Association, the California Chiropractic Association, the Texas Chiropractic Association, the British Columbia Chiropractic Association, the Ontario Chiropractic Association, L'Association des Chiropraticiens du Québec, the Foundation for Chiropractic Education and Research, and the Chiropractic Foundation for Spinal Research.

The Quebec association and the Chiropractic Foundation for Spinal Research did not distribute patient brochures. Of the remaining nine groups, researchers found that 100 percent distributed materials that included unsubstantiated claims. These claims come from groups that have "high visibility and are among the most authoritative spokespersons for chiropractic in North America. Collectively, they constitute an important voice for chiropractic on this continent," say the study's authors.

What are they telling prospective patients? The claims are wide-ranging and significant, including the idea that chiropractic can be an effective alternative to drugs and surgery for many conditions; treat scoliosis; prevent painful conditions; prevent disease and other organ dysfunction; help chronic pain; safely and effectively treat a variety of childhood illnesses; improve athletic performance; and remove subluxations, which can cause nerve irritation and disease. Not one of these claims is supported by scientific evidence, say the authors, and some claims are so general and vague that they are untestable.

Despite claims from Canadian Chiropractic Association leaders that they support evidence-based chiropractic, the study showed that the CCA is guilty of distributing brochures with unjustified or unsubstantiated claims. Here is a sample of the CCA claims the study noted. Below each claim are the study's authors' comments in bold.

"Would it surprise you to learn that up to 80 percent of all headache sufferers obtain substantial relief from chiropractors?"

Manipulation for patients with headache has found increasing experimental support in recent years. However, this literature does not substantiate the claim that 80% of all patients with headaches will benefit from manipulation.

"For the Young" — "The spine ... should get the same regular check-ups as your teeth, not just when you've got pain. As chiropractors, we can work out an effective treatment program for you ...Your youthful bodies respond best to chiropractic care. Early treatments may prevent many painful conditions later."

The prophylactic value, if any, of chiropractic care is unproven and largely unstudied. The value of "regular check-ups" by chiropractors is also unknown.

"Why Chiropractic is a Safe and Healthy Choice" — "... when compared to other therapies, chiropractic is safer and more effective ... chiropractic care is safe and effective with less risk than many medications or medical interventions."

These assertions do not specify any particular health problem. Claims for the relative safety and effectiveness of one form of healing versus another should be judged with respect to the particular health problems for which care is provided. There are very few controlled trials that compare chiropractic (manipulative) and medical (pharmacological) intervention methods.

"Recent studies have illustrated the importance of proper spinal alignment and mechanics on athletic performance in a variety of sports ... with many vertebral subluxations going undetected, there are many athletes not performing at their top capabilities. Spinal subluxations and deviations can alter the function of the athlete's neuromuscular and skeletal system ... For baseball and golf players spinal subluxations will alter swing mechanics."

The effects, if any, of spinal subluxations upon athletic performance have not been scientifically validated.[5]

The authors' conclusions fly in the face of the chiropractic party line regarding false and misleading claims by their members. They found that a "significant segment of 'official chiropractic' in Canada and the United States publishes uncritical and scientifically unvalidated claims for the chiropractic healing art."[6]

And The Provinces Are No Better

On the surface, chiropractors in Canada and the United States appear to have most of the trappings of a legitimate health care profession. Two of the most important of these are licensure and the ability to self-regulate. These provisions put chiropractic in an elite group of health care workers, along with medical doctors, dentists, optometrists, dietitians, and pharmacists, among others.

In Canada, the responsibility to regulate health care providers rests with the provinces. Each province has its own legislation regulating chiropractic and a provincial regulatory board, which has a mandate to regulate the profession in the public interest. In Canada, the regulatory boards are: British Columbia College of Chiropractors, College of Chiropractors of Alberta, Chiropractors' Association of Saskatchewan, Manitoba Chiropractors' Association, College of Chiropractors of Ontario, Ordre des Chiropraticiens du Quebec, New Brunswick Chiropractors Association, Nova Scotia Chiropractic Board, Prince Edward Island Chiropractic Association, and the Newfoundland and Labrador Chiropractic Board. In 1978, the Canadian Federation of Chiropractic Regulatory Boards (CFCRB) was established by chiropractors and mandated to provide education, support, and information on licensing, testing, and discipline. The college in British Columbia has not participated in the federation's activities since 1995.[7]

Each provincial organization has detailed rules governing the practice of chiropractors in the province, including regulations on advertising, billing, record keeping, sexual harassment, and more. They have the power to investigate complaints and discipline members for professional misconduct. And they do. Each year, the colleges publish records of complaints, how they were handled, and what punishments were meted out to their members. Records indicate that chiropractors are disciplined for improper billing, for sexually harassing or assaulting patients, for false advertising, for lack of professionalism, and for other infractions. To lawmakers and the public, it looks as though chiropractors are policing their members and regulating their profession. But a closer examination of the situation reveals a different story.

In 1998, the Canadian Federation of Chiropractic Regulatory Boards asked the provincial bodies to send it a list of all disciplinary cases that resulted in a significant outcome, that is, cases that, in their view, "amounted to significant effort and consequence on the part of the regulatory board to the registrant."[8] The federation received ninety-nine cases covering the years 1990 to 1997. Of that number, there were six complaints of practicing outside the scope of practice, and sixteen complaints regarding advertising issues. A closer look at the cases reveals that all six scope-of-practice cases came from Alberta. Of the sixteen cases involving unauthorized advertising, the cases came from several jurisdictions, but not one came from Ontario. There are about 760 chiropractors in Alberta. In Ontario, there are 2,800 working chiropractors. Anyone at the regulatory offices with a computer and a half-hour could find Ontario chiropractors' Web sites that break the advertising rules in the province. A visit to chiropractic offices in any city or town in the province would reveal pamphlets, posters, and newsletters that make unsubstantiated claims for chiropractic.

In fact, regulators might want to take a few minutes and look at their own Web sites in their search for infractions. All anyone has to do is visit one of the official chiropractic sites across Canada to find example after example of false and misleading claims, claims that are not backed by scientific evidence or claims that, by their very nature, cannot be verified.

Let's take a tour of some official chiropractic Web sites as they appeared in July 2002.

Ontario Chiropractic Association (www.chiropractic.on.ca):

Research supports the effectiveness of chiropractic in the treatment of back pain, neck pain, and neck aches, however, many chiropractic patients have found that it also helps in promoting overall health.

Research does not support chiropractic for any of those problems, and patients' subjective opinion about what may or may not be affecting their health is of little scientific value.

British Columbia College of Chiropractors (www.bcchiro.com):

Each of us is born with the ability to heal and recover from illness. Our bruises heal, cuts mend and common colds are overcome. Your nervous system regulates this inborn healing ability.

Think of your brain as a central command post sending and receiving information through telephone wires (your nerves) which branch out to connect all areas of a city (your body). A short circuit in a wire cuts off communication just like misalignments in your spine can put pressure on the nerves. This pressure interferes with your nervous system, affects your ability to self-heal and may prolong injury or illness.

There is no evidence that misaligned vertebrae or subluxations put pressure on nerves and interfere with nerve flow affecting overall health.

From professional athletes to homemakers, engineers to electricians, infants to seniors, chiropractic care has been the answer to optimum health. Many people see a Doctor of Chiropractic for back, neck or joint problems, while others may seek relief from the discomfort caused by headaches, high blood pressure, asthma or other conditions. Still others find that regular visits to their chiropractor keep them in peak condition.

There is no evidence that chiropractic improves overall health or is effective in the treatment of high blood pressure or asthma or other organic diseases. Finally, there is no evidence that regular chiropractic adjustments have any effect on health.

College of Chiropractors of Alberta Web site (www.ccoa.ab.ca):

The chiropractic adjustment is thought to restore the body's powerful ability to heal itself, so it is not surprising that many patients say they sleep better and have more energy following their treatments.

Chiropractors can play a major role in preventative care, protecting against future pain and health problems. A wealth of independent studies supports the effectiveness of chiropractic care.

There is no evidence that chiropractic adjustments speed healing or increase energy. There is no evidence that chiropractic can prevent health problems. The claim that chiropractic is effective cannot be tested because the conditions are not specified.

Nova Scotia College of Chiropractors Web site (wwwmedianet.ca/nsca/):

Chiropractic is concerned with the preservation and restoration of health, and focuses particular attention on the subluxation. A subluxation is a complex of functional and/or structural and/or pathological articular changes that compromise neural integrity and may influence organ system function and general health.

The idea that subluxations produce symptoms or affect general health has not been scientifically established.

Newfoundland and Labrador Chiropractic Board Web site
(www.nfldchiro.com):

> Chiropractic's approach to health tries to use the body's natural
> powers of healing, and philosophically does not employ drugs or
> surgery as the primary intervention…The scientific basis of chiro-
> practic has been, and continues to be, demonstrated by quality
> research and scientific investigation.

Chiropractic does not have a scientific basis and research has demonstrated
the benefit in some cases of spinal manipulative therapy, not chiropractic.

Many of the Web sites of the official chiropractic organizations in Canada
are riddled with unsubstantiated claims about the benefits of chiropractic.
These boards and associations have been granted the power and responsibility
to regulate their members, but they cannot even regulate themselves. It seems
unlikely that the regulatory bodies would take any kind of proactive action
against chiropractors making false claims. As evidence, all you need to do is
take a look at the Chiropractic Awareness Council.

The C.A.C. — Breaking the Rules in a Big Way

It's impossible to understand how regulators can miss something like
the Chiropractic Awareness Council (C.A.C.), a Canadian organization of
chiropractors dedicated to "promoting public awareness of Chiropractic life
principles by promoting awareness of the devastating effects of the Vertebral
Subluxation Complex on the expression of Human Potential."[9]

It is difficult to enumerate the false claims made by C.A.C. because virtually every statement they make in relation to chiropractic and health is
unsubstantiated and unsupported.

They recommend chiropractic adjustments for babies immediately after
birth and regularly thereafter for all kinds of childhood illnesses. *(See "The
Not-So-Well Adjusted Child")* But children are not their only targets. The
C.A.C. Web site also makes false claims aimed to entice adults. One Web
page is titled, "Chiropractic can improve your sex life!" Below this tantalizing
headline, the C.A.C. claimed that vertebral subluxations could interfere with
nerve flow to the testicles, vagina, penis, prostate, and uterus. If the nerve
flow is affected negatively by subluxations, they warn that the following
problems may occur: infertility, decreased energy/vitality, impotence,
decreased libido, and sexual or reproductive dysfunction. Again, there is no
evidence that any of these claims is true.

The council headquarters is in Guelph, Ontario. The names of the members of the board of directors are listed on the site, as is a list of the council's full membership. The C.A.C. site breaks numerous provisions of the College of Chiropractors of Ontario Standards of Practice, including the prohibition against making claims that are false or misleading, making claims that cannot be verified, and using testimonials outside the chiropractor's office.

So though chiropractors are quick to inform lawmakers, academic institutions, and the public that they are one of a small group of self-regulated health professions in Canada, their self-regulation appears to be non-existent, at least in terms of advertising and promotion. Perhaps individual Canadian and American chiropractors are merely taking their lead from the top. As researchers have shown, the leading institutions for chiropractors in both countries publish uncritical and scientifically unvalidated claims with no apparent repercussions at all from the myriad state and provincial regulatory agencies, even though those claims are in flagrant contravention of written policy.

The unsubstantiated claims that chiropractors and their organizations make are a problem, but they are more importantly a symptom of a much deeper problem — a lack of consensus around what chiropractors do, a lack of agreement around what chiropractors can legitimately claim to do, and, more profoundly, a systemic lack of understanding and acceptance of the basic concepts of science.

Beyond the Scope of Practice

An important part of being a regulated health profession is having a defined scope of practice. This protects the public from practitioners who might perform procedures or manage conditions for which they are neither trained nor competent. It also provides the profession with guidelines for the proper regulation and discipline of their own members.

Chiropractors are regulated in all the provinces of Canada (and every American state), usually by statutes in an act passed by the provincial government and named for the profession.

The chiropractic acts vary slightly province to province (and more widely from state to state), but they are generally consistent in their description of the profession and its rules of practice. Some, like Ontario's, explicitly define scope of practice, while others, like the act in New Brunswick, do not. The problem with chiropractic lies in the gap between what legislators intended when they wrote the acts and what chiropractors believe the acts empower them to do.

Manitoba legislators were clear that chiropractic is "the examination and treatment principally by hand and without the use of drugs or surgery of the spinal column, pelvis and extremities and associated soft tissues..."[10]

The Chiropractic Act of Quebec is broader, describing chiropractic as "any act the object of which is to make corrections to the spinal column, pelvic bones, or to other articulations of the human body, by use of the hands..."[11]

The 1991 Ontario Chiropractic Act says:

> The practice of chiropractic is the assessment of conditions related to the spine, nervous system and joints and the diagnosis, prevention and treatment primarily by adjustment, of dysfunctions or disorders arising from the structures or functions of the spine and the effects of those dysfunctions or disorders on the nervous system; and dysfunctions or disorders arising from the structures or functions of the joints.[12]

The key phrase is "and the effects of those dysfunctions or disorders on the nervous system." Those dozen words opened the door for chiropractors. For many chiropractors, those "disorders" are subluxations, and they interfere with healthy nerve flow, leading to sickness and disease. That means they believe they can treat virtually any illness that might befall a human being.

Based on this thinking, many chiropractors feel their scope of practice is unlimited, as is their right to make claims of benefit and cure. As chiropractic scholar Joseph Keating Jr. points out:

> Thousand of chiropractors world-wide have and continue to base their manipulative approaches to patient care on subluxation. In the United States both national professional organizations are vocal adherents to the concept of subluxation."[13]

Not surprisingly, chiropractors cannot agree on what chiropractic is, what chiropractors do, and, more importantly for patients, what they *cannot* do.

Chiropractor Herbert Vear examined all state chiropractic practice acts in the United States. What he found was a mess. Reading them "adds to the confusion of the problems in definition facing the profession. To reach agreement on defining 'subluxation,' 'adjustment,' and 'manipulation,' three terms fundamental to all chiropractic physicians, may prove to be a monumental task."[14]

This lack of definition leads to a more serious problem, says Vear. "The ... practice Acts only confuse the question further when statutory scope of practice is examined. The diversity of interpretation of what constitutes scope of chiropractic practice is bewildering at best and professional suicide at worst."[15]

The situation in Canada is similar. This lack of consensus among chiropractors means that they do not have clearly defined standards of practice or scope of practice. Chiropractors and their leadership have consistently misrepresented this reality to lawmakers, health commissions, universities, and the public.

Former Canadian Chiropractic Association president Ronald Carter admitted that chiropractic is facing a crisis, a crisis that goes to the core of the profession. "While we face professional crisis our energies and dollars are invested in marketing programs depicting subluxation."[16] Carter openly discusses how adherence to the unproven theory of subluxation creates serious ethical issues around diagnosis and treatment:

> Its [sic] more than a word, it represents belief systems, different philosophies, it challenges our ethics, it provides different factions an issue to fight about. Our own justification of this word allows us to keep, and observe our peers breaking, the Eleventh Commandment: Thou shalt not take advantage of the sick.[17]

Studies show a majority of chiropractors subscribe to the notion that the chiropractic subluxation may be related to the cause of most disease.[18] Their belief in subluxation leads inevitably to exceeding their prescribed scope of practice and misleading patients. Chiropractor Lon Morgan says that chiropractors have to justify their claims of being able to treat various illnesses by invoking what he calls a "mystical model of subluxation silliness."

He describes the identification and removal of subluxations — the core of the practice of many chiropractors — like this:

> We then proceed with an infinite number of incoherent and conflicting methods to identify these spinal "boo-boos". We follow that up with an equal number of exotic "techniques" to excoriate [sic] these "spinal demons."[19]

What Morgan is describing is a profession in disarray. Because chiropractors cannot agree on what they are treating, how they treat it, or what works, they find it impossible to describe their scope of practice or to enforce consistent standards of practice. Most of this infighting and confusion is carefully covered up by the profession's leadership, but occasionally, when their internal arguing and feuding gets loud enough, these contradictions and inconsistencies become apparent to the public.

The Activator — Nonsense in Saskatchewan, Fine Elsewhere

The Activator is one of the most common gadgets in chiropractic practice. *(See "Gizmos, Parlour Tricks, and Nonsense")* It is a small, hand-held device that delivers a spring-loaded adjustment to the patient's spine. The Activator has become a popular tool among Canadian chiropractors.

More than a third of chiropractors in Canada use the device to fix subluxations and treat a host of ailments in children and adults. But the Chiropractors' Association of Saskatchewan (CAS) believes the device is ineffective. Since 1978, the CAS has banned the Activator's use in its home province. The organization's bylaws prohibit administering a chiropractic adjustment with a mechanical device. But late in 2001, that prohibition was challenged by fifteen Saskatchewan chiropractors who used the Activator in their practices.

In the fractious court battle that ensued, the divisiveness that characterizes chiropractic broke out in a very public fight about the supposed science-based nature of the profession. The CAS argued that there was no scientific evidence to suggest the Activator was effective. Through their lawyer, Jay Watson, the fifteen chiropractors disagreed and then brought out the profession's dirty laundry, arguing that much of chiropractic in general lacks scientific validation.

"They can't deny and their witnesses didn't deny at trial that there are many chiropractic techniques used by all chiropractors in North America that have no scientific proof behind them such as extremity adjustments or thoracic spine adjustment. There's no scientific evidence to support that it helps people," said Mr. Watson.

However, the Saskatchewan Court of Appeal upheld the CAS ban on the Activator on February 15, 2002. The Activator is used by about 50 percent of all chiropractors in all other provinces and in the United States, according to the manufacturer.

The public battle — it was covered by the Saskatchewan media — revealed that chiropractors couldn't agree on what is proper and efficacious treatment. While the Saskatchewan association bans the use of the Activator, chiropractors in other provinces are free to use the device, billing provincial health insurance plans and patients for the treatments.

A similar situation exists around Applied Kinesiology, which is used by about one-third of Canadian chiropractors.[20] Applied Kinesiology (AK) is a form of pseudo-scientific muscle testing used to detect disease and organ dysfunction by its proponents. There is no scientific evidence to support the claims of the practitioners of AK, and there have been several controlled tests that have shown it to be useless.[21, 22] While other chiropractors across the country use AK and charge patients for the service, chiropractors in British Columbia are prohibited from using the technique.[23] *(See "Gizmos, Parlour Tricks, and Nonsense")*

Despite efforts to sanitize the profession, it continues to have a poor reputation and to be marginalized among health science professionals. A few chiropractic researchers say that is the case partly because of its "dogmatic orientation to theory and refusal to clearly delimit the range of conditions for which clinical services may be appropriate."[24] Translation: Chiropractors have beliefs that are divorced from evidence and, in some cases, from reality. This makes any real self-regulating of chiropractic almost impossible, as the next case demonstrates.

The Complaint That Went Nowhere

On February 4, 2001, a Windsor-based physician named Dr. Anthony Hammer sent a letter of complaint to the College of Chiropractors of Ontario, the regulatory body for the province's twenty-eight hundred chiropractors. Dr. Hammer had come across a chiropractor's Web site that appeared to be in contravention of several of the CCO's regulations. His complaint against chiropractor Brian J. Nantais D.C. of Tecumseh, Ontario was clear and concise. In it, Dr. Hammer noted:

> Dr. Nantais lists 46 conditions on his Web site (www.nantaischiro.com) that he claims chiropractic commonly helps. Among these are:
> - shingles
> - stomach ulcers
> - asthma
> - bed-wetting
> - frequent ear infections
> - poor circulation.
>
> In the absence of any credible scientific evidence that chiropracty conducted within the legislative context of the scope has any effect, beneficial or harmful, on nearly all the conditions he mentions, particularly those cited above, he is in breach of the 1991 Chiropractic Act. He is practicing outside the limits of professional and personal competence because none of the conditions cited above are related to the spine or joints. He is also acting unethically and in breach of a section of The Act by misleading the general public into believing that chiropractic is an effective treatment for a large number of medical conditions that neither have any plausible scientific connection to chiropracty nor

any scientifically credible studies to support the establishment of a therapeutic relationship. In fact, in the case of asthma, studies indicate the opposite; that chiropracty is actually ineffective as a form of treatment. He has failed to comply with the advertising standards of The College by distributing testimonials on his internet (www.nantaischiro.com). I look forward to a response from Dr. Nantais and The College.

The College contacted Nantais about the complaint on May 17. Nantais expressed surprise that a medical doctor "would take the time and effort to forward a complaint about a very professional and accurate and vital Web site."[25] Regarding the patient testimonials, Nantais noted that the CCO has no rules regarding Web sites and added that he considered his site an in-office information program. Chiropractors are allowed to post or offer for view patient testimonials in their office.

Nantais defended his claims: "In my own practice, I believe I have seen every one of those conditions helped through chiropractic care. As a matter of fact, I believe there is wonderfully scientifically sound evidence that chiropractic, or more specifically, the restoration of normal nervous system function, has the ability to help these conditions. Again it is through the restoration of NORMAL NERVE SYSTEM FUNCTION that the body can use its own reparative process to regain proper health."[26]

Dr. Hammer filed a more detailed complaint on August 14, calling attention to a Yellow Pages advertisement by Nantais that invited people to call a phone number to hear him reciting patient testimonials.

On September 13, 2001, Nantais sent a letter to the CCO saying that he had changed his Web site from "Chiropractic Commonly Helps" to "Chiropractic May Help." But in October, Dr. Hammer checked the site and found the language unchanged. Hammer wrote the CCO again.

Months passed. Dr. Hammer called the CCO in January 2002 and was told it had heard the complaint in November 2001 but had deferred finalizing it pending the acceptance in writing of an undertaking by the chiropractor to change his advertising. Dr. Hammer would get a copy of the committee's decision as soon as possible.

That month, Dr. Hammer informed the CCO that Nantais's site remained unchanged and told them that the chiropractor had recently sent out with the local newspaper a flyer that contained patient testimonials — a clear violation of CCO regulations.

Nantais was still using a recorded phone message containing patient testimonials. The CCO complaints officer had not listened to it, so Dr. Hammer sent her a tape. This new information had gone to the complaints committee and to Nantais. A decision would be made as soon as possible. Weeks of silence followed.

Frustrated, Dr. Hammer sent a letter on March 12, 2002, to the Health Professions Appeal and Review Board (HPARB), the body that oversees regulated health professions in the province. The college said the new information sent by Dr. Hammer had slowed the process down.

On March 18, 2002, Dr. Hammer sent the CCO a new Nantais flyer. Another month passed. In late April, the HPARB told Dr. Hammer the CCO had given Nantais until April 23 to comply with three provisions regarding advertising. On May 7, 2002, the college would finalize their decision, if possible.

Another month passed. Hammer wrote the HPARB. It informed him on June 3 that the CCO had indeed heard the complaint on May 7, 2002. They were still working on the decision. He would get a copy as soon as possible.

On July 30, 2002, the committee sent a letter to Dr. Hammer informing them that they had ruled on his complaint. The committee found that Nantais had failed to remove testimonials from his office phone greeting until prompted by the committee and that he did not submit a revised Yellow Pages advertisement despite agreeing to do so. The committee referred these alleged infractions and the allegation that Nantais engaged in unprofessional conduct to the Discipline Committee.

The committee found Nantais's Web site claim that "Chiropractic May Help" a long list of ailments acceptable. More importantly, they dismissed Dr. Hammer's complaint that Nantais was operating beyond the scope of practice. The committee stated that there is evidence that appropriate chiropractic care may help patients with asthma, and that though it would be inaccurate to state that chiropractic care cures epilepsy, there are case studies citing improvement or abatement of epileptic symptoms for patients under chiropractic care. The committee itself provided more than a dozen references to studies on chiropractic and its effect on a wide range of diseases and disorders including epilepsy, asthma, otitis media, seizure disorders, as well as athletic ability and general health. The committee told Dr. Hammer that he either did not understand the chiropractic paradigm or he simply disagreed with it but, in their view, there is evidence in the chiropractic literature that improvement in neuro-spinal integrity may have an effect on other illnesses.

Nantais is not the only chiropractor making such claims. Other Canadian chiropractors are also making outrageous statements about the benefits of chiropractic.

> Have you have taken your child to a pediatrician and have not received good results through traditional medical care? Is your child

suffering from a life-threatening disorder? Does your child suffer from attention deficit disorder? Is your child on Ritalin? If so, consider chiropractic care as an alternative to the traditional model of medicine. Our focus is to enhance your child's nervous system and immunological system via gentle hands-on chiropractic spinal adjustments.

This is from the Web site of chiropractor Jeffrey Needham (www.need-hamfamilychiro.com). The site is filled with false and misleading statements. Needham also engages in scare tactics, trying to frighten parents into bringing their children in for chiropractic treatment.

"Why should I take them to a chiropractor?"

"Well, just like the dentist a spinal check-up performed by a chiropractor could prove to be valuable in the life of your child. With not only the trauma of childbirth itself, children are constantly falling, jumping and running. These normal childhood activities are just a few of the many methods for vertebral subluxations to occur. If not detected these subluxations can have serious health consequences for the future ... Many pediatric visits to the chiropractor are due to ear infections, allergies, asthma, attention problems, bed-wetting, back/neck pain and headaches. Although, chiropractic does not treat specific symptoms, we find that a healthy immune system results in an effective defense mechanism. Such complications can arise when a subluxation within the vertebra of the spine impair communication of the messages traveling from your brain via the spinal cord to the body.

"Pediatric chiropractors are specifically trained to examine and adjust children of all ages. Even for newborns it's important to remove subluxations to ensure the future health of your child."

These statements are unsupported, and most chiropractors know it — or should know it. Just last year, a widely discussed journal paper stated, "Currently available experimental data do not justify claims for the value of chiropractic care in populations of children."[27]

Needham then goes on to make a series of unproven claims, including the idea that chiropractic preventative adjustments are necessary to keep children healthy.

Often, subluxations exist without the signs and symptoms, yet they can produce colic, ear infections, asthma etc. We stress that chiropractic is not a treatment for signs and symptoms, a healthy spine and nervous system creates a strong defense mechanism to battle against sickness. This is why we promote that people without signs and symptoms be checked for subluxations.

Nothing in this statement is backed up by evidence. Again, chiropractors themselves have made this clear in their writings, stating, "The prophylactic value of chiropractic care and of subluxation correction are unproven."[28] While the profession discreetly debates about the science and ethics of these beliefs and tactics, parents and children are deluded into thinking that they need their spines adjusted to avoid terrible future deformation and disease.

Denials, Evasions, and Threats

The chiropractic leadership in Canada is aware, or should be aware, that chiropractors are making unsupported claims and operating outside the scope of practice. They have received formal letters from physicians at the Hospital for Sick Children in Toronto, from the Canadian Pediatric Society, and from a group of concerned neurologists, all telling them that chiropractors are making false claims, treating children, and operating far beyond their scope of practice by treating or claiming to treat organic disease. Those letters were rebuffed by the chiropractic regulatory agencies and professional associations, which, rather than investigate the concerns, issued denials or demanded retractions and threatened action against the physicians raising the issues. Often the message was ignored, while the messenger was attacked.

Dr. John Wedge experienced that first-hand when he and three colleagues at Toronto's famous Hospital for Sick Children sent a letter of concern to the Ministry of Health in Ontario about chiropractors treating babies and children.

Dr. Wedge is an orthopedic surgeon and the hospital's surgeon in chief. He had had, in the past, little interest in chiropractic and had never engaged in chiro-bashing, as he called it. When he worked at University Hospital in Saskatoon, he allowed chiropractic students to observe during rounds. But in the fall of 2001, he was growing worried about the increasing number of parents he was seeing who had their children under the care of a chiropractor for non-musculoskeletal problems such as ear infections, asthma, and bed-wetting. He and his colleagues were also concerned about chiropractors doing preventative manipulation to remove so-called subluxations, and counselling parents about the dangers of immunization.

On May 11, 2001, he sent a letter outlining these concerns, which he and three other colleagues had signed, to Mary Beth Valentine, director of the program policy branch of the Integrated Policy and Planning Division of the

Ministry of Health and Long-Term Care of Ontario. They raised their concerns regarding pediatric chiropractic and asked her to look into them. In October, after the media reported on the doctors' letter, Jo Ann Wilson, the registrar and general counsel for the College of Chiropractors of Ontario (CCO), the regulatory body for the province's chiropractors, sent a five-page letter to Dr. Wedge. It was marked "Without Prejudice" at the top. In it she questioned why the doctors contacted the government without first contacting the college. She demanded that he provide details of any incident involving a chiropractor acting improperly and she wanted it all in writing immediately. She closed the letter with a warning that the college would not be letting the issue drop and that if Dr. Wedge could not substantiate the allegations made in his letter, the college wanted a written apology and retraction.

The letter, and what he perceived to be its threatening tone, perplexed Dr. Wedge. The college is the body that regulates chiropractic in Ontario in the public interest, but it seemed more interested in defending chiropractors than in investigating the doctors' concerns, he thought. Dr. Wedge is a polite, soft-spoken man, but his letter back to the CCO was firm and direct. He took exception to the threatening tone of their letter and then made it clear that the CCO had no authority to question his right to correspond with whomever he saw fit. He repeated that his concerns came out of his own experience with children and their parents and the claims that chiropractors were making regarding the ability to successfully treat disorders such as ear infections, bed-wetting, asthma, attention deficit disorder, and much else.

To reinforce his point, he provided a recent advertisement from an Oakville, Ontario newspaper, in which chiropractors were claiming to be able to help a list of childhood disorders. Dr. Wedge told the CCO that such claims were inappropriate and that no scientific evidence existed to support them. As a start, he suggested the CCO investigate the chiropractors who took out the advertisement, something that should not be too difficult, as their names were printed on the ad. He also suggested that the CCO might want to spend less time "attacking critics" and more time policing its profession. He noted in closing that they seemed more concerned with disseminating chiropractic propaganda than with being a regulatory body.

Then Dr. Wedge added his own warning — he did not want to be pestered with anymore threatening letters from the CCO. "I never heard from them again," he said.[29]

A position paper on chiropractic care for children issued by the Canadian Pediatric Society in February 2002 met with the same kind of defensiveness and evasion that greeted the doctors at Sick Kids. The position paper states, among other things, that children do not need chiropractic adjustments to be healthy, that there is no evidence that chiropractic care is effective for asthma, bed-wetting, ear infections, learning disabilities, or a host of other disorders, and that the Canadian Paediatric Society supports childhood immunization, a treatment some chiropractors counsel against. *(See "The Not-So-Well-Adjusted Child")* In response to the paper, the chiropractic leadership skated around the issues, implying that chiropractors treat children for musculoskeletal problems.

"One of the effects that chiropractors find in clinical practice is that as we treat spinal problems, what we see is improvement generally in the health of patients across the board," Stan Gorchynski, chairman of the Ontario Chiropractic Association, told a *National Post* reporter. "And as a result, parents will bring their children in."[30]

In another press report, Gorchynski suggested the same thing — that chiropractic effectiveness, not marketing, was drawing in parents. "What we're seeing is that patients attend because they get benefit," Gorchynski said. "And these are people who pay, out of their pocket."

He then went a step further, noting that there was a great deal of anecdotal evidence that supported chiropractic for kids.

> He recounted such an anecdote. An adult patient asked him to treat her 18-month old daughter, who had been on antibiotics for ear infections since she was three weeks old. "Within three weeks of care, the child was off antibiotics and that was about 10 years ago and (she) hasn't been on them since," he noted. "The issue here is: What did I treat? I didn't treat her ear problems. I treated her spine. And she improved. We can split hairs as to what I treated. But I didn't treat her ears. I didn't even come near her ears."[31]

He also assured reporters and the public that The Canadian Chiropractic Association does not espouse an anti-immunization policy. He said chiropractors who urge parents not to immunize their children could be disciplined. Then, in a moment of candour, Gorchynski admitted that some chiropractors do not believe in using drugs or other artificial means such as vaccination to promote the body's immune system. Those chiropractors, he said, might be compelled to explain their views to their patients so that they could make an informed decision.[32]

But even that admission falls short of the reality of the situation. Though official chiropractic maintains that their membership merely informs parents about the pros and cons of immunization, it is difficult, if not impossible, to find a single chiropractic pamphlet, Web site, book, or article that is supportive of childhood vaccination.

Another person who found out first-hand how the chiropractic professional associations react to criticism is Toronto physician Dr. Greg Dubord. Dubord co-coordinated a seminar on alternative medicine, including chiropractic, for the continuing education of doctors across Canada. The Review of Alternative Medicine Institute (RAM), of which Dubord is a director, organized the seminar, which was accredited by the College of Family Physicians of Canada.

A chiropractic representative attended the seminar at the Toronto Airport Hilton in October 1999, and he didn't like what he heard. Montreal physician Dr. Murray Katz did a thirty-minute presentation on chiropractic. It was frank and critical.

About a month later, Dr. Dubord received a letter from David Chapman-Smith, a lawyer and the general counsel for the Ontario Chiropractic Association. Along with the letter, Chapman-Smith attached a formal letter he had sent to Dr. Calvin Gutkin, the executive director and chief executive officer of the College of Family Physicians of Canada, which questioned whether the seminars should be accredited in the future and questioned the backgrounds and suitability of Dr. Dubord and co-director Dr. Wallace Sampson to run the seminar. "Under their joint leadership the RAM seminar has highly unreliable health information," wrote Chapman-Smith.[33]

He suggested a chiropractor would be a more appropriate speaker and he cautioned that the college "risks considerable embarrassment through continued association with this program." He encouraged the college to look into the issues and copied the letter to the College of Physicians and Surgeons of Ontario and the Ontario College of Family Physicians, both regulatory bodies for physicians.

Dr. Dubord responded by sending a letter to Jean Moss, the president of the Canadian Memorial Chiropractic College, who had received a copy of Chapman-Smith's original letter. In it, he addressed the not-too-subtle tactics the chiropractors had employed:

> Chiropractic is a much younger profession than medicine, and youth is forgivably awkward at times. With all due respect to them, the Ontario Chiropractic Association was a tad misinformed to recruit Mr. Chapman-Smith, a lawyer, to attempt to influence the content of a scientific symposium. Science doesn't work that way. Not in Canada.[34]

Despite the defensive tactics, the evasions, and the public denials, it's clear that most chiropractic leaders are well aware of the problems in the profession. Unfortunately, some seem to view the issue not as a fundamental problem but as a media relations matter.

In October 2000, the Ontario Chiropractic Association President's Letter spoke about the upcoming inquest. It issued the same warning:

> We are aware that chiropractic detractors are again going to prac-
> titioners' offices posing as patients in order to pick up promo-
> tional materials which can be used against the profession. I cau-
> tion you that public materials on display in your office should
> reflect the chiropractic scope of practice as outlined in The
> Chiropractic Act. The further away from The Chiropractic Act
> that your materials are, the greater the likelihood that you will be
> challenged on them. All available OCA materials are appropriate
> for public consumption.[35]

The chiropractic leadership wants the profession to appear legitimate for the public and the media, who occasionally take a slightly closer look at chiropractic claims. Most of the efforts of the professional leadership are, like these appeals, not aimed at actually cleaning up chiropractic, but only cleaning up its appearance.

Clinical Practice Guidelines — More Window Dressing

In 1994, the Canadian Chiropractic Association commissioned the production of a set of clinical practice guidelines that would assist chiropractors in delivering appropriate care for specified clinical circumstances. Earlier, American chiropractors had produced a set of guidelines that were not very good, in part because they failed to address the whole controversy surrounding the vertebral subluxation and its treatment implications.[36] Guidelines based on an entity that may or may not exist just don't work very well.

In comparison, the Canadian guidelines did better, but they too had serious flaws in the areas of use of evidence and editorial independence. Two researcheers gave the CCA document low marks in important areas — 39 percent for identification and use of evidence, 46 percent for stakeholder involvement, and zero for editorial independence. More worrisome was the CCA document's weakness in linking evidence to recommendations about treatment.[37] None of that really mattered, because regardless of what the document said, Canadian chiropractors were unlikely to agree on it or follow it.

That's what sociologist Leslie Biggs discovered when she polled chiropractors on their beliefs and attitudes. She found that chiropractors had such divergent opinions about chiropractic philosophy and scope of practice that implementing standards of practice would not work, nor were they likely to change clinical behaviour.

She followed that study with another that looked at chiropractors' attitudes toward standards of care. Standards of care define appropriate treatment based on well-founded scientific evidence. Guidelines provide a framework for clinical practice that should be followed in most circumstances, but standards of care "represent the highest level of clinical scrutiny which, in essence, represents core elements of clinical knowledge."[38] She found that chiropractors in Canada could not agree on any definition of standards of care. Because of that, there is little chance they would implement or accept them. "We concluded that it would be difficult to implement national CPGs [clinical practice guidelines] given the competing views of chiropractic philosophy and scope of practice," wrote Biggs.[39]

One third of Canadian chiropractors are what Biggs calls "empiricists." They see chiropractic as an alternative form of health care. They subscribe to the traditional chiropractic philosophy as espoused by D.D. and B.J. Palmer, and they support a broad scope of practice. They are the Canadian version of American "straight" and "super straight" chiropractors. This group supported a narrow definition of standards of care, limiting it to issues of safety and diagnosis. They did not believe that standards of care were related to the validation of chiropractic methods. Most favoured standards set by an expert panel of chiropractors with no outside input from doctors or other experts.

The chiropractors Biggs surveyed worried that standards of care could represent a "new form of policing the chiropractic profession," and so they rejected any organization or group outside of chiropractic being involved in setting the standards. In the end, chiropractors could not agree on who should set standards of care, but most favoured the Canadian Chiropractic Association, which is seen as best representing the interests of the entire profession.

Most telling was that chiropractors were least interested in having chiropractic research organizations set the standards. "Only 40% of chiropractors would entrust the setting of standards of care to chiropractic research funding agencies, which arguably represent the more scientific approach to chiropractic but do not represent the mainstream view within chiropractic."[40] This is an extremely important point, because if standards of care are to be based on well-founded scientific evidence, who better to help set them than chiropractic researchers? What the survey reveals is that when it comes to setting guidelines and standards, the majority of chiropractors do not believe in a science-based practice. Chiropractic organizations are aware of this fact, yet they continue to market chiropractic to the public as a science-based health care system.

Biggs optimistically speculates that rationalist chiropractors — the one-fifth of the profession that supports a scope of practice limited to musculoskeletal disorders — and moderates could reach a compromise. But, she wrote, overall consensus appeared impossible:

> ...it is unlikely that an agreement over standards of care could be reached between empirically-oriented chiropractors and rationalists and moderates even if the standards were developed by a chiropractic organization(s). The data in this article and our earlier study consistently indicate that empiricist chiropractors have a different vision of chiropractic than rationalists and moderates.[41]

Regulation — Appearance and Reality

The fact that chiropractors have separate and distinct visions of chiropractic is well known within chiropractic. The profession understands that the schisms among their membership present a problem when dealing with the public and with government and insurers.

Though these divisions make regulation of the profession a practical impossibility, the chiropractic leadership is unwilling or unable to do anything substantive about it. Instead, the leadership has focused on damage control in the media and in the presentation of the profession to the public. If reality cannot be managed, then perception will be.

In a 1997 Ontario Chiropractic Association newsletter, vice president Glenn Yates spoke to the issue directly. His words reveal the reality behind the façade of chiropractic.

> A discussion of OCA direction would be incomplete without a strong reference to philosophy. The OCA and individual OCA board members are sometimes accused of pursuing an evidence based "medical" model at the expense of chiropractic philosophy in pursuit of its goals. While evidence has its place in dealing with groups ands organizations which make decisions based on evidence, the OCA and its individual board members are representative of the strongly principled chiropractor.[42]

Here, Yates expresses the attitude toward evidence held by many members of the profession. He also reveals the leadership's open admission that their presentation of chiropractic is purely expedient: for people interested in evidence, they will be evidence-based, if that's what it takes to succeed.

But Yates goes on to assure the philosophy-based members that their brand of chiropractic will be well represented where it is likely to be beneficial — in front of the public.

The concern and fear of loss of voice in terms of not using chiropractic language in our materials and in not addressing and educating the public about the vertebral subluxation complex is acknowledged and understood. You will see materials currently being procured for future release that this issue has not only been addressed but it also being pursued.[43]

While it's true that the OCA is a professional association that must reflect the opinions and interests of its membership, the same cannot be said of the College of Chiropractors of Ontario. It is the regulatory body, mandated to act in the public interest. But a report from the CCO in 2001 addressing the issue of scope of practice reveals a profession in a profound state of confusion about what it is, what it does, and what responsibility it has to the public.

In an October 2001 CCO newsletter, Alan Gotlib, former vice president of the organization, told the province's chiropractors that he was concerned that chiropractors were operating beyond the scope of practice without fully informing the patient. This practice "has continued to cloud professional growth and brought pressure to the concepts of public safety and protection," he wrote. Gotlib then went on to say that the profession was working with stakeholders to develop standards of practice designed to raise the level of enforceability and to reinforce the importance of chiropractors operating within the scope of practice. Gotlib emphasized the idea that the province only licenses certain controlled acts, and that the profession must define its scope of practice by setting out policies, guidelines, and standards within their statutory mandate and by articulating them to the profession and the public. He then proposed an extraordinary idea: that the scope of practice is essentially what chiropractors say it is.

Our scope of practice statement is not a license. It is a description setting out an explanation to the public about what we commonly do and what they may expect when attending a chiropractor."[44]

Informing the patient is the most important thing, said Gotlib, and he then provided an outline of what chiropractors may do that is breathtaking in its inclusiveness.

To insure [sic] consent is fully informed and voluntarily given, chiropractors must clearly explain the following to their patients:
- a service being provided is in your capacity as a chiropractor and conforms to the current standards of practice of chiropractic; or
- a service being provided is in your capacity as a chiropractor

but does not conform to the usual and customary standards of practice of the profession of chiropractic and the patient may not have the benefit of malpractice liability protection in the event of an adverse outcome. In this scenario, the chiropractor may receive the patient's consent to undertake a short therapeutic trial of treatment for a particular condition currently not well-supported in the scientific literature with clear, convincing and cogent evidence, but supported by experts in clinical opinion or case studies in peer-reviewed scholarly chiropractic literature;

- a service being provided is not in your capacity as a chiropractor but simply as a practitioner operating in the public domain, does not conform to the standards of practice of the profession of chiropractic, and the patient may not have the benefit of malpractice liability protection in the event of adverse outcome. In this scenario, services that are not controlled acts, such as iridology or ear candling, could be provided if the member has appropriate training and expertise.

This outline empowers chiropractors to treat everything with any technique they choose, as long as they inform the patient. Though Gotlib invoked professional standards of practice, not only do chiropractors in Canada not agree on any standards of practice, examination of those standards reveals they do not address the fundamental issues in the profession. The bottom line? Chiropractors can do pretty much anything within chiropractic, and even engage in more pseudo-scientific practices such as ear candling and iridology, and it's okay with the regulators.

Gotlib then provides chiropractors with a blanket excuse that allows them to treat virtually any human ailment. He wrote:

Confusion arises when patients with serious conditions, such as allergies, cancer or AIDS, believe they are being treated for those particular conditions when, in fact, the treatment focuses on concurrent secondary neuro-musculoskeletal problems. There is a clear distinction in treating a patient for a condition as opposed to treating a patient with a condition.[45]

Notice it's the patient who is "confused" about what the chiropractor is treating. The idea that chiropractors can treat allergies and other serious disorders is not something invented by confused patients, as Gotlib glibly asserted, but rather a notion strongly promoted by some chiropractors and their official bodies from coast to coast.

Gotlib then addressed a major controversy in modern chiropractic and amazingly dismissed the entire issue in a sentence. He wrote:

> ...the treatment of pediatric conditions, such as colic, enuresis, asthma, otitis media, attention deficit hyperactivity disorder, commonly referred to as non-neuro-musculoskeletal, has yet to be based on unequivocal cogent evidence beyond the expert clinical opinion or case report levels. Also, characterizing some of these conditions as non-neuro-musculoskeletal as opposed to neuro-musculoskeletal is in dispute. These academic arguments are not relevant to the patient — what is relevant is safety and competent, ethical chiropractic care.[46]

The distinction between "neuro-musculoskeletal" and "non-neuro-muskuloskeletal" is fundamental to any real understanding and enforcement of a chiropractic scope of practice. It is not a mere academic argument. It is extremely relevant to the patient. If all conditions are neuro-musculoskeletal, as subluxuation-based chiropractors claim, then any human ailment — from asthma to multiple sclerosis to learning disabilities — falls within the chiropractic scope of practice.

Chiropractors present themselves as experts in the handling of back pain and other musculoskeletal problems when addressing lawmakers and academics. But they don't really see themselves that way at all. Gotlib told the chiropractors of Ontario:

> Clearly, the scope of practice statement does not restrict or limit us to only musculoskeletal conditions. The purpose of the Regulated Health Professions Act (RHPA), was to provide for the evolution in the role that all regulated professionals, including chiropractors, play in the health care system.[47]

The CCO is well aware of the crisis bubbling just below the surface in chiropractic. Many chiropractors are hostile to the notion of a science-based practice that focuses on musculoskeletal problems and leaves behind the dogma of the Palmers. They are a vocal element within chiropractic, and when Gotlib sought to dispel some myths about the regulatory body, he spoke to the issue that sits at the core of the controversy:

> **CCO would like to take the opportunity to set the record straight on a number of issues that have arisen and may be causing concerns to some members:**

CCO is not out to get subluxation-based chiropractors

Subluxation-based or evidenced-based, limited care or full-spectrum care, the CCO could not care less, as long as members comply with all CCO standards of practice, policies and guidelines. A range of practitioners serves on CCO Council and committees, and participate as examiners and peer assessors.[48i]

Coming from the former vice president of the body policing the largest group of chiropractors in the country, the statement that the CCO "could not care less" whether chiropractors practice "subluxation-based or evidence-based" care is astonishing.

It contrasts dramatically with the way the profession presents itself to the public, revealing the ongoing misrepresentation of the profession on the one hand, and the lack of any real self-regulation on the other. The two kinds of chiropractic Gotlib lists could not be more different, and to abdicate responsibility for dealing with the difference is to forfeit in any real way the regulation of the profession.

These issues within chiropractic seem to evaporate when it's time to talk about the profession to doctors or to the public. Less than a year before the CCO outlined the scope of practice issues in their October report, David Leprich, chairman of the board of governors of the Canadian Chiropractic Association, wrote a letter to *The Medical Post* in defense of chiropractic. In it he posed and then answered a series of questions, one of which was, Is chiropractic scientific?

He wrote, "What began as a poorly understood form of treatment more than 100 years ago has evolved into a healing discipline firmly grounded in science." Answering the question of what chiropractors treat, Leprich mentioned disorders of the spine and its associated nervous system, as well as back pain, neck pain, and headache. When he addressed the issue of chiropractic for children, he stated that chiropractors treated children for pretty much the same things that they treated adults — musculoskeletal problems, particularly low-back pain."[49]

This primer was, at best, incomplete and unrepresentative of the modern chiropractic profession in Canada. At worst, it was an utter misrepresentation of chiropractic, a whitewash that grossly misrepresents the state of the profession today.

CMCC: School as Saviour?

The notion that CMCC is turning out a new generation of science-based chiropractors who will, by their attitudes and education, reform the profession, appears to be more public relations than fact.

Though CMCC claims it conducts a science-based program, its graduates don't seem to be very scientific. They account for about 75 percent of licensed chiropractors in Canada, and they seldom run science-based practices. Many of them use unscientific and pseudo-scientific modalities — most of which have been shown to be bogus — on their patients.

A 1993 survey of Canadian chiropractors by the National Board of Chiropractic Examiners found that:

- 27.4 percent used homeopathic remedies
- 31 percent used applied kinesiology
- 66.3 percent used acupressure/meridian therapy.[50]

Studies show that CMCC students form an interest in unscientific ideas long before they graduate. A recent survey of CMCC students found that 80 percent of those surveyed favoured more emphasis on the philosophy of chiropractic. They felt that chiropractic philosophy was a "very important part of their chiropractic education."[51] This sounds benign enough, unless you know what chiropractic philosophy is. It's an outdated, irrational dogma, a set of unscientific ideas and principles handed down as a form of divine wisdom from the founders of chiropractic. Chiropractor and historian Joseph Donahue calls chiropractic philosophy an "unscientific relic of D.D. Palmer's personal religious beliefs."[52] It is a body of unproven and unprovable doctrine.

But CMCC students want more of it, not less, and they told their teachers as much. More than 90 percent of them thought that chiropractic philosophy was "important for a successful practice." In fact, students at CMCC can't seem to get enough of what several chiropractic scholars consider the scourge of the profession:

> The recent proliferation of student philosophy clubs and the increasing popularity of extracurricular philosophy seminars presented by self-styled experts in this domain suggests that students' needs in this area have not been fully addressed by the traditional approach to teaching the philosophy of chiropractic."[53]

The young students should be more science-oriented than their teachers, but they're actually more interested in the philosophy of chiropractic than their instructors – although not by much.

At what is touted as one of the most science-oriented chiropractic schools in the world, 61 percent of all faculty members and 83 percent of clinical education faculty members "felt that the philosophy of chiropractic should be part of all aspects of the college's education process."[54] Rather than abandon what some chiropractors have called pseudo-scientific nonsense, CMCC's teachers are recommending more of it in the program.

The reason for that may originate in the beliefs held by the teachers themselves. The same survey revealed that 79 percent of the faculty believed philosophy should play a part in the school clinic's patient management program and that 67 percent "disagreed with only treating a patient chiropractically when there is current scientific evidence to support the treatment."[55]

That means that the instructors teaching the great majority of Canada's chiropractors believe in applying irrational, unscientific beliefs to patient care. As well, they support treating patients with chiropractic in the absence of scientific evidence in support of its use. Real clinical practice guidelines and standards of care must be based on science in order to be valid and valuable. The inability of chiropractors to define their profession or their scope of practice or to agree on profession-wide, evidence-based standards of practice is not surprising when you examine what they've been taught at CMCC.

Another survey of CMCC students shows how Canada's chiropractors-in-training are becoming less, rather than more, scientific.

CMCC students have a great interest in what chiropractic calls "Brand Name," or simply "Name," techniques. These techniques — and there are dozens and dozens of them —have little or no scientific evidence to support their underlying theory or their efficacy. *(See "Gizmos, Parlour Tricks, and Nonsense")*

Nonetheless, students are clamouring to learn them, and 87 percent of those surveyed wanted increased exposure to Name techniques.[56] They are so interested that students at CMCC have formed their own "Technique Clubs" under the purview of the Student Administrative Council.

The students' appetite for Name techniques is most likely simply a reflection of their popularity among practicing chiropractors in Canada. The problem? CMCC students want more training in Name techniques that have little, if any, evidence of effectiveness. As well, most Name techniques are based upon unscientific ideas such as vitalism, subluxation, and Innate. The entrepreneurs promoting and marketing the techniques "can make virtually any unsubstantiated claim they want without fear of professional censure."[57]

As chiropractor Lon Morgan wrote: "These methods of 'analysis' and treatment of the holy subluxation are more dependent on the promotional personality of the 'technique' peddler than they are upon credible evidence. All too often these 'analysis' and 'technique' methods and gadgets are sold to students and practitioners with messianic fervor that obscures their lack of credible verification."[58]

How can educators introduce students to Name techniques that make claims with little evidence to back them up and integrate that teaching with the model of chiropractic presented at CMCC? A CMCC faculty member looking at the question came up with a remarkable observation — except for acute low back pain and certain types of headaches, there are few studies that support the efficacy of the model of chiropractic the college teaches anyway.[59] Putting Name techniques onto the CMCC curriculum, many of which are incompatible with one another, let alone the college's core approach, is fraught with difficulties. But introduction of Name techniques has occurred and will likely expand. Why?

Brian Gleberzon, an assistant professor at CMCC, couldn't be clearer about it:

> When considering curricular integration of Name techniques, it is possible for CMCC to be responsive to student desires, which cannot be ignored when one remembers that college revenues are so highly tuition dependent. This should not be interpreted as a suggestion to pander to student's every whim. However, a curriculum that reflects current practice activities of Canadian chiropractors (including CMCC graduates) may ultimately have a positive influence on alumni membership.[60]

Gleberzon acknowledges that the acceptance of these techniques comes with some dangers and that the school will have to try to "prevent outlandish techniques from taking hold among students through exploitation of their inexperience."[61] He also admits that some of the techniques already taught at CMCC, such as Palmer HIO (Hole-in-One), support a vitalistic paradigm of chiropractic. That's a polite way of saying the technique is unscientific and depends upon pre-scientific, irrational beliefs.

How can all this be reconciled in what purports to be a science-based academic institution? It can't be, and Gleberzon admits it. But he says science has also punched some holes in the general curriculum, noting that the "hard science approach" has been used to "refute aspects of the Diversified model which are simultaneously taught to students."[62] Not only are CMCC students confronted with science challenging the main form of chiropractic therapy they're taught, but now they have to balance the dogmatic, unscientific approach of Name techniques too. Most of those are incompatible with each other and with the Diversified model they are taught at CMCC.[63] It must all be quite confusing for the undergraduates at the college.

Strip away the obfuscating language of chiropractic journal articles, and the reality is that CMCC students are presented with a hodge-podge of unscientific, incompatible, irrational therapies, all under the umbrella of chiropractic. They have no real way to differentiate the effective, evidence-based, scientific therapies from the nonsense.

How will the school's administrators make rational, evidence-based decisions about teaching name techniques in the absence of evidence? They won't. They will just fulfill their mandate to present a "practice-related" curriculum, which means, like most colleges, they will prepare students to get a job by reflecting the job market they will enter.

So CMCC will not lead chiropractic. Rather, it will reflect the current state of chiropractic, even if the mirror shows a practice awash in unscientific and pseudo-scientific techniques.

CMCC will graduate 150 new chiropractors each year. Projections indicate that 5,000 chiropractors will join the ranks in Canada by 2005, pushing the total to 10,000. The balance of new chiropractors will come from a variety of chiropractic colleges, mostly American-based schools. Those schools, said Gleberzon, "provide extensive exposure to a wide variety of Name techniques either in the core curriculum or within an elective program."[64] The result, from both CMCC and elsewhere, is more brand new chiropractors practicing more unproven and unscientific forms of chiropractic on Canadian patients.

The Corvaro Suit

One of those patients was Petronilla Corvaro. On August 17, 2000, the thirty-eight-year-old student went to the CMCC's outpatient clinic complaining of lower back pain and a tension headache. According to a statement of claim filed with the Superior Court of Justice in Ontario by Corvaro, that visit was the beginning of a nightmare. The claims in the statement have not been proven in a court of law. According to the statement, during her August 17 visit she was not x-rayed, nor did the CMCC chiropractor give her a proper examination or make an appropriate diagnosis before he adjusted her neck. She was not asked to sign any informed consent form. Immediately after the adjustment, Nilla, as she's called, experienced significant pain on the right side of her neck. Her headache only got worse, she felt dizzy, and her back pain didn't disappear. Over the next ten months, Nilla received over twenty chiropractic back adjustments from CMCC staff and students and from a chiropractic clinic not associated with CMCC. The CMCC chiropractors, including faculty members, repeatedly suggested additional neck adjustments, which Nilla consistently declined. Her condition did not improve.

On June 12, 2001, she felt a sharp and frightening pain in her lower back as she dressed. Concerned, for the first time she left the sphere of chiropractic treatment and went to the emergency department of the Toronto East General Hospital. Nilla had an MRI scan done the next day. It revealed a prolapsed disc at L4-5 and a herniated disc at L5-S1, which compressed the right S1 nerve root.

According to the statement of claim, Nilla refused surgery for the disc problems on the advice of an associate professor at the CMCC. She is now disabled and may require back surgery in the future. Nilla continues to experience pain and decreased mobility. She is suing the CMCC and others for $6.5 million for lost income and damages.

So, according to the statement of claim, practitioners at the CMCC, including CMCC staff, repeatedly treated a patient without detecting prolapsed and herniated discs. Amani Oakley, the lawyer representing Ms Corvaro, says that after she filed the statement of claim the CMCC asked her for clarification fo some points. Ms Oakley says she supplied the additional information, but CMCC officials have yet to file a Statement of Defence in this case. We asked CMCC for their comments about Corvaro's suit but they did not provide us with a response. Ironically, Nilla was a student at the CMCC when she went for her first treatment in August 2000. She has since left the college, disillusioned. She now has serious concerns about what she and other students were taught about how the body functions and how to treat it.

Anti-vaccination Thinking at the CMCC

Finally, the claim that CMCC is turning out more science-oriented chiropractors took a hard blow this year with the publication of a study looking at what CMCC students thought about vaccination. Today, a significant proportion of chiropractors continue to reject vaccination, and it remains a subject of contention in the chiropractic community. In Canada, both the CCA and the CMCC officially endorse vaccination, but practicing chiropractors are allowed to counsel their patients on its pros and cons, allowing them freedom of choice on the matter. *(See "The Not-So-Well-Adjusted Child")*

Surely, young chiropractic students at CMCC would be better informed than their older colleagues. Actually, a little more than half agreed with vaccination, and they became more negative the longer they stayed at CMCC. By fourth year, only 39.5 percent of students were in favour of vaccination. What's wrong? The authors blame guest speakers and anti-vaccination books and magazine articles. But they also note that fundamental chiropractic philosophy is antithetical to the concept of vaccination.

In any case, the evidence speaks for itself. After years of telling universities, the press, and the public that CMCC is a modern, science-based institution, its leadership has produced a school that has utterly failed to dispel unscientific ideas about vaccination in its students, and has failed to "vaccinate" them against pseudo-scientific thinking.

Undefined, Unproven, and Unmanageable

When the CCA and the CMCC wrote their submission to the Commission on the Future of Health Care in Canada in June 2002, they called for chiropractic to be raised up to be a full partner in the Canadian health care team. They carefully presented chiropractic as a treatment for musculoskeletal problems (particularly back pain) that was scientific and evidence-based.[65]

That's not the picture painted by chiropractor Paul Carey in a 1999 issue of *Communique*, a chiropractic newsletter he edits. In a forum designed to be read by chiropractors, Carey responded to a letter writer and provided an accurate and candid evaluation of chiropractic in Canada, based on his thirteen years of experience with the Canadian Chiropractic Protective Association, the profession's largest insurer in Canada. He wrote:

> There is no common, agreed upon definition of chiropractic. If there is, I would like you to forward it to me. I would also like to see any such definition embraced by the majority of chiropractors as I have not been able to find this definition or to see this kind of agreement among chiropractors. In fact, over the years, in dealing with over a thousand legal claims, I have not yet had two chiropractors give me the same definition of chiropractic. I find that interesting. Some of them give definitions of which I am completely unfamiliar. Others make a good attempt to explain and define themselves, but again, unanimity is lacking.[66]

This problem, as Carey was quick to point out, is not some mere academic debate. Not having any agreement around the nature of your profession, particularly in the field of health care, presents some serious issues. Carey then addressed the explosive problem so carefully avoided by the regulatory bodies — vitalistic chiropractic, or practitioners who subscribe to a "philosophy-based" practice. Here, he eschewed the obfuscating language used in so many chiropractic research papers and addressed the issue in plain English:

> I have been in the job of defending chiropractors of all philosophies and techniques for thirteen years. In that time I have had to deal with

hostile lawyers (lots of them), judges (a few) and many p...
them, as well). All these, combined with many chir...
obliged me in the defense of chiropractic, have attempte...
what can be proven, what is scientific and what is sustaina...

Unfortunately, no matter how sincere and well ...
belief systems are, they lack any ability to defend or help ...
ropractor in the court system. In fact, many times they ...
diance to the credibility and acceptance of chiropractic bu...
the variety and range of the belief systems that chiropractors ...
some of them bordering on the absurd. That is not just my ...
sonal opinion. This is the opinion of most persons who have h...
them. We have many cases where we have not been able to get c...
single chiropractor to come to the defense of another chiroprac...
Even when the chiropractor was given the option of getting an...
chiropractor he could find or choose to defend him, none would.
...I would suggest to you that vitalistic chiropractic is not very
well defined or supportable and I would ask you, if you have any
solid academic proof, to please supply it to me as I do not see it as
being supported by research or "increasingly embraced by the ever
demanding public." I would certainly invite you to objectively
support that statement.[67]

Carey's comments recall the old chiropractic joke; "For every chiropractor there is an equal and opposite chiropractor." But the problem is no joke. The situation he described in 1999 is not better, it's worse.

Chiropractic students want more philosophy, not less. They want more exposure to unproven, vitalistic NUCCA techniques, not less. And practicing chiropractors, rather than moving toward the solid, scientific footing Carey yearns for, continue to make unsubstantiated claims and are using unproven techniques more and more each year.

While chiropractors debate these issues in private, and worry aloud about the future of their profession, who is looking out for the patient? Who is looking after the interests of regular Canadians? Who is policing the ad campaigns and the pamphlets and the Web sites?

Asleep at the Wheel

In each province, the ministry of health is responsible for overseeing the self-regulated health professions. Usually, a committee or board is in place to monitor the regulatory bodies that police each profession. The general view, though, is that self-regulated professions are just that; they've earned the right to regulate themselves and to discipline their own members. And the government counts on them to do just that.

The provincial health insurance agencies that pay out for chiropractic treatment operate the same way. They refer all questions about scope of practice or billing to the regulators. Their job is to pay out, not to police the profession, they say. But what if the profession is not regulating itself very well? What happens when concerns about a profession are brought to the ministry officials? Not much, it seems.

We have learned of several attempts by concerned physicians, parents, and others to alert government officials to the serious problems within the chiropractic profession. In each case, the attempt was met with silence or inaction. We've described the efforts of Dr. Wedge and Dr. Hammer. Here are more examples of people trying to alert the government to a serious health issue.

In May 1999, Dr. Murray Katz made a formal presentation to medical consultants with the Ontario Ministry of Health in Kingston, Ontario about pediatric chiropractic in the province. On June 4, 1999, W.G.G. Fisher, the district medical consultant coordinator, wrote back to thank Dr. Katz. "Your presentation on the practice of chiropractors in Ontario was most enlightening. The written material that was distributed to the medical consultants was also of great interest, and a typical response has been '*I had no idea this was going on.*' It remains to be seen if my colleagues and I will have any opportunity to influence future decisions in the areas of practitioner funding."[68] On June 29 of that year, Dr. Katz received a letter from Susan Fitzpatrick, the acting director of the Health Services Division. She too thanked him for the presentation and assured him that the ministry closely scrutinized the services it funds and promised, "The ministry will research further the efficacy of chiropractic treatment for children." She closed the letter by saying that Dr. Katz's suggestions would be "thoroughly researched and recommendations made as appropriate."

Dr. Katz never heard from the ministry again.

In the fall of 1999, Sharon Mathiason and her husband, Allan, had a meeting with then minister of health for Saskatchewan Pat Atkinson. The Mathiasons had lost their twenty-year-old daughter, Laurie, after she suffered a stroke following chiropractic neck manipulation. Mrs. Mathiason briefed the minister for forty-five minutes regarding her concerns about pediatric chiropractic. According to Mathiason, the minister said she would contact the other four provinces that funded chiropractic to discuss the idea of potentially de-listing pediatric chiropractic from the province's health insurance program. Mathiason says she has heard nothing further from the government. Saskatchewan continues to pay for pediatric chiropractic.

In the fall of 1998, an Alberta radiologist, Dr. Marvin Levant, was getting more and more worried about chiropractic. He was concerned that many x-rays ordered by chiropractors — particularly for children — seemed in his opinion, and the opinion of other experts, to be unnecessary and inappropriate. Then he heard about the death of Laurie Mathiason. Dr. Levant did further research into the treatment of children by chiropractors and thought it was time to talk to the government.

He wrote Deputy Minister of Health Lyle Ford and requested a meeting. Dr. Levant met with Ford and several other Ministry of Health officials. During the three-hour session, Dr. Levant briefed them on pediatric chiropractic. "I brought a small doll, the size of newborn. I showed them the height of the neck of a newborn baby, roughly one inch. Chiropractors claim to be able to selectively manipulate the seven segments of that neck. And I told them that it is ludicrous. Baby's heads virtually sit on their shoulders, they virtually have no neck," said Levant.

The doctor also showed them the textbook on pediatric chiropractic used by chiropractic students, and presented the officials with a folder of other articles and pediatric chiropractic material, outlining the claims they make regarding childhood illnesses. He noted that at the time the government paid about $3.5 million to chiropractors for the treatment of children. They thanked him for the presentation. Dr. Levant says he is not aware of any action taken by the Ministry of Health on the issue of pediatric chiropractic.

In May 2001, four senior physicians at Toronto's Hospital for Sick Children wrote a letter to Mary Beth Valentine at the Ontario Ministry of Health. Valentine is the director of the program policy branch and oversees the self-regulating health professions in the province. The four doctors expressed their concern about pediatric chiropractic. They were direct about why they were writing:

> We understand that these chiropractors are responsible to the College of Chiropractic of Ontario, yet the CCO seems either unable or unwilling to enforce and ensure a strict adherence to its legally mandated scope of practice. As appeals to the CCO have met with silence in these regards, we trust that you and your ministry will expeditiously rectify this situation which has the potential to affect the health of the children of Ontario.[69]

The doctors say that, to their knowledge, nothing has been done.

The authors met with Mary Beth Valentine and her staff in June 2001 in the ministry offices in Toronto. Valentine told us that her department monitored all the health professions and that they had seen no "red flags" for chiropractic. They seemed unaware of the position statement on pediatric chiropractic by the Canadian Paediatric Society and of the 1998 position taken by the Alberta Society of Radiologists. We presented a file folder that included the statements and a variety of other material documenting false claims, anti-immunization statements, and other apparent infractions of the CCO rules. We followed up in the following weeks with several calls as to the status of the review of the material.

We received no response to our calls.

Conclusion

Chiropractic has no future, just a past it can't escape. Its survival into the twenty-first century is remarkable, but it has nothing to do with its importance as a health care profession. Its only value is face value. When anyone, anywhere, at any time has made the effort to penetrate the façade, what they find isn't a solid, coherent foundation, but a jumble of lies, misconceptions, and delusion.

In Palmer's hometown of Davenport, Iowa, a young *Quad-City Times* reporter, Mark Brown, decided to do a special report on the profession that made the mid-west town famous. As part of his investigation, Brown visited dozens of chiropractors, simply presenting himself as a new patient. He was repeatedly x-rayed; one chiropractor found his left leg longer than the other, while the next said it was the other way around. One chiropractor used a potato and a magnet to determine what kind of supplements he needed. Though healthy, Brown was told he had a hiatus hernia, a compression fracture of a cervical vertebra, illeocecal valve syndrome, and something called "ocular lock" — he was even told his ears stuck out to act as antennae for "nerve energy". His back was adjusted, his head was adjusted, and he was sold a drawer full of pills and a set of arch supports. One chiropractor even photographed his bum. In his thirty-six-page special report, Brown found all the same problems we did: outdated Palmerian dogma, unproven gadgets and gizmos, a blizzard of nonsensical techniques, chiropractors who treated babies and even animals, an ongoing war with science and medicine, and unscrupulous practice-building techniques. The difference? He was writing in 1981.

When we re-read Brown's piece, we were disturbed that so little has changed. And it convinced us even more strongly that the profession seems incapable of real progress, despite its protestations to the contrary. Chiropractors, even those critical of the profession, harbour hope that it will discard its past, reform itself, and move into the ethical and scientific future. As non-members of the chiropractic community, we hold no such hope.

We have spoken to rational chiropractors such as Americans Charles DuVall Jr. and Samuel Homola, who have publicly renounced the pseudo-science of subluxation, the insanity of Name techniques, and quasi-religious concepts like Innate. They, and a few chiropractors like them, treat a limited range of musculoskeletal problems with the conservative application of mobilization and manipulation. A very small group of reformists have set up associations for chiropractors who wish to practice scientifically. Members follow guidelines that specifically reject subluxation, nerve interference, outrageous claims, preventative maintenance, unproven chiropractic techniques, and unscientific alternative treatments. The National Association for Chiropractic Medicine (NACM), in the United States, and the Canadian Orthopractic Manual Therapists Association (COMTA) have only managed to attract about five hundred members between them. There are at least sixty-six thousand chiropractors in North America.

We see no indication that any major chiropractic association in Canada or the United States is seriously interested in reform. Ironically, the Chiropractic College of Ontario, the regulatory body for the province with the largest number of chiropractors in Canada, prohibits its members from joining COMTA. And no chiropractic organization in Canada, including the Canadian Memorial Chiropractic College, has renounced subluxation, nonsensical techniques, or pediatric chiropractic. Without these first, fundamental steps, any chance of real reform is impossible.

Within the rarified world of chiropractic academia, a few critics, like Lon Morgan and Joseph Keating Jr., call for reform and despair at the unmitigated nonsense that surrounds them. They are vilified or ignored by most of those who read their work, and the rest of the profession appears to be utterly unaware of their ideas. They openly worry about the future of chiropractic. But from our point of view, the fate of the profession, for its own sake, is unimportant.

What really matters is that chiropractic has betrayed its patients' trust. The chiropractic profession is always playing what is best for the patient against what is best for chiropractic. Most often, the patient loses. For example, Applied Kinesiology testing for allergies is utter bunk, but the chiropractic profession does not publicly reject it. Why not? Like us, chiropractic organizations should be perfectly aware that chiropractors are using Interro and Vegatest machines in Canada, machines that have been shown to be completely useless diagnostic tools. Yet they continue to be used. Why? How is that in the best interest of patients?

Chiropractic officials are aware, or should be aware, that every day chiropractors are charging Canadian patients and the government for treatments that are, in some cases, breathtaking in their stupidity. In fact, it's difficult to read about some chiropractic techniques in use today without bursting out laughing. While officials go on radio and television claiming that the profession is scientific, chiropractors are squeezing patient's skulls, checking their leg lengths, and treating children's reading problems by adjusting their spines.

And chiropractic officials are well aware that many chiropractors routinely operate beyond the scope of practice intended by the legislation governing them. In fact, chiropractic officials actively fuel government administrators' delusion that chiropractors only treat spinal conditions — meaning back problems — and not everything from high blood pressure to multiple sclerosis.

Let us be clear about this point: Almost everything, every criticism of chiropractic, raised in this book has been available to chiropractic officials for years, and we have little doubt they've read them. You may have been shocked or surprised by some of the things chiropractors claim, believe, or do, but for officials, it should be old news. They've known about the problems, in some cases for decades, and they've just let it happen.

If that wasn't bad enough, those same officials in Canada publish or distribute patient brochures and Web sites that make unsubstantiated claims. If the leadership promotes false claims, who is going to lead the reform? We've come to the conclusion that the idea of reformation from within is as fanciful as the subluxation.

Other health care professions that were once considered mainstream — such as homeopathy and naturopathy — but that couldn't take the heat of scientific scrutiny have fallen by the wayside. They now exist on the fringe, excluded from government insurance programs and lacking the legitimacy of self-regulation. Chiropractic has, by its own admission, made no major contribution to the body of scientific knowledge in the last one hundred years. Nothing specific to chiropractic has been shown to be of any health benefit. Spinal manipulative therapy that may be effective in the treatment of a small range of low-back pain can be done by other therapists who are better educated, just as skilled, and not encumbered by decades of anti-scientific dogma and irrational beliefs.

There is no place for unscientific health care in the twenty-first century. Chiropractors should not be allowed to call themselves doctors. They should not be allowed to bill provincial health plans for their unscientific treatments. It's a charade to have them licensed and self-regulated. They're unregulatable, and no one in the government appears to be paying attention to what they do. Chiropractors who are bilking patients and private and public insurance plans by using bogus treatments and testing should be prosecuted for health fraud.

One of the saddest stories we heard in the course of writing this book was told to us by Sharon Mathiason. After her daughter Laurie had her neck manipulated by a chiropractor, she complained of severe neck pain. She had booked an appointment to see the chiropractor again the next day. Concerned, Sharon told her daughter she should see a doctor. "But mom," her daughter replied, "she *is* a doctor." Laurie went to the chiropractor, had her neck adjusted, and had a fatal stroke on the adjustment table.

Laurie's assumption was understandable. We have to trust legislators to ensure that a government-approved profession that can bestow the title "doctor" is a valid, science-based health care system. Chiropractic is not.

Chiropractors like to suggest that the battle is between chiropractic and medicine. That's untrue. The real battle is between science and science fiction. Medical doctors are not in an economic "turf war" with chiropractors. Neurologists don't need more patients with strokes, orthopedic surgeons are so busy they cannot keep up, and there aren't enough family doctors in Canada to serve all its citizens. Doctors sometimes speak out against the claims of chiropractic because those claims are false. Brave physicians take action against chiropractors when they mislead or harm patients. And medical organizations speak out against chiropractic quackery — like claims for pediatric chiropractic — because it *is* quackery.

Chiropractors are in a battle with science and reality — and with themselves. While they argue endlessly about philosophy and subluxation, the world of scientific medicine is rapidly leaving them behind. In 2002, Life Chiropractic College was de-certified for its weak curriculum. Its founder, Sid Williams, was an indefatigable promoter of subluxation-based chiropractic. And Canadian neurologists issued a major statement strongly denouncing unproven claims and unscientific chiropractic treatments.

The chiropractic profession faces huge problems. It has not been able to attract more than about 10 percent of the population with its hard-to-swallow paradigm and treatments. In the meantime, chiropractic colleges have continued to graduate new chiropractors struggling to pay off student loans and start their practices. Even the Canadian Memorial Chiropractic College, which prides itself on being based in science, has failed to inoculate those new students against nonsense. As Joseph Keating Jr. points out, "Cut off from the wider health science community, the gobbledygook so often encountered among chiropractors has usually gone unchallenged within chiropractic institutions."[1] Newly minted chiropractors, convinced that "Chiropractic works!", lacking skepticism, and enchanted with all kinds of unscientific, irrational notions, are likely to make outrageous claims and engage in questionable practices. In a highly competitive environment, and faced with a public seemingly more open to magical thinking and holistic hooey, the temptation to engage in chiro-nonsense is almost irresistible. Keating warns that it could be a "a recipe for quackery, health fraud, and student loan defaults."[2]

As we finished this book, we found ourselves considering the following questions:

Why should Canadian citizens, governments, and private health care plans pay for chiropractic treatments that are unproven and far beyond any reasonable interpretation of their scope of practice?

Why doesn't the government clamp down on chiropractic organizations that stoop to quackery in their publications and refuse to stamp out bogus treatments in their profession?

Why do government bodies in Canada continue to take chiropractic at face value when proof of its divisiveness, quackery, and lack of evidence and efficacy are easy to uncover?

Why are chiropractors allowed to treat healthy babies and children who have nothing wrong with their spines?

Why do health insurance plans pay chiropractors without knowing what they are treating children for?

Why should ordinary Canadians be expected to untangle the morass of chiropractic treatments when chiropractors can't?

We think the existence of government-legitimized and government-funded chiropractic in Canada is the health story of the decade. Chiropractic organizations aren't just guilty of misrepresenting unproven treatments for gain — that would be just simple quackery or health fraud. They're guilty of misrepresenting the entire profession, and government has been asleep at the wheel, leaving ordinary Canadians vulnerable to exploitation.

Chiropractic's founder, D.D. Palmer, was born in Canada. He was a deeply religious man who believed that without the flow of intelligence through the nerves, disease could rise up in the body. In Canada, the body chiropractic is riddled with sickness. Strong medicine is required.

Afterword

HOW TO CHOOSE A CHIROPRACTOR IF YOU DECIDE TO CONSULT ONE
Stephen Barrett, M.D.

F inding a competent chiropractor can be difficult because the majority of chiropractors are involved in unscientific practices.[1,2] Most problems that are suitable for chiropractic care can be managed as well or better by medical doctors, osteopaths, or physical therapists. If you do decide to consult a chiropractor, begin with a telephone interview during which you explore the chiropractor's attitudes and practice patterns.

Positive Signs

Try to find a chiropractor whose practice is limited to conservative treatment of back pain and other musculoskeletal problems. Ask your medical doctor for the names of any who fit this description and appear to be trustworthy.

Membership in the National Association for Chiropractic Medicine or the Canadian Academy of Manipulative Therapists (CAMT) is a very good sign, but the number of chiropractors who belong to these groups is small. CAMT's "orthopractic guidelines" describe a science-based approach to manipulative therapy. The Chirobase Web site (http://www.chirobase.org) has posted more detailed guidelines and maintains a directory of chiropractors who subscribe to them.

In addition to manual manipulation or stretching of tight muscles or joints, science-based chiropractors commonly use heat or ice packs, ultrasound treatment, and other modalities similar to those of physical therapists. They may also recommend a home exercise program. For most conditions that chiropractic care can help, significant improvement should occur within a few visits.

Negative Signs

Avoid chiropractors who advertise about "danger signals that indicate the need for chiropractic care," make claims about curing diseases, try to get patients to sign contracts for lengthy treatment, promote regular "preventive" adjustments, use scare tactics, or disparage scientific medical treatment or preventive measures such as immunization or fluoridation.

Avoid chiropractors who purport to diagnose or treat "subluxations," who have waiting room literature promoting "nerve interference" as an underlying cause of disease, or who post charts or distribute literature suggesting that chiropractic might help nearly every type of health problem.

Avoid any chiropractor who routinely performs or orders x-ray examinations of all patients. Most patients who consult a chiropractor do not need them. Be especially wary of full-spine x-ray examinations. This practice has doubtful diagnostic value and involves a large amount of radiation.

Avoid chiropractors who "prescribe" dietary supplements, homeopathic products, or herbal products for the treatment of disease or who sell any of these products in their offices. For dietary advice, the best sources are physicians and registered dietitians.

Avoid chiropractors who offer Biological Terrain Assessment, body fat analysis, computerized "nutrient deficiency" testing, contact reflex analysis, computerized range-of-motion analysis, contour analysis (also called moire contourography), cytotoxic testing, electrodermal testing, Functional Intracellular Analysis (FIA), hair analysis, herbal crystallization analysis, inclinometry, iridology, leg-length testing, live blood cell analysis (also called nutritional blood analysis or Hemaview), testing with a Nervo-Scope or similar spinal heat-detecting device, Nutrabalance, NUTRI-SPEC, pendulum divination, reflexology, saliva testing, spinal ultrasound testing to "measure progress, surface electromyography (SEMG), thermography, a Toftness device, weighing on a twin-scale device called a Spinal Analysis Machine (S.A.M.), or any other dubious diagnostic procedure identified on Quackwatch.

Avoid chiropractors who utilize acupuncture, Activator Methods, allergy testing, applied kinesiology, Bio Energetic Synchronization Technique (B.E.S.T.), chelation therapy, colonic irrigation, cranial or craniosacral therapy, laser acupuncture, magnetic or biomagnetic therapy, Neuro Emotional Technique (NET), or Neural Organization Technique (NOT), or who exhibit a dogmatic attachment to any other specific chiropractic technique or school of thought.

Understand that some chiropractic treatments involve significant risk. Spinal manipulations involving sudden movements have greater potential for injury than more conservative types of therapy. Be aware that chiropractic neck manipulation can cause serious injuries. Neck manipulation should be done gently and with care to avoid excessive rotation that could damage the patient's vertebral artery. It should never be used unless symptoms indicate a specific need for it. A small percentage of chiropractors advocate neck manipulation to "balance" or "realign" the spine no matter where the patient's problem is located. I recommend avoiding such chiropractors.

Additional Safeguards

Never consult a chiropractor unless your problem has already been diagnosed by a competent medical practitioner. Don't rely on a chiropractor for a diagnosis. Although some chiropractors know enough to avoid diagnostic difficulty, there is no simple way for a consumer to determine who can do so. As an additional safeguard, ask any chiropractor who treats you to discuss your care with your medical doctor.

Remember that although manipulative therapy has value in treating back pain and may relieve other musculoskeletal conditions, chiropractors are not the only source of manipulative therapy. Physical therapists, many osteopathic physicians, and a small number of medical doctors also do it. The Canadian Association of Manipulative Therapists is a good referral source for Canadian practitioners.

———

Dr. Barrett, a retired psychiatrist who resides in Allentown, Pennsylvania, operates the Quackwatch and Chirobase Web sites and is vice president of the National Council Against Health Fraud.

NOTES

CHAPTER 1

1   Joseph Keating Jr., "Old Dad Chiro Comes to Portland," *Chiropractic History*, 13, 2 (1993), p. 37.

2   H. Vear, "The Canadian Genealogy of Daniel David Palmer," *Chiropractic Journal of Australia,* 27, 4 (1997), p. 138.

3   D.D. Palmer, *The Chiropractic Adjuster: Science and art and philosophy of chiropractic* (1910), p. 17.

4   D.D. Palmer, *The Chiropractic Adjuster*, 1, 1 (1908), p. 4., 28, 4 (1950-51), p. 452.

5   J. Cross, "Thomas J. Palmer, frontier publicist," *The Chronicles of Oklahoma*, 28, 4 (1950–51), p. 452

6   E. Harrison, "A Brief History of D.D. Palmer," *The American Chiropractor*, (Jan.-Feb. 1995), p. 30.

7   Anton Mesmer, *Propositions Concerning Animal Magnetism* (1779).

8   Anton Mesmer, *Propositions.*

9   E. Harrison, "A Brief History of D.D. Palmer," *The American Chiropractor*, (Jan-Feb 1995), p. 31.

10   E. Harrison, "A Brief History of D.D. Palmer," *The American Chiropractor*, (Mar-Apr 1995), p. 42., http://www.vcu.edu/engweb/eng372/intro.htm.

11   N. Scott, "Evangelicalism, Revivalism, and the Second Great Awakening," *National Humanities Centre Web Site,* www.nhc.rtp.nc.us, October, 2000.

12   A. Woodlief, "American Romanticism," *Victoria Commonwealth University Web site,* http://www.vcu.edu/engweb/eng372/into.htm.

13   B. Floyd, "From Quackery to Bacteriology," *University of Toledo Web site,*

http://www.cl.utoledo.edu/canaday/quackery/quack1.html.

14   J. Childress, "Dr. Samuel Overton Vintage Medical Ledgers Perused,"
      TXGenWeb Project Web site,
      http://www.rootsweb.com/~txsmith/Pioneers/Childress/treatment.html.

15   D.D. Palmer, *The Chiropractor's Adjuster: Science and art and philosophy of
      chiropractic* (1910), p. 18.

16   D.D. Palmer, *The Chiropractor's Adjuster: Science and art and philosophy of
      chiropractic* (1910), p. 18.

17   B. Westbrooks, "The Troubled Legacy of Harvey Lillard: The
      Black Experience in Chiropractic," *Chiropractic History*, 2, 1 (1982), p.
      48.

18   Andrew Still, *Philosophy of Osteopathy*, (1899), Chapter XV, reproduced on
      http://www.meridianinstitute.com/eamt/files/still2/st2ch15.html.

19   Andrew Still, *Philosophy of Osteopathy*, (1899), Chapter XV.

20   D.D. Palmer, *The Chiropractor*, (March 1897).

21   N. Gevitz, *The D.O.'s — Osteopathic Medicine in America*, p. 20.

22   Quoted in W. Wardell, *Chiropractic —History and Evolution of a New
      Profession* (1992), p. 59.

23   Joseph Keating Jr., "Old Dad Chiro Comes to Portland: Rediscovering DD in
      Oregon, 1908-10," *Chiropractic History*, 13, 2 (1993), p. 37.

24   Joseph Keating Jr., "Heat by Nerves and Not by Blood: the First Major
      Reduction in Chiropractic Theory, 1903," *Chiropractic History*, 15, 2 (1995)
      p.73.

25   Joseph Keating Jr., *Philosophical Constructs for the Chiropractic Profession*, 2, 1
      (1992) p. 9.

26   D. Richards, "The Palmer Philosophy of Chiropractic —An Historical
      Perspective," *Chiropractic Journal of Australia*, 21, 2 (1991), p. 65.

27   D.D. Palmer, *The Chiropractor's Adjuster*, (1909), p. 3.

28   D.D. Palmer, Letter to P.W. Johnson, May 4, 1911.

29   D.D. Palmer, *The Chiropractor*, (1914), p. 11.

30   D.D. Palmer, *The Chiropractor*.

31   D.D. Palmer, *The Chiropractor*, p. 4.

CHAPTER 2

1   B.J. Palmer, *The Science of Chiropractic: Its Principles & Adjustments* (1906), p.
     407.

2   B.J. Palmer, *The Science of Chiropractic: Its Principles & Adjustments*.

3   B.J. Palmer, *The Science of Chiropractic: Its Principles & Adjustments,* p. 407.

4   B.J. Palmer, *Fountain Head News*, (November 1999).

5   B.J. Palmer, *Fight to Climb*, p. 58.

6   R. Gibbons, "BJ in 1906: predictions and personal reflections," *Chiropractic
     History*, 14, 12 (June1994), p.12.

7   B.J. Palmer, *Fight to Climb*, p. 87.

8   B.J. Palmer, *Conflicts Clarify* (1951), p. 94.

9 Quoted in W. Wardell, *Chiropractic – History and Evolution of a New Profession,* (1992), p. 77.
10 Quoted in W. Wardell, *Chiropractic – History and Evolution of a New Profession,* (1992), p. 72.
11 Joseph Keating Jr., "Shhhh!!! . . . Radiophone station WOC is on the air: chiropractic broadcasting 1922-1935", *European Journal of Chiropractic,* 43 (1995), p. 21-37.
12 R. Gibbons, "B.J. and the 'Long Blue Shadows,'" *Chiropractic History,* 19, 2 (1999), p. 15.
13 B.J. Palmer, *Fountain Head News* (1924).
14 B.J. Palmer, Letter to the Field, (May 1923).
15 J. Moore, "The Neurocalometer: Watershed in the Evolution of a New Profession," *Chiropractic History,* 15, 2. p. 51.
16 Quoted in Joseph Keating Jr., *B.J. of Davenport,* p. 192.
17 B.J. Palmer, *The Hour Has Struck.*
18 B.J. Palmer, *Fountain Head News* (1924).
19 B.J. Palmer, *The Hour Has Struck.*
20 B.J. Palmer, *The Hour Has Struck.*
21 B.J. Palmer, *Fountain Head News,* (October 11 1924).
22 B.J. Palmer, *The Hour Has Struck.*
23 B.J. Palmer, *Fountain Head News,* (Sept 27 1924).
24 B.J. Palmer, *Fountain Head News,* (1924).
25 Joseph Keating Jr., "Introducing the Neurocalometer: a view from the Fountain Head," *Journal of the Canadian Chiropractic Association,* 35, 3 (1991), p. 177.
26 Joseph Keating Jr., "Introducing the Neurocalometer: a view from the Fountain Head."
27 Joseph Keating Jr., *B.J. of Davenport,* p. 286.

CHAPTER 3

1 D. Nansel and M. Szlazak, "Letters to the Editor," *Journal of Manipulative and Physiological Therapeutics,* 20, 3 (1997), p. 221.
2 M. Gatterman, *Foundations of Chiropractic: Subluxation* (St. Louis, Missouri, 1995), p.16.
3 Joseph Keating Jr., "Letters to the Editor," *Journal of Canadian Chiropractic Association,* 44, 3 (2000), p. 190.
4 M. Gatterman, *Foundations of Chiropractic: Subluxation,* p. 54.
5 S. French et al, "Reliability of Chiropractic Methods Commonly Used to Detect Manipulable Lesions in Patients with Chronic Low-Back Pain," *Journal of Manipulative and Physiological Therapeutics,* 23, 4 (2000), p. 237.
6 S. French et al, "Reliability of Chiropractic Methods Commonly Used to Detect Manipulable Lesions in Patients with Chronic Low-Back Pain," p. 237.
7 G. Magner, *Chiropractic: The Victim's Perspective* (1995), p. 35.
8 S. French et al, "Reliability of Chiropractic Methods Commonly Used to

Detect Manipulable Lesions in Patients with Chronic Low-Back Pain,"
p. 237.

9   Joseph Keating Jr., "Science and Politics and the Subluxation," *American Journal of Chiropractic Medicine*, 1, 3 (1998), p. 108.

10 P. Brodal, *The Central Nervous System – Structure and Function* (1992), p. 54.

11 D.D. Palmer, *The Chiropractor* (1914), p. 23.

12 George Magner, *Chiropractic – The Victim's Perspective* (1995), p. 13.

13 D.D. Palmer, *The Chiropractor* (1914), p. 48.

14 Joseph Keating Jr., "Introducing the Neurocalometer: a view from the Fountain Head," *The Journal of the Canadian Chiropractic Association*, 35 (1991) p. 3.

15 P. Bolton, "The 'Wet Specimen,'" *Chiropractic Journal of Australia*, 24, 4 (1994), p. 147.

16 D.D. Palmer, *The Chiropractor's Adjuster: A Text-Book of the Science Art and Philosophy of Chiropractic* (1910).

17 D. Nansel and M. Szlazak, "Somatic dysfunction and the phenomenon of visceral disease simulation" [Letter], *Journal of Manipulative and Physiological Therapeutics*, 20 (April 1997), p. 389.

18 R. Schafer and L. Sportelli, *Opportunities in Chiropractic Health Care Careers* (1994), p. 48.

19 D. Nansel and M. Szlazak, "Somatic Dysfunction and the Phenomenon of Visceral Disease Simulation: A Probable Explanation for the Apparent Effectiveness of Somatic Therapy in Patients Presumed to be Suffering from True Visceral Disease," *Journal of Manipulative and Physiological Therapeutics*, 18, 6 (1995), p. 385.

20 M. Gatterman, *Foundations of Chiropractic: Subluxations* (1995), p. 54.

21 R. Leach, *The Chiropractic Theories: Principles and Clinical Applications* (1994), p. 43.

22 D. Nansel and M. Szlazak, "Somatic Dysfunction and the Phenomenon of Visceral Disease Simulation: A Probable Explanation for the Apparent Effectiveness of Somatic Therapy in Patients Presumed to be Suffering from True Visceral Disease," *Journal of Manipulative and Physiological Therapeutics*, 18, 6 (1995), p. 383.

23 Lon Morgan, "Innate intelligence: its origins and problems," *Journal of the Chiropractic Association*, 42,1 (1998), p. 38.

24 Lon Morgan, "Innate intelligence: it's origins and problems," *Journal of the Chiropractic Association*.

25 Joseph Keating Jr., "The Meanings of Innate," *Journal of the Canadian Chiropractic Association*, 46,1 (2002), p. 10.

26 T. Jordan, "Letters to the Editor," *Journal of the Canadian Chiropractic Association*, 42, 3 (1998), p. 179.

27 M. Whitney, "Letters to the Editor," *Journal of the Canadian Chiropractic Association*, 42, 3 (1998), p. 181.

28 T. Preston, "Letters to the Editor," *Journal of the Canadian Chiropractic Association*, 42, 3 (1998), p. 178.

29 K. Dick, "Letters to the Editor," *Journal of the Canadian Chiropractic Association*, 43, 3 (2000), p. 190.

30 D. Nansel and M. Szlazak, "Letters to the Editor," *Journal of Manipulative and Physiological Therapeutics*, 20, 3 (1997), p. 221.

31 D. Nansel D and M. Szlazak, "Letters to the Editor," *Journal of Manipulative and Physiological Therapeutics*, p. 221.

32 Joseph Keating Jr., "Letters to the Editor," *The Journal of the Canadian Chiropractic Association*, 35, 4 (1991), p. 246.

33 Joseph Donahue, "Philosophy of Chiropractic: lessons from the past – guidance for the future," *The Journal of the Canadian Chiropractic Association*, 34, 4 (1990) p. 194.

34 Tom Preston, "Letters to the Editor," *Journal of the Canadian Chiropractic Association*, 42, 3 (1998), p.178.

35 L. Biggs, D. Hay and D. Mierau, "Canadian chiropractors' attitudes towards chiropactic philosophy and scope of practice: implications for the implementation of clinical practice guidelines," *Journal of the Canadian Chiropractic Association*, 41, 3 (1997), p. 146-154.

36 L. Biggs, D. Hay and D. Mierau, "Canadian chiropractors' attitudes towards chiropactic philosophy and scope of practice: implications for the implementation of clinical practice guidelines," p. 152.

37 Craig Nelson, "Letters to the Editor," *Journal of Manipulative and Physiological Therapeutics,* 16, 4 (1993), p.281.

38 Joseph Keating Jr., "A survey of philosophical barriers to research in chiropractic," *The Journal of the Canadian Chiropractic Association*, 33, 4 (1989), p. 186.

CHAPTER 4

1 C. Anrig and G. Plaugher, *Pediatric Chiropractic* (1997), p. 292.

2 Chiropractic Life Centre Web site, http://www.chiroforlife.com/newsletter.htm, June 12, 2002.

3 Chiropractic Life Centre Web site, http://www.chiroforlife.com/newsletter.htm, June 12, 2002.

4 Chiropractic Life Centre Web site http://www.chiroforlife.com/ChiroInfo/whoneedschiro.htm, June 12, 2002.

5 J. Winchester, Bridgeport Family Chiropractic Web site http://www.family-chiropractor.org/, June 13, 2002.

6 Turner Head Injury and Wellness Centre Web site http://www.turnerwellness.com/children/children-main.htm, June 12, 2002.

7 Ontario Chiropractic Association, brochure, *Chiropractic and Children: Infants and Toddlers*, undated.

8 M. Verhoef and C. Papadopoulos, "Survey of Canadian chiropractors' involvement in the treatment of patients under the age of 18," *Journal of the Canadian Chiropractic Association,* 43,1 (1999), p. 53.

9 M. Verhoef and C. Papadopoulos, "Survey of Canadian chiropractors' involvement in the treatment of patients under the age of 18," p. 54.

10   M. Verhoef and C. Papadopoulos, "Survey of Canadian chiropractors' involvement in the treatment of patients under the age of 18," p. 56.

11   M. Verhoef and C. Papadopoulos, "Survey of Canadian chiropractors' involvement in the treatment of patients under the age of 18," p. 56.

12   Chiropractic Awareness Council (C.A.C.) Web site, www.ca4life.com, Statement of Purpose, Dec. 17, 1999.

13   Chiropractic Awareness Council (C.A.C.) Web site, www.ca4life.com, Statement of Purpose, Dec. 17, 1999.

14   A. Gotlib and M. Beingessner, "Annotated bibliography of the biomedical literature pertaining to chiropractic, pediatrics and manipulation in relation to the treatment of health conditions," *Journal of the Canadian Chiropractic Association*, 39, 3 (1995), p. 159.

15   J. Balon et al, "A Comparison of Active and Simulated Chiropractic Manipulation as Adjunctive Treatment for Childhood Asthma," *New England Journal of Medicine*, 339, 1013 (1998), p. 20.

16   J. Wiberg, J. Nordsteen and N. Nilsson, "The short-term effect of spinal manipulation in the treatment of infantile colic: A randomized controlled clinical trial with a blinded observer," *Journal of Manipulative and Physiological Therapeutics*, 22 (1999), p. 517-22.

17   Canadian Paediatric Society, "Chiropractic Care for Children: Controversies and Issues," *Paediatrics & Child Health*, 7, 2 (2002), p. 85-89.

18   E. Olafsdottir, et al, "Randomised controlled trial of infantile colic treated with chiropractic spinal manipulation," *Archives of Diseases in Childhood*, 84 (2001), p.138-141.

19   J. Grod et al, "Unsubstantiated Claims in Patient Brochures From the Largest State, Provincial and National Chiropractic Associations and Research Agencies," *Journal of Manipulative and Physiological Therapeutics*, 24, 8 (2001), p. 517.

20   Chairmen of the Departments of Pediatrics of Pediatrics Hospitals in Canada, "Children and chiropractors," *The Canadian Journal of Paediatrics*, 2, 1(1994) p. 1.

21   J. Winchester, "Drug Companies Lie," Letter to the Editor, *The Kitchener-Waterloo Record*, (Dec. 29, 1998), p. A10.

22   K. Kulhay, "Vaccination Risk Awareness Evenings," Advertisement, *Vitality magazine*, (1999).

23   Stirling Chiropractic Family Wellness Centre Web site, http://www.stirlingchiropractic.com/Vaccinations/vaccinations.shtml, (June 15, 2002).

24   College of Chiropractors of Ontario Web site, "Information on Immunization, Policy P–033, Executive and Quality Assurance Committees," http://www.cco.on.ca/information_on_immunization1.htm, June 15, 2002.

25   The Canadian Chiropractic Association, *Position Statement Vaccination and Immunization*, (April 2002).

26   D.D. Palmer, *The sick get well by magnetism*. Brochure, 1889.

27   D.D. Palmer, *The Chiropractic Adjuster*, (1915), p. 35.

28   B.J. Palmer, *The Science of Chiropractic: Its Principles and Adjustments*, (1906), p. 17.

29 B.J. Palmer, *The Philosophy of Chiropractic*, 1909.

30 B.J. Palmer, *The Science of Chiropractic: Its Principles and Philosophies*, (1906).

31 L. Morgan, "Pertussis immunization: an update," *Journal of the Canadian Chiropractic Association*, 41, 2 (1997), p. 90.

32 Letters to the Editor, *Journal of the Canadian Chiropractic Association*, 41,4, (1997), p. 240.

33 Letters to the Editor, *Journal of the Canadian Chiropractic Association*, p. 241.

34 Letters to the Editor, *Journal of the Canadian Chiropractic Association*, p. 244.

35 J. Busse et al, "Attitudes toward vaccination: a survey of Canadian chiropractic students,"*Canadian Medical Association Journal*, 166,12, (2002), p. 1534.

36 J. Busse et al, "Attitudes toward vaccination: a survey of Canadian chiropractic students,"*Canadian Medical Association Journal, p.1544*.

37 M. Verhoef and C. Papadopoulous, "Survey of Canadian chiropractors' involvement in the treatment of patients under the age of 18," *Journal of the Canadian Chiropractic Association*, 43, 1 (1999), p. 53.

38 C. Anrig and G. Plaugher, *Pediatric Chiropractic*, (1997), back cover.

39 Future Perfect Web Site, http://www.webvalence.com/sites/stuartwarner/Chiropediatrics/Conference.html, (June 15, 2002).

40 R. Smith, *At Your Own Risk*, (1970), p. 50.

41 The Art of Management Inc. Web site, http://www.amican.com/chiropro-file.htm, (June 17, 2002).

42 The Art of Management Inc. Web site, http://www.amican.com/chiroarti-cles.htm, (June 17, 2002).

43 Transcript, patient interview with chiropractor.

44 The Art of Management Inc. Web Site, http://www.amican.com/chiroarti-cles.htm, (June 17, 2002).

45 Transcript, phone conversation with chiropractor.

46 The Art of Management Inc. Web Site, http://www.amican.com/chiroarti-cles.htm, (June 17, 2002).

47 Today's Chiropractic Web site, "Women in Chiropractic: Claudia Anrig," http://www.todayschiropractic.com/052001/women02.html, (June 18, 2002).

48 Koren Publications Web site, http://www.korenpublications.com/0901pn_1_.htm, (June 18, 2002).

49 Koren Publications Inc., *Infants and Babies*, brochure, undated.

50 Canadian Chiropractic Association Web site, http://www.ccachiro.org/, (June 18, 2002).

CHAPTER 5

1 *Coroner's Inquest into the Death of Laurie Jean Mathiason: Transcript of Inquest.* Saskatoon, Saskatchewan: Meyer Compu Court Reporting; (1998).

2 Dan Zabreski, "Probe link between chiropractic therapy, stroke, jury urges," *The Star Phoenix* [Saskatoon], September 12,1998.

3 CBC Radio, *As It Happens*, September 13, 1998.

4   Canadian Chiropractic Association, "Press Release: Canadian Chiropractic Association to act upon recommendations set out by coroner's inquest," October 6, 1998.

5   Canadian Chiropractic Association, "Information Sheet," undated.

6   Dynamic Chiropractor, "Chiropractic Acquitted in Canada: Patient's Death after Manipulation Not Attributed to DC," *Dynamic Chiropractic* November 2, 1998.

7   Circle Centre Chiropractic Clinic, "Patient Letter," November 1, 1998.

8   Tony Anziano, "Letter to the Editor," *The Hamilton Spectator,* November 10, 1999.

9   advertisement. "The Truth About Chiropractic And Neck Adjustment," *The Burlington Post,* March 5, 2000.

10   H.R. Pratt-Thomas and K.E. Berger, "Cerebellar and spinal injuries after chiropractic manipulation," *Journal of the American Medical Association,* 133 (1947), p. 600-603.

11   A.G.J Terrett, *Current Concepts in Vertebrobasilar Complications following Spinal Manipulation,"* (Des Moines, Iowa: NCMIC Group Inc., (2001) p. 9.

12   A.G.J Terrett, *Current Concepts,* p. 10.

13   World Chiropractic Alliance, *Chiropractic and the Risk of Stroke,* http://www.worldchiropracticalliance.org/positions/stroke.htm, July 9, 2002.

14   V. Dabbs and W. J. Lauretti, "A Risk Assessment of Cervical Manipulation vs.NSAIDs for the Treatment of Neck Pain," *Journal of Manipulative and Physiological Therapeutics* 18, 8 (1995) p. 530-536.

15   P.F. Carey, "A report on the occurrence of cerebral vascular accidents in chiropractic practice," *The Journal of the Canadian Chiropractic Association,* 37, 2, (1993), p.104-106.

16   S. Haldeman and P. Carey, M. Townsend, and C. Papadopoulas, "Arterial Dissections following cervical manipulation: the chiropractic experience," *Canadian Medical Association Journal,* 165, 7 (2001), p.905-6.

17   N. Klougart, C. Leboeuf-Yde and L.R. Rasmussen, "Safety in chiropractic practice. Part 2: Treatment of the upper neck and the rate of cerebrovascular incidents," *Journal of Manipulative and Physiological Therapeutics,* 19 ,9 (1996), p. 563-9.

18   J. Dvorak and E. Orelli, "How dangerous is manipulation of the cervical spine?" *Manual Medicine,* 2 (1985), p.1-4.

19   A. Vickers and C. Zollman, "The manipulative therapies: osteopathy and chiropractic," *British Medical Journal,* 319 (1999) p. 1176-9.

20   I. Coulter, "Efficacy and Risks of Chiropractic Manipulation: What Does the Evidence Suggest?" *Integrative Medicine,* 1, 2, (1998), p. 61-66.

21   V. Dabbs and W. J. Lauretti, "A Risk Assessment of Cervical Manipulation vs. NSAIDs for the Treatment of Neck Pain," *Journal of Manipulative and Physiological Therapeutics* 18, 8 (1995) p. 530-536.

22   A.G.J. Terrett, *Current Concepts,* p. 120.

23   M.T.Y Chan, N.G. Zurab, and J.W Norris, "Diagnostic Strategies in Young Patients with Ischemic Stroke," *The Canadian Stroke Consortium,* 1999.

24 J.W.Norris, V. Beletsky and N.G. Zurab, "Sudden neck movement and cervical artery dissection,"*Canadian Medical Association Journal*, 63, 1, (2000), p 38-40.

25 Norris J. Personal correspondence, June 5, 2002.

26 E. Ernst, "Manipulation of the cervical spine: a systematic review of case reports of serious adverse events," *Medical Journal of Australia*, 176, 8 (2002), p. 376-380.

27 E. Ernst, "Spinal manipulation: its safety is uncertain," *Canadian Medical Association Journal*, 166, 1, (2002), p. 40-41.

28 E. Ernst, "Spinal manipulation: its safety is uncertain," p. 40-41.

29 D.M. Rothwell, S.J. Bondy and I. Williams, "Chiropractic Manipulation and Stroke, A Population-Based Case-Control Study," *Stroke*, 32 (2001), p.1054-1060.

30 A.G.J Terrett, *Current Concepts*, p. 142.

31 N. Klougart, C. Leboeuf-Yde and L.R. Rasmussen, "Safety in chiropractic practice: Part 2:Treatment of the upper neck and the rate of cerebrovascular incidents," *Journal of Manipulative and Physiological Therapeutics*, 19, 9 (1996) p. 563-9.

32 S. Haldeman, P. Carey, M. Townsend and C. Papadopoulas, "Arterial Dissections following cervical manipulation: the chiropractic experience," . *Canadian Medical Association Journal*, 165, 7 (2001), p.905-6.

33 P.F. Carey, "A report on the occurrence of cerebral vascular accidents in chiropractic practice," *The Journal of the Canadian Chiropractic Association*, 37, 2, (1993), p.104-106.

34 R.S. Hosek et al, "Letter to the Editor," *Journal of the American Medical Association*, March 6, 1981.

35 N. Klougart, C. Leboeuf-Yde and L.R. Rasmussen, "Safety in chiropractic practice: Part 2: Treatment of the upper neck and the rate of cerebrovascular incidents," *Journal of Manipulative and Physiological Therapeutics*, 19, 9, (1996) p. 563-9.

36 E.L. Hurwitz, I.E Coulter, A.H. Adams, B.J Genovese and P.G. Shekelle, "Use of Chiropractic Services from 1985 Through 1991 in the United States and Canada," *American Journal of Public Health*, 88, 5, (1998).

37 J. Keating Jr., "Shhh! ... Radiophone station WOC is on the air: chiropractic broadcasting 1922-1935," *European Journal of Chiropractic* , 43, 29, 1995, p. 21- 37.

38 J. Keating, "Introducing the Neurocalometer: a view from the Fountain Head," 35, 3 (1991) p.165.

39 J. Nash, C. Johnson and B. Green, "Hole In One: A History of Its Founding," *Chiropractic History*, 16, 2 (1996), p.77.

40 J. Moore, "The Neurocalometer: Watershed in the Evolution of a New Profession," *Chiropractic History*, 15, 2 (1995), p. 51.

41 B.J. Palmer, "Hole-in-One Theory Absolutely Right," *Fountain Head News*. 18, 3 (1933).

42 S. Bolton, "The 'Wet Specimen,'" *Chiropractic Journal of Australia*, 24, 4,

(1994), p.147.

43 I. Coulter, E. Hurwitz, A. Adams, W. Meeker, D. Hansen, R. Mootz, P. Aker, B. Genovese and P. Shekelle, "The appropriateness of manipulation and mobilization of the cervical spine," RAND, 1996.

44 I. Coulter et al, "The appropriateness of manipulation,"1996.

45 I. Coulter et al, "The appropriateness of manipulation,"1996.

46 G. Bove, N. Nilsson, "Spinal Manipulation in the Treatment of Episodic Tension-Type Headache," *Journal of the American Medical Association*, 280,18, (1998), p.1576.

47 I. Coulter et al, "The appropriateness of manipulation,"1996.

48 I. Coulter, "Efficacy and Risks of Chiropractic Manipulation: What Does the Evidence Suggest?" *Integrative Medicine*, 1,2 (1998), p. 61-66.

59 Kim Barton, "Personal letter," undated.

50 A.G.J Terrett, "Misuse of the Literature by Medical Authors in Discussing Spinal Injury," *Journal of Manipulative Therapy*, 18, 4 (1995).

51 World Chiropractic Alliance, "Chiropractic and Risk of Stroke," www.world-chiropracticalliance.org/positions/stroke.htm

52 I. Coulter, "Efficacy and Risks of Chiropractic Manipulation: What Does the Evidence Suggest?" *Integrative Medicine*, 1, 2, (1998), p. 61-66.

53 Chiropractic Canada, "Why Chiropractic is a Safe and Healthy Choice," pamphlet, 1999.

54 A. Terrett, *Current Concepts*, p.65-66.

55 B.J. Gleberzon, "Chiropractic Care of the Geriatric Patient: Clinical Diagnosis: Treatment, Management and How to Err on the Side of Caution: A Primer/ Workbook for the CD 410 courses at the CMCC," 1998.

56 A. Terrett, *Current Concepts*, p.40.

57 *Coroner's Inquest into the Death of Laurie Jean Mathiason: Transcript of Inquest,* Saskatoon, Saskatchewan: Meyer Compu Court Reporting, (1998).

58 A. Terrett, *Current Concepts*, p. 63.

59 Paul Carey, "Letters to the Editor," *Journal of the Canadian Chiropractic Association*, 39, 3 (1995), p. 188.

60 Igor Steiman, "Letters to the Editor," *Journal of the Canadian Chiropractic Association*, 39, 3 (1995), p. 188.

61 David Chapman-Smith, "Cervical Adjustment: Rotation is Fine, Pre-testing is Out, but Get Consent," *The Chiropractic Report*. 13, 4 (July 1999).

62 G.N. Dunn, "Managing Risk in Your Chiropractic Practice 2001," *Journal of the Canadian Chiropractic Association*, 45,4 (2001), p . 248-255.

63 A. Terrett, *Current Concepts*, p. 10.

CHAPTER 6

1   Greg Dunn, "There's Going to be an Inquest," *Canadian Chiropractor*, 5, 3 (June, 2000) p. 48.

2   Murray Naiberg, Affidavit to Lana Dale Lewis Inquest Court, (April 12, 2001).

3   John Deck, Letter, (June 16, 1999).

4   Murray Naiberg, Letter, (October 24, 1999).

5   Paul Carey, "Informed consent – the new reality," *Journal of the CCA*, 32, 2 (1998), p. 91.

6   David Chapman-Smith, "Trust Me, I'm a Doctor," *The Chiropractic Report*, 15, 5 (2001), p. 1.

7   Joseph Keating Jr., "The Meanings of Innate," *Journal of the CCA*, 4,1 (2002) p. 5.

8   Ronald Carter, "Letter to the Editor," *Calgary Herald New Media*, undated.

9   "The Truth About Chiropractic and Neck Adjustment," advertisement, *Burlington Post*, March 20, 2000.

10 R. Bryans, Letter to the Editor, *Montreal Gazette*, April 10, 2000.

11 Greg Dunn, "Guest Editorial: There Is Going To Be An Inquest," *Canadian Chiropractor*, 5, 3 (2000), p. 4.

12 Ontario Chiropractic Association newletter, (January 2001), p. 2.

13 Murray Naiberg, "Affadavit to Lana Dale Lewis Inquest Court," (April 12, 2001).

14 Michael Ford, "Affidavit, Coroner's Inquest Court," (April 12, 2001).

15 Murray Naiberg, "Letter to Investigations and Resolutions, The College of Physicians and Surgeons of Ontario," (March 18, 2002).

16 Dr. John Richardson, "Report to Amani Oakley," undated.

CHAPTER 7

1   *York University Centre for Health Studies report*, (May 5, 1998) p. 4.

2   York University, *Proposal for the Establishment of a Doctor of Chiropractic Degree.* (April 27, 1998).

3   Donald Livingstone, Personal Letter, (Nov. 30, 1998).

4   Richard Hu, Personal Letter, (Dec. 8, 1998).

5   Harry Shulman, Personal Letter, (Sept. 29, 1998).

6   James Waddell, Personal Letter, (Jan. 6, 1999).

7   James Waddell, Personal Letter, (Nov. 10, 1998).

8   Ken Yong-Hing, Personal Letter, (Sept. 15, 1998).

9   P. Shekelle et al, "Spinal manipulation for low-back pain," Annals of Internal Medicine, 117, 7 (1992) p. 590-8.

10 *Responses to APPC's Preliminary Inventory of Questions Based on Notes from the APPC-Sponsored Open Forum on CMCC*, (February 12, 1998).

11 D. Brown, "CMCC's persistent pursuit of university affiliation Part I," *Journal of the Canadian Chiropractic Association*, 36, 1 (1992), p. 33-37.

12 D. Brown, "CMCC's persistent pursuit of university affiliation Part II," *Journal of the Canadian Chiropractic Association*, 38, 1 (1994), p. 42.

13 D. Brown, "CMCC's persistent pursuit of university affiliation Part II," p. 43.

14 D. Brown, "CMCC's persistent pursuit of university affiliation Part II," p. 53.

15 Charles Picciotto, Personal Letter, (December, 1998).

CHAPTER 8

1   Donald Sutherland, "Trial by Fire: Canadian Royal Commissions Investigate Chiropractic," *Chiropractic History*, 5, 27 (1985), p. 29.

2   Donald Sutherland, "Trial By Fire," p. 29.

3   Donald Sutherland, "Trial By Fire," p. 29.

4   Donald Sutherland, "Trial By Fire," p. 29.

5   I. Coulter, "Is chiropractic care primary health care?" *The Journal of the Canadian Chiropractic Association*, 35, 2 (1992), p. 96-101.

6   Canadian Chiropractic Association, "Synopsis of Studies – 1997," www.ccachiro.org, July 12, 2002.

7   Rachel Moore, Yang Mao, Jun Zhang and Kathy Clarke, "Economic Burden of Illness 1993," Health Protection Branch, Health Canada, 1993.

8   M. Gatterman, "Letters to the Editor," *The Journal of the Canadian Chiropractic Association*, 36, 4 (1992), p. 231-232.

9   Joseph Donahue, "Philosophy of chiropractic: lessons from the past – guidance for the future," *The Journal of the Canadian Chiropractic Association*, 34, 4 (1990), p. 194-205.

10   Canadian Chiropractic Association, "Synopsis of Recent Studies 1997," www.ccachiro.org, July 12, 2002.

11   Ontario Chiropractic Association. *Chiropractic and Low Back Pain*, Pamphlet, Undated.

12   T.W. Meade, S. Dyer, W. Browne, J.O. Townsend and A. Frank, "Low back pain of mechanical origin: randomized comparison of chiropractic and hospital outpatient treatment," *British Medical Journal*, 300 (1990), p.1431-1437.

13   B.W. Koes, W.J.J. Assendelft, G.J.M.G. van der Heijden, L.M. Bouter and P.G. Knipschild, "Spinal manipulation and mobilization for back and neck pain: a blinded review," *British Medical Journal*, 303 (1991), p.1298-1303.

14   B.W. Koes, W.J.J. Assendelft, G.J.M.G. van der Heijden and L.M. Bouter, "Spinal manipulation for low back pain: an updated systematic review of randomized clinical trials," *Spine*, 21 (1996), p. 2860-73.

15   B.W. Koes et al, "Spinal manipulation for low back pain," p. 2860-73.

16   P.G. Shekelle, A.H. Adams, M.R. Chassin, E.L. Hurwitz and R.H. Brook, "Spinal manipulation for low-back pain," *Annals of Internal Medicine*, 117, 7 (1992), p. 590-598.

17   Paul Shekelle, Reed Phillips, Daniel C. Cherkin and William C. Meeker, "Chiropractic in the United States: Training, Practice, and Research. Chapter XI: Benefits and Risks of Spinal Manipulation," (Sept., 1997).

18   Joseph Keating Jr., "Chiropractic: Science and Antiscience and Pseudoscience Side by Side," *Skeptical Inquirer*, July/August 1997.

19   P.G. Shekelle, A.H. Adams, M.R. Chassin, E.L. Hurwitz and R.H. Brook, "Spinal manipulation for low-back pain," *Annals of Internal Medicine*, 117, 7 (1992), p. 590-598.

20   P.G. Shekelle, et al, "Spinal manipulation for low-back pain," *Annals of Internal Medicine*, 117, 7 (1992), p. 590-598.

21 Paul Shekelle, "RAND Misquoted," *ACA Journal of Chiropractic*, 30, 7 (1993), p. 59-63.

22 Paul Shekelle, Reed Phillips, Daniel C. Cherkin and William C. Meeker "Chiropractic in the United States: Training, Practice, and Research. Chapter XI: Benefits and Risks of Spinal Manipulation," (Sept., 1997).

23 D.C. Cherkin, R.A. Deyo, M. Battie, J. Street and W. Barlow, "A Comparison of Physical Therapy, Chiropractic Manipulation and Provision of an Educational Booklet for Treatment of Patients with Low Back Pain," *New England Journal of Medicine,* 8, 339 (1998), p. 1021-1029.

24 Tim Carey, "The Outcomes and Costs for Acute Low Back Pain Patients Seen by Primary Care Practitioners, Chiropractors and Orthopedic Surgeons," *New England Journal of Medicine,* 333, 14 (Oct. 5, 1995), p. 913-917.

25 S.J. Bigos et al, "Acute Low Back Pain Problems in Adults, Clinical Practice Guideline No. 14," AHCPR Publication No. 95-0642, Rockville, MD, Agency for Health Care Policy & Research, 1994.

26 Chiropractic College of Alberta, "Chiropractors : Here to help you Get Back into Action!" www.ccoa.ab.ca, June 15, 2002.

27 P. Manga, D.E. Angus, C. Papadopoulos and W. Swan, "The Effectiveness and Cost Effectiveness of Chiropractic Management of Low-Back Pain: Executive Summary," Ontario Ministry of Health, August, 1993.

28 B.W. Koes et al, "Spinal manipulation for low back pain," p. 2860-73.

29 P. Manga et al, "The Effectiveness and Cost Effectiveness of Chiropractic Management of Low-Back Pain: Executive Summary, Ontario Ministry of Health, August, 1993, p.2.

30 Paul Shekelle, Reed Phillips, Daniel C. Cherkin and William C. Meeker "Chiropractic in the United States: Training, Practice, and Research. Chapter XI: Benefits and Risks of Spinal Manipulation," (Sept., 1997).

31 Daniel Cherkin and Robert Mootz, "Chiropractic in the United States: Training, Practice, and Research. Chapter XII: Synopsis, Research Priorities, and Policy Issues" (Sept., 1997).

32 T.S. Carey, J.M. Garett, A. Jackman, and N. Hadler, "Recurrence and care seeking after acute back pain: Results of a long-term follow-up study," *Medical Care,* 37, 2 (1999), p.157-164.

33 D.R. Smucker, T.R. Konrad, P. Curtis and T.S. Carey, "Practitioner self-confidence and patient outcomes in acute low back pain," *Archives of Family Medicine,* 7 (1998), p. 223-228.

34 T.S. Carey, "Commentary," *ACP Journal Club*, March-April, 1999, p. 130-42.

35 D.R. Smucker, T.R. Konrad, P. Curtis and T.S. Carey, "Practitioner self-confidence and patient outcomes in acute low back pain," *Archives of Family Medicine,* 7 (1998), p. 223-228.

36 V. Lawrence, "Commentary," *Annals of Internal Medicine,* 118, 2 (1993).

37 S.J. Bigos et al, "Acute Low Back Pain Problems in Adults, Clinical Practice Guideline No. 14," AHCPR Publication No. 95-0642, Rockville, MD, Agency for Health Care Policy & Research, 1994.

38 S. Homola, *Inside Chiropractic: A Patient's Guide*, (Amherst, New York: Prometheus Books, 1999), p. 69.

39 J. Grod, D. Sikorski and J. Keating Jr., "Unsubstantiated claims in patient brochures from the largest state, provincial, and national chiropractic associations and research agencies," *The Journal of the Canadian Chiropractic Association*, 24, 8 (2001), p. 514-519.

40 L. Biggs, D. Hay and D. Mierau, "Canadian chiropractors' attitudes towards chiropractic philosophy and scope of practice: implications for the implementation of clinical practice guidelines," *The Journal of the Canadian Chiropractic Association*, 41, 3 (1997), p.145-154.

41 B.J. Gleberzon, "Name Techniques in Canada: current trends in utilization rates and recommendations for their inclusion at the Canadian Memorial Chiropractic College," *Journal of the Canadian Chiropractic Association*, 44, 3 (2000), p. 161.

42 J.R.E. Jamison and R.L. Rupert, "Maintenance care: towards a global description," *The Journal of the Canadian Chiropractic Association*, 45, 2 (2001), p. 100.

43 J.R.E. Jamison, R.L. Rupert, "Maintenance care: towards a global description," p. 101.

44 L. Hestoek and C. Leboeuf-Yde, "Are chiropractic tests for the lumbo-pelvic spine reliable and valid? A systematic critical literature review," *Journal of Manipulative Physiological Therapeutics*, 23, 4 (2000), p. 258-275.

45 E. Ernst, "Commentary: Chiropractors' use of X-rays," *The British Journal of Radiology*, 71 (1998), p. 250.

46 E. Ernst, "Commentary: Chiropractors' use of X-rays," p. 249-252.

47 Paul Shekelle, Reed Phillips, Daniel C. Cherkin and William C. Meeker, "Chiropractic in the United States: Training, Practice, and Research. Chapter XI: Benefits and Risks of Spinal Manipulation," (Sept., 1997).

48 Canadian Memorial Chiropractic College, "Mission Statement: The philosophy of chiropractic," 1999.

49 Oak Bay Family Chiropractic Centre, "Pamphlet," Calgary, Alberta, undated.

50 Ogi Ressel, "Letter to the Editor," *The Medical Post*, 35, 29 (September 7, 1999).

51 Ontario Chiropractic Association, "Pamphlet: Chiropractic and Low Back Pain," undated.

52 Troy J. Jordan, "Letter to the Editor," *Journal of the Canadian Chiropractic Association*, 42, 3 (1998), p. 179.

CHAPTER 9

1 Leslie Biggs, "'Hands off Chiropractic': Organized Medicine's Attempts to Restrict Chiropractic in Ontario, 1900-1925," *Chiropractic History*, 5 (1985) p. 13.

2 Ralph Lee Smith, *At Your Own Risk: The Case Against Chiropractic*, (Richmond Hill: Simon & Schuster of Canada Ltd., 1969), p. 158.

3   Joseph Keating Jr., Letter to the Editor, *The Journal of the Canadian Chiropractic Association*, 35, 4 (1991), p. 246.
4   Jarolslaw P. Grod, David Sikorski and Joseph Keating Jr., "Unsubstantiated Claims in Patient Brochures From the Largest State, Provincial, and National Chiropractic Associations and Research Agencies," *The Journal of Manipulative and Physiological Therapeutics*, 24, 8 (2001), p. 518.
5   Donald C. Sutherland, "Trial By Fire: Canadian Royal Commissions Investigate Chiropractic," *Chiropractic History*, 5 (1985), p. 30.
6   Donald C. Sutherland, "Chiropractic: From rejection to acceptance 1900-1980," *The Journal of the Canadian Chiropractic Association*, 42, 3 (1998), p. 168.
7   Sutherland, "Trial By Fire," p. 33.
8   Sutherland, "Trial By Fire," p. 35.
9   Leslie Biggs, "'Hands off Chiropractic,'" p. 16.
10 Leslie Biggs, "Chiropractic Education: A Struggle for Survival," *Journal of Manipulative and Physiological Therapeutics*, 14, 1 (1991), p. 22.
11 Leslie Biggs, "Chiropractic Education," p. 27.

CHAPTER 10

1   Samuel Homola, *Inside Chiropractic: A Patient's Guide* (Amherst, New York: Prometheus Press, 1999), p. 131-132.
2   David Leprich, "ALTERNATIVE PRACTITIONERS: All you ever wanted to know about chiropractors…," *The Medical Post*, (February 8, 2000).
3   Joseph Keating Jr., Letter, May 28, 1993.
4   Brian Gleberzon, "Name techniques in Canada: current trends in utilization rates and recommendations for their inclusion at the Canadian Memorial Chiropractic College," *The Journal of the Canadian Chiropractic Association*, 44, 3 (2000), p.164.
5   Brian Gleberzon, "Chiropractic 'Name Techniques': a review of the literature," *The Journal of the Canadian Chiropractic Association*, 45, 2 (2001), p. 93.
6   Joseph Keating Jr., "System for classifying the acceptability of clinical treatment methods," *The Journal of the Canadian Chiropractic Association*," 35, 1 (1991), p. 13.
7   Lon Morgan, "Letters to the Editor," *The Journal of the Canadian Chiropractic Association*, 42, 3 (1998), p. 184.
8   Carolyn Green, Craig Martin, Ken Bassett and Arminee Kazanjian, "A Systematic Review And Critical Appraisal of the Scientific Evidence on Craniosacral Therapy," *British Columbia Office of Health Technology Assessment*, (May, 1999), p. 39.
9   George Magner, *Chiropractic: The Victim's Perspective*, (Amherst, New York: Prometheus Books, 1995), p. 25.
10 Ray H. Gin and Bart N. Green, "George Goodheart, Jr., D.C., and a History of Applied Kinesiology," *Journal of Manipulative and Physiological Therapeutics*, 20, 5 (1997), p. 333.

11   Dennis M. Richards, "The Activator Story: Development of a New Concept in Chiropractic," *Chiropractic Journal of Australia*, 24, 1 (1994), p. 30.

12   Robert Cooperstein, "Thompson Technique, *Chiropractic Technique*, 7, 2 (1995), p. 63.

13   George Magner, *Chiropractic: The Victim's Perspective* (Amherst, New York: Prometheus Books, 1995), p. 25.

14   Ted Morter, "The Theoretical Basis and Rationale for the Clinical Application of Bio-Energetic Synchroniztion," *The Journal of Vertebral Subluxation*, 2, 1 (1998), p. 31.

15   Brian Gleberzon, "Chiropractic 'Name Techniques': a review of the literature," *The Journal of the Canadian Chiropractic Association*, 45, 2 (2001), p. 93.

16   Brian Gleberzon, "Name techniques in Canada: current trends in utilization rates and recommendations for their inclusion at the Canadian Memorial Chiropractic College," *The Journal of the Canadian Chiropractic Association*, 44, 3 (2000), p.166.

17   Brian Gleberzon, "Name techniques in Canada," p. 164.

18   Mike Milne, "Special Report: Are physicians' opinions about chiropractors changing?," *Canadian Medical Association Journal*, 138, (June 1, 1988), p. 1053.

19   Consumer Reports, "Chiropractors: Can They Help? Do They Harm?," *Consumer Reports,* (June, 1994), p. 388.

20   Samuel Homola, "Chiropractic Nutrition: The good, the bad, and the patently false," *Nutrition Forum*, (May/June, 1998), p. 21.

21   Joseph Keating Jr., "Chiropractic: Science and Antiscience and Pseudoscience Side by Side," *Skeptical Inquirer*, (July/August 1997), p.40.

22   Joseph Keating Jr., "Chiropractic: Science and Antiscience," p. 42.

23   "What we teach," *The Chiropractic Journal*, (October, 1993), p. 35-37.

24   Keating Jr., "Chiropractic: Science and Antiscience," p. 42.

25   Joseph Keating Jr., *B.J. of Davenport*, p. 69

26   George Magner, *Chiropractic: The Victim's Perspective* (1995), p. 35-36.

27   P. Pierse, Pediatric Section of the Alberta Medical Association, "Positions of Endorsement," (December 15, 1998).

28   D. Tunney, RifeBare Web site http://www.rifetechnology.com/qa.htm (June 28 2002).

29   D. Tunney, RifeBare Web site http://www.rifetechnology.com/qa.htm (June 28,2002).

CHAPTER 11

1   R. Harvey, "Chiropractic Claims: A survey of offices across Toronto found most offered more than back and neck relief," *Toronto Star*, October 22, 1999.

2   C. Milne, "Oh, your achey, breaky back: Despite an antagonistic medical establishment and some areas of controversy, scientific evidence is securely on the side of chiropractic for back and neck pain," *The Globe and Mail*, November 30, 1999, p. R11.

3   C. Milne, "Oh, your achey, breaky back," *The Globe and Mail*, November 30, 1999, p. R11.

4   J.P. Grod, D. Sikorski, and JC. Jr Keating, "Unsubstantiated Claims in Patient Brochures From the Largest State, Provincial, and National Chiropractic Associations and Research Agencies," *Journal of Manipulative and Physiological Therapeutics*, 24, 8 (2001), p. 514-519.

5   J.P. Grod et al, "Unsubstantiated Claims," p. 515.

6   J.P. Grod et al, "Unsubstantiated Claims," p. 514.

7   A.E. Toth, D.M. Lawson, and J. W. Nykoliathon, "Chiropractic complaints and disciplinary cases in Canada," *Journal of the Canadian Chiropractic Association*, 42, 4 (1998), p. 229-242.

8   A. E. Toth et al, "Chiropractic complaints," p. 240.

9   Chiropractic Awareness Council (C.A.C.) Web site, "Statement of Purpose," www.ca4life.com, Dec. 17, 1999.

10   Federation of Chiropractic Licensing Boards, "Official Directory 2002," Updated February, 2002.

11   National Assembly of Quebec, Fourth Session, Twenty-Ninth Legislature, "Bill 269:Chiropractic Act," Charles-Henri Dube, Quebec Official Publisher, 1973.

12   Chiropractic Act, Regulated Health Professions Act, 1991. Statutes of Ontario, (1991), Queens Printer of Ontario, Chapter 18.

13   J. C. Keating Jr., "Science and Politics and Subluxation," American Journal of *Chiropractic Medicine*, 1, 3 (September, 1988), p. 107-110.

14   H. J. Vear, "Quality assurance: standards of care and ethical practice," *Journal of the Canadian Chiropractic Association*, 35, 4 (December, 1991), p. 215-220.

15   H. J. Vear, "Quality assurance," p. 217.

16   R. Carter, "Commentary: Subluxation – the silent killer," *Journal of the Canadian Chiropractic Association*, 44, 1 (2000), p. 9-18.

17   R. Carter, "Commentary. Subluxation," p. 13.

18   W. H. Quigly, "Chiropractic's Monocausal Theory of Disease," *American Chiropractic Association Journal*, 18, 6 (1981), p. 52-60.

19   L. Morgan, "Letter to the Editor," *Journal of the Canadian Chiropractic Association*, 44, 3 (2000), p. 182-183.

20   M.G. Christensen and D.R.D. Morgan, "Job Analysis of Chiropractic in Canada: A Report, Survey, Analysis, and Summary of Practice of Chiropractic within Canada," (Greeley, CO), National Board of Chiropractic Examiners, 1993.

21   J.J. Kenny, R. Clemens and K.D. Forsythe, "Applied kinesiology unreliable for assessing nutritional status," *Journal of the American Dietetic Association*, 88 (1988), p. 698-704.1988.

22   J.J. Triano, "Muscle testing response to provocative vertebral challenge and spinal manipulation: a randomized controlled trial to construct validity," *Journal of Manipulative and Physiological Therapeutics*, 17 (1994), p.141-148.

23   British Columbia College of Chiropractors, "Professional Conduct Handbook," A-3-11. July 24, 2000.

24 J.P. Grod et al, "Unsubstantiated Claims," p. 514.

25 B.J. Nantais, Letter, May 17, 2001.

26 Nantais, Letter, May 17, 2001.

27 J.P. Grod et al, "Unsubstantiated Claims," p. 517

28 J.P. Grod et al, "Unsubstantiated Claims," p. 517

29 Dr. John Wedge, Personal interview, June 28, 2002.

30 Brad Evenson, "Pediatricians warn against chiropractors : Latest salvo in turf war: Children are being treated for asthma, colds, bedwetting," *National Post* (Toronto), February 27, 2002.

31 H. Braswell, "Pediatricians' society urges doctors to do their homework on chiropractic," *Canadian Press*, March 1, 2002.

32 Braswell, "Pediatricians' society," March 1, 2002.

33 David Chapman-Smith, Letter to Dr. Calvin Gutkin, November 12, 1999.

34 Greg Dubord, Letter to Jean Moss, December 6, 1999.

35 Ontario Chiropractic Association, "OCA President's Letter," October 10, 2000.

36 Ontario Chiropractic Association, "OCA President's Letter," October 10, 2000.

37 M. Brouwers and M. Charette, "Evaluation of clinical practice guidelines in chiropractic care: A comparison of North American guideline reports," *Journal of the Canadian Chiropractic Association*, 45, 3 (2001), p. 141-153.

38 L, Biggs, D. Hay, D. Mierau, "Standards of care: what do they mean to chiropractors and which organizations should develop them," *Journal of the Canadian Chiropractic Association*, 43, 4 (1999), p. 249-257.

39 L. Biggs et al, "Standards of care," p. 250.

40 L. Biggs et al, "Standards of care," p. 254.

41 L. Biggs et al, "Standards of care," p. 256.

42 G.R. Yates, "OCA Vice-President's Letter," *Ontario Chiropractic Association*, May 30, 1997.

43 Yates, "OCA Vice-President's Letter," May 30, 1997.

44 Yates, "OCA Vice-President's Letter," May 30, 1997.

45 Yates, "OCA Vice-President's Letter," May 30, 1997.

46 Yates, "OCA Vice-President's Letter," May 30, 1997.

47 Yates, "OCA Vice-President's Letter," May 30, 1997.

48 Yates, "OCA Vice-President's Letter," May 30, 1997.

49 D. Leprich, "Alternative practitioners: All you ever wanted to know about chiropractors...," *The Medical Post*, 36, 6 (February 8, 2000).

50 M.G. Christensen and D.R.D. Morgan, "Job Analysis of Chiropractic in Canada: A Report, Survey, Analysis, and Summary of the Practice of Chiropractic within Canada," (Greeley, CO), National Board of Chiropractic Examiners, 1993.

51 D. Waalen , T. Watkins and R. Saranchuk, "The philosophy of chiropractic: an action research model of curriculum review," *The Journal of the Canadian Chiropractic Association,* 43, 3 (1999), p.149.

52 J. Donahue, "Philosophy of chiropractic: lessons from the past – guidance for

the future," *The Journal of the Canadian Chiropractic Association*, 34, 4 (1990), p.194-204.

53 D. Waalen , T. Watkins and R. Saranchuk, "The philosophy of chiropractic: an action research model of curriculum review," *The Journal of the Canadian Chiropractic Association,* 43, 3 (1999), p. 150.

54 D. Waalen et al, "The philosophy of chiropractic," p. 155.

55 D. Waalen et al, "The philosophy of chiropractic," p. 155.

56 B. J. Gleberzon, "Name techniques in Canada: current trends in utilization rates and recommendations for their inclusion at the Canadian Memorial Chiropractic College," *Journal of the Canadian Chiropractic Association*, 44, 3 (2000), 157-167.

57 B. J. Gleberzon, "Name techniques in Canada," p. 166.

58 L. Morgan, "Letter to the Editor," *Journal of the Canadian Chiropractic Association,* 44, 3 (2000), p.182-183.

59 Gleberzon, "Name techniques in Canada," p. 166.

60 Gleberzon, "Name techniques in Canada," p. 166.

61 Gleberzon, "Name techniques in Canada," p. 166.

62 Gleberzon, "Name techniques in Canada," p. 165.

63 Gleberzon, "Name techniques in Canada," p. 166.

64 Gleberzon, "Name techniques in Canada," p. 163.

65 Canadian Memorial Chiropractic College and Canadian Chiropractic Association, "Sustaining and Improving our Healthcare: A Call for Action: Submission to the Commission on the Future of Healthcare in Canada," June, 2002.

66 P. Carey, "Dr. Carey Replies…," *Communique*, March 1, 1999.

67 P. Carey, "Dr. Carey Replies…," *Communique*, March 1, 1999.

68 W.G.G. Fisher, Letter to Murray Katz, June 4, 1999.

69 M. Levis, R. Barlow, J. Wedge and H. O'Brodovich, "Letter to Mary Beth Valentine," May 11, 2001.

CONCLUSION

1 Joseph Keating Jr., "Chiropractic: Science and Antiscience and Pseudoscience Side by Side," *Skeptical Inquirer*, July/August, 1997, p. 40.

2 Keating, "Chiropractic: Science and Antiscience," p.40.

AFTERWORD

1 Christenson MG, Morgan DRD. *Job Analysis of Chiropractic: A Report, Survey Analysis, and Summary of the Practice of Chiropractic within the United States.* Greeley, Colorado: National Board of Chiropractic Examiners, 1993. This report is based on the responses by 4,835 full-time chiropractors who responded to a 1991 NBCE survey about their practices during the previous two years. The figures included: Activator Methods, 51.2 percent; applied kinesiology,

37.2 percent; acupressure/meridian therapy, 65.5 percent; acupuncture, 11.8 percent; cranial adjusting, 27.2 percent; and homeopathic remedies, 36.9 percent. "Nutritional counseling, etc." was listed by 83.5 percent. Although the data does not indicate what this involved, it is clear that a large percentage of chiropractors are inappropriately prescribing dietary supplements.

2   Chiropractors. *Consumer Reports* 59:383-390, 1994. This included a survey of 476 chiropractors chosen randomly from the American Chiropractic Association membership directory. Nearly one quarter of the 274 who responded sent material stating that spinal misalignments and "interferences" threatened overall health, and 35 percent implicated the spine in disorders of the body's organs.